Frontiers in Spinal Neurosurgery

Edited by James Jin Wang, Xianli Lv, Guihuai Wang, Kiran Sunil Mahapure and Zhenxing Sun

Published in London, United Kingdom

Frontiers in Spinal Neurosurgery
http://dx.doi.org/10.5772/intechopen.1000270
Edited by James Jin Wang, Xianli Lv, Guihuai Wang, Kiran Sunil Mahapure and Zhenxing Sun

Contributors
Ghazwan Abdulla Hasan, Mustafa Hayder Qatran, Aloysius Bambang Darwono, Volodymyr Radchenko, Jincai Yang, Yong Hai, Peng Yin, Bo Han, Honghao Yang, Jixuan Huang, Pablo Pazmiño, João Paulo Machado Bergamaschi, Marcelo Botelho Soares de Brito, Ariel Falbel Lugão, Thiago Queiroz Soares, Gustavo Vitelli Depieri, Edgar Takao Utino, Fábio da Silva Forti, Kai-Uwe Lewandrowski, Fernanda Wirth, Noor Us Saba, Mohd Faheem, Punita Manik, Kee D. Kim, Charles C. Lee, Kung-Chia Li, Yu-Chieh Hsieh, Ching-Hsiang Hsieh, Ting-Hua Liao, Armando Armas-Salazar, Fátima Ximena Cid-Rodríguez, José Luis Navarro-Olvera, Edgar Abarca-Rojano, Noé Tellez-León, María de la Luz Montes-Castillo, Ana Isabel García-Jerónimo, José Damián Carrillo-Ruiz, Raj Kumar Manas, Om Prasad Biswal, Smita Nayak, Rajesh Kumar Das, Sheng Yang, Chunyang Xia, Bhoresh Dhamija, Steven Tominey, Shabin Joshi, Rahim Hussain, Dheeraj Batheja, Birender Balain, Claudio Irace, Peihai Zhang, Xuejun Yang, Yuzeng Liu, Yong Hai, Hongtao Ding, Mingzheng Zhao, Pragya Kumar, Jasmine Kaur Chawla

First published in London, United Kingdom, 2023 by IntechOpen
IntechOpen is the global imprint of INTECHOPEN LIMITED, registered in England and Wales, registration number: 11086078, 5 Princes Gate Court, London, SW7 2QJ, United Kingdom

British Library Cataloguing-in-Publication Data
A catalogue record for this book is available from the British Library

Additional hard and PDF copies can be obtained from orders@intechopen.com

Frontiers in Spinal Neurosurgery
Edited by James Jin Wang, Xianli Lv, Guihuai Wang, Kiran Sunil Mahapure and Zhenxing Sun
p. cm.
Print ISBN 978-1-83769-631-4
Online ISBN 978-1-83769-630-7
eBook (PDF) ISBN 978-1-83769-632-1

Meet the editors

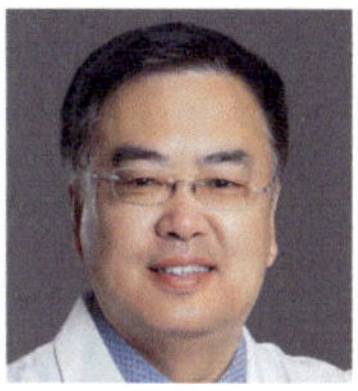

Dr. James Wang is Professor of Neurosurgery, Beijing Tsinghua Changgung Hospital, School of Clinical Medicine, Tsinghua University, Beijing, China, and Clinical Professor of Neurosurgery, University of Washington, Seattle, USA. He graduated from Beijing Capital Medical College, China in 1983. He completed his neurosurgery training at Ohio State University Hospital, USA in 1999 and became a board-certified neurosurgeon in 2003. Dr. Wang then served as the chief physician of neurosurgery at Group Health Hospital and Providence Hospital in Seattle. Since 2015, he has been a professor and the associate dean of the Institute of Clinical Neurosciences, Tsinghua University.

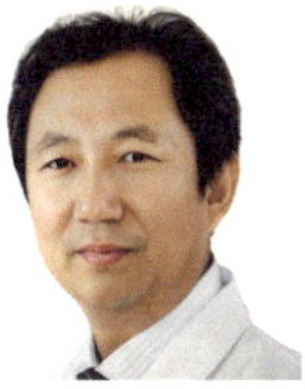

Dr. Guihuai Wang is a professor and the director of the Department of Neurosurgery, Beijing Tsinghua Changgung Hospital, School of Clinical Medicine, Tsinghua University, Beijing, China. He serves as the chairman of the Spinal Cord and Spine Expert Committee of the Neurosurgeon Branch of the Chinese Medical Doctor Association, the deputy chairman of the Neuro-Oncology Committee of the Chinese Anti-Cancer Association, and the deputy chairman of the Spinal Cord and Peripheral Nerve Repair Materials and Application Professional Committee of the Bone Repair Materials and Devices Branch of the Chinese Society of Biomaterials. He is also deputy secretary-general and member of the Standing Committee of the First Committee of the Neuro-Tumor Branch of the Chinese Society of Neuroscience, a member of the World Federation of Neurosurgery (WFNS), and an editorial board member of the *Journal of Translational Neuroscience and Clinics.*

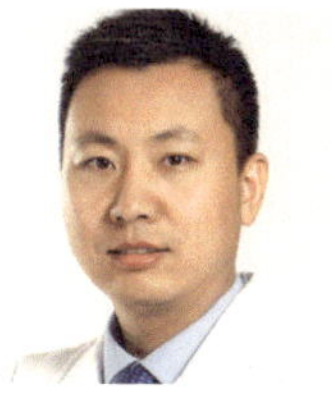

Dr. Xianli Lv, MD, is an associate professor in the Department of Neurosurgery, Beijing Tsinghua Changgung Hospital, School of Clinical Medicine, Tsinghua University, Beijing, China. His research focuses on neuroendovascular therapy of intracranial aneurysms, cerebral arteriovenous malformation, intracranial dural arteriovenous fistula, spinal vascular malformation, and pediatric cerebrospinal vascular malformation. He has one national invention patent to his credit. He has authored 195 peer-reviewed articles and edited 6 books He is a deputy editor of *Neuroscience Informatics* and *Frontiers in Neurology*. He is also an editorial member of *Interventional Neuroradiology*, *Stroke and Vascular Neurology*, *Journal of Neuroradiology*, *The Neuroradiology Journal* and *World Journal of Radiology*. Dr. Lv is a member of the World Stroke Organization (WSO) and the World Federation of Interventional Therapeutic Neuroradiology (WFITN). He was the cover person for the *World Journal of Radiology* in 2022 and the *Journal of China Science and Technology Achievements* in 2023.

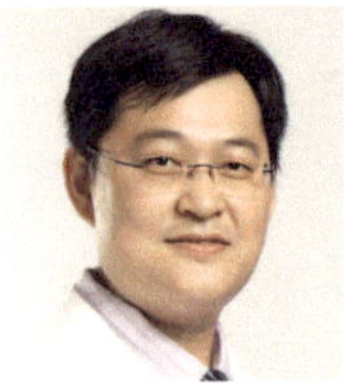

Dr. Zhenxing Sun, MD, is from the Department of Neurosurgery, Beijing Tsinghua Changgung Hospital, School of Clinical Medicine, Tsinghua University, Beijing, China. He has published numerous SCI articles and four invention patents. His research focuses on the treatment of spinal diseases such as Chiari malformation, syringomyelia, atlantoaxial dislocation, basilar indentation, tethered cord syndrome, and spinal cord tumor; cervical and lumbar spondylosis, especially the surgical treatment of cervical posterior longitudinal ligament ossification (OPLL) and failed back surgery syndrome (FBSS); and comprehensive treatment of primary and metastatic spinal tumors.

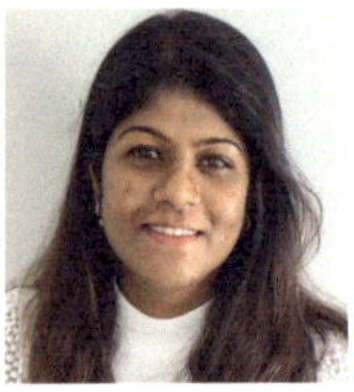

Kiran Mahapure is a board-certified plastic surgeon trained in India with more than a decade of experience in general and plastic surgery. She holds a master's degree in General Surgery and Plastic Surgery. She is ECFMG certified and currently pursuing a pediatric plastic surgery fellowship at the University of Tennessee, USA. Dr. Mahapure has rich experience in laparoscopic surgery, colon surgery, breast surgery, vascular surgery, aesthetic surgery, cleft and craniofacial surgery, aesthetic surgery, trauma surgery, general reconstruction, and gender reassignment surgery. She is actively involved in research and has published more than twenty manuscripts. She is a peer reviewer for several journals, volume editor for an upcoming book series, and review editor for a reputed group of journals.

Contents

Preface

Spinal neurosurgery is among the fastest-growing subspecialties in both neurosurgery and orthopedics. New spinal surgery techniques, equipment, and implants have revolutionized spinal surgery in the past two decades. With the aging population worldwide, surgical treatments for degenerative spinal disease will certainly become more popular.

This book includes contributions from internationally renowned spinal surgeons from more than 10 countries that reflect the status of spinal surgery in both developing and developed countries. Section 1 covers the ever-growing and popular minimally invasive spinal (MIS) surgery techniques, including endoscopic spinal surgery. This section provides a better understanding of when to use MIS decompression without fusion to preserve motion and when to consider MIS-assisted fusion and fixation. Section 2 deals with surgery for congenital spinal disorders, like neural tube defects. Section 3 discusses the common procedures for spinal and peripheral nerve trauma. Section 4 includes some miscellaneous spinal procedures and techniques, like spinal rehabilitation, spinal surgery navigation, and some controversial topics like how to manage complicated spinal metastatic lesions.

This book is a useful reference for surgeons or medical school students who are interested in these spinal topics. It will improve knowledge and understanding of spinal surgery. We would like to acknowledge the encouragement, motivation, and assistance from the Beijing Municipal Administration of Hospitals Incubating Program (PX2020039), Beijing, China, and Tsinghua Precision Medicine Foundation (20219990008), Tsinghua University, Beijing, China. Finally, we would like to thank IntechOpen and Publishing Process Manager Mr. Josip Knapic for his dedication and hard work throughout the publication process.

James Jin Wang, Guihuai Wang, Xianli Lv and Zhenxing Sun
Department of Neurosurgery,
Beijing Tsinghua Changgung Hospital,
School of Clinical Medicine,
Tsinghua University,
Beijing, China

Kiran Sunil Mahapure M.D. M.Ch
Pediatric Plastic Surgery Fellow,
University of Tennessee Health Science Centre,
Memphis, TN, United States

Section 1

Minimum Invasive Spine Surgery/Endoscopic Surgery

Chapter 1

Endoscopic Spine Surgery: The Next Golden Standard Technique in Spinal Surgeries

Ghazwan Abdulla Hasan and Mustafa Hayder Qatran

Abstract

Minimally invasive surgeries continue to advance at an immensely fast pace, moving from open discectomy surgeries to microscopic ones using tubular systems, to do fusions, to correct deformities, until we reached a place where we are tackling most spinal pathologies in a minimally invasive fashion, For many spine surgeons, the field of spine endoscopy, whether uniportal or biportal, is still unexplored, to some extent due to their mastery in open and microscopic techniques, and to another extent the learning curve that it takes to master endoscopic spine, as well as a lack in well-structured clearcut data regarding its indications and limitations, and this chapter will hopefully shed the proper lighting on the field of spinal endoscopy, making surgeons understand its utility in treating different pathologies, discussing the research and data comparing spinal endoscopy with more traditional techniques, as well as understanding endoscopic spine surgery's learning curve, and how to overcome the timeline in mastering its basic techniques.

Keywords: spine endoscopy, interlaminar approach, transforaminal approach, MIS, uniportal endoscopy, biportal endoscopy

1. Introduction

In the 70s, Hijikata, a Japanese surgeon, who was famous for performing diagnostic discographies. He developed tubes to introduce this approach to the posterolateral annulus under fluoroscopic control. He could incise the annulus, and, using pituitary rongeurs; he could remove the nucleus of the disc in what he described to be a "percutaneous necluotomy".

He published this procedure in the Japanese language. This was one of the reasons why this procedure did not gain widespread attention among the surgical community, but it was definitely the starting point [1, 2].

Forst and Hausmann [3] described the use of an arthroscope to visualize the contents of the intervertebral disc in 1983, and the first description of an endoscopic discectomy by Kambin et al. followed soon after in 1988 [4]; however, a spine surgery still stayed behind other specialties in the inclusion of indirect visualization. Nonetheless, the need for less invasive spine procedures and surgeon drive to provide these solutions and improve care quality has driven the global advancement of spinal endoscopy [5].

And keeping up with such the swift pace and such great advances, spine surgeons should be open and ready to tackle the field of endoscopic spine surgeries, as it is only a matter of time (and research papers) that stand between us now, and between standardizing spinal endoscopy as a potential gold standard technique in most spinal pathologies.

2. Nomenclature of spinal endoscopy

The endoscope will be defined as a visualization device placed into the body with an integrated working channel that provides a surgical corridor for tools to manipulate, ablate, and resect tissue [6].

There are two different approaches to divide the world on spinal endoscopy [7].

1. According to the property of the endoscopy used:

    - A full endoscopic system (percutaneous endoscopic system), which is the most commonly used system in endoscopic spine surgery, the working channel and the optics being in the same tubular device with utilization of a monoportal approach with continuous saline irrigation.

    - A microendoscopic system, which is the second most frequently used endoscopic device, this category involves using a rigid endoscope (microendoscope) attached to a tubular retractor with tissue dilators, which help minimize muscle retraction, and unlike the other endoscopic systems; this system is not a water-based procedure, and constant saline irrigation is not used. So it's more of a MIS microscope than an endoscope.

    - Biportal endoscopic system, which is the third category of endoscopic spine surgery, with separate optical and working channels. The endoscopic portal is used for viewing the surgical field with constant saline irrigation, whereas the instrumental portal is used for surgical instrumentation and procedure.

2. According to the method of approach:

    - The transforaminal approach refers to a posterolateral minimally invasive approach to the disc or epidural space through the foraminal window.

    - Interlaminar approach, which is similar to the usual open or microscopic approach.

    - Anterior/Posterior approach to the cervical spine.

    - Caudal or trans-sacral approach.

So as the technology and techniques have advanced, the terminology used to describe these procedures has developed organically and has become heterogeneous and sometimes confusing to patients, providers, and payors [7]. Because of that issue, a formal consensus regarding the proper naming of such newly developed procedures had to be implemented to clear up the confusion and avoid any miscommunication. This was why the AOSpine minimally invasive spine surgery taskforce developed the definitions and nomenclature consensus in 2020 (**Figure 1**). They developed the concept "full- endoscopic" to describe procedures performed with a working-channel endoscope.

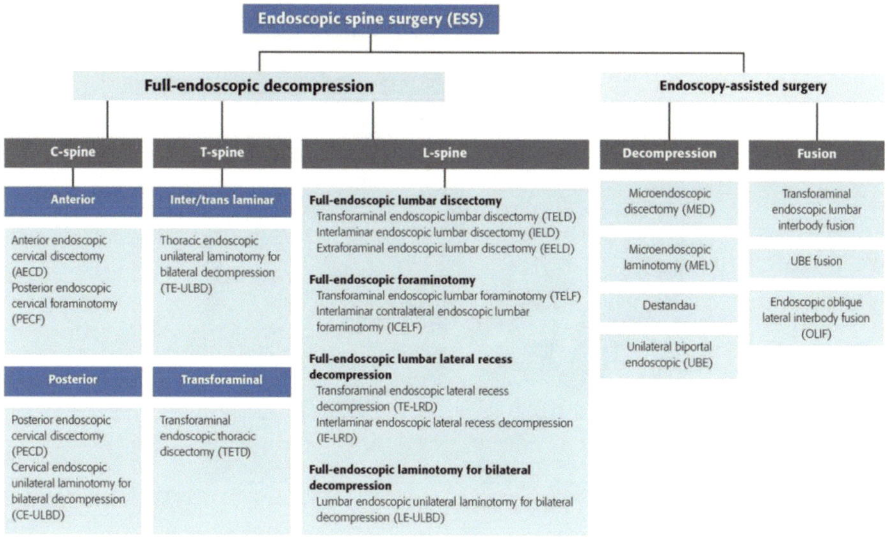

Figure 1.
The AOspine endoscopic spine surgery nomenclature consensus.

This distinguishes those procedures from "endoscope-assisted"operations, where tools are passed through trajectories separate from the working endoscopic channel [7] and according to the consensus guidelines, the procedures are named according to the following formula:

Approach corridor/Visualization/Segment of spine/Procedure

3. Clinical applications and outcomes

There are three important main indications in endoscopic spinal surgery:

- Discectomies.
- Spinal stenosis decompression.
- Fusions.

Let us begin by dividing the endoscopic indications according to spinal regions and their approach:

3.1 Lumbar spinal endoscopy

3.1.1 Transformational lumbar discectomy

A. Indications:

- Soft lumbar disc herniation (LDH) of various types, the advancement in technology and experience, and its practical application have widened to include migrated, recurrent, foraminal, extraforaminal, and even partially calcified LDH (**Figures 2** and **3**) [8].

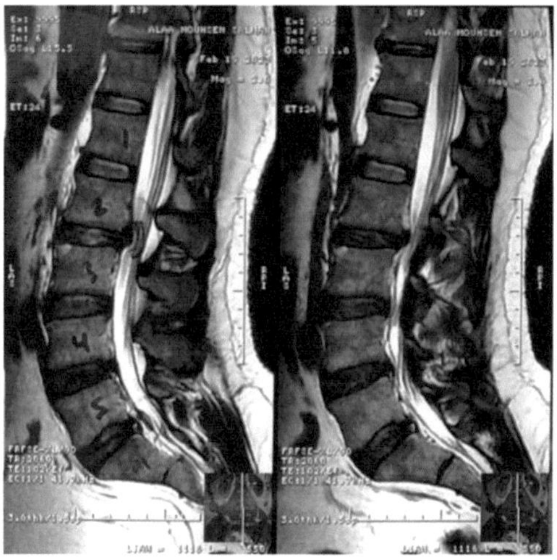

Figure 2.
Sagittal MRI view of L2–3 soft disc herniation.

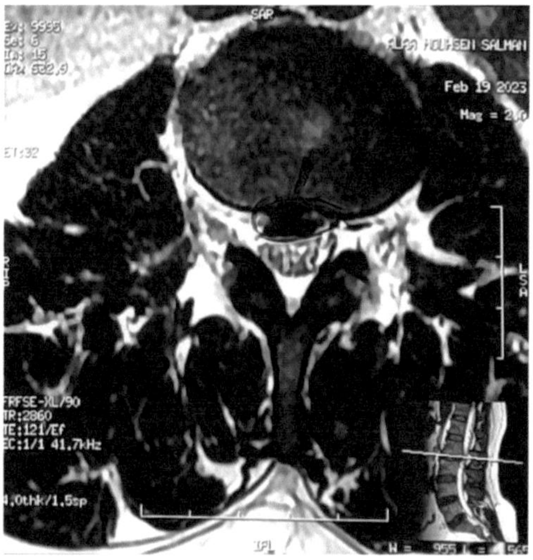

Figure 3.
Axial MRI view of L2–3 soft disc herniation.

B. Contraindications [8]

- Extensive migrated LDH.
- Calcified discs.
- L5-S1 level (male patients, high iliac crests). (Relative contraindication as expert level can do it)
- Multilevel pathology. (Relative contraindication as expert level can do it)

- Spinal canal central stenosis.
- Spondylolisthesis or instability (**Figure 4**)
- Nerve root anomalies such as conjoined root.
- Profound motor deficit.
- Cauda equine syndrome.

C. Technique [9]:

- The patient is positioned prone on a radiolucent table with a pelvic and a thoracic roll.
- The desired level's midline, inferior, and superior vertebral plates are marked under visualization of the image intensifier, and lateral markings to the midline of 8, 10, and 12 cm will be the possible entry points.
- The patient is submitted to light sedation, and at the point of entry, an infiltration with local anesthetic without a vasoconstrictor is performed. The sedation should be light since the patient must be aware of being alert if some nerve root is stimulated during the procedure.
- The entire procedure is performed through the intervertebral foramen between the exiting and traversing nerve roots (Kambin's safety triangle) without needing to resect bony or ligamentous structures (**Figures 5** and **6**).
- The intervertebral disc is punctured, and discography with methylene blue or indigo carmine, associated with non-ionic contrast, is done.
- Through the guides, the endoscope is inserted into the intervertebral disc, and an indirect intervertebral disc decompression is performed (**Figure 7**) (inside-out technique), followed by a thermal nucleoplasty.

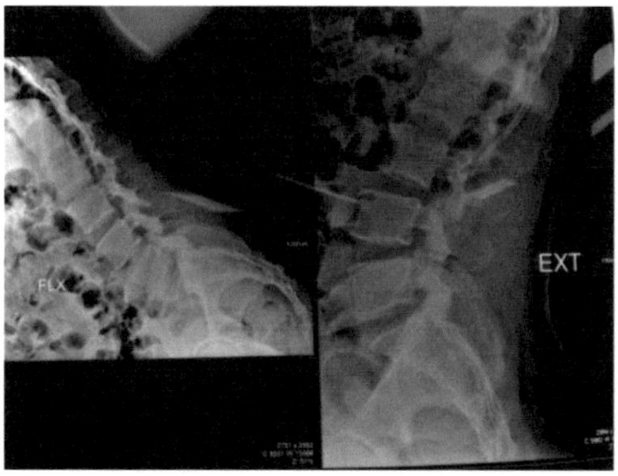

Figure 4.
Assessment of instability by flexion extension X-ray shows no contraindication to such approach.

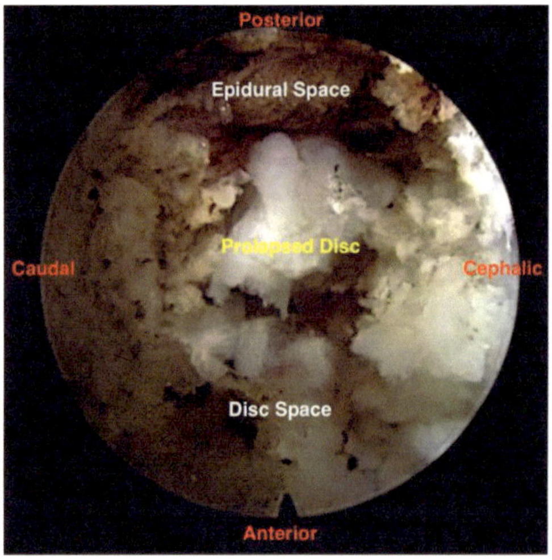

Figure 5.
Disc extraction using the transforaminal approach.

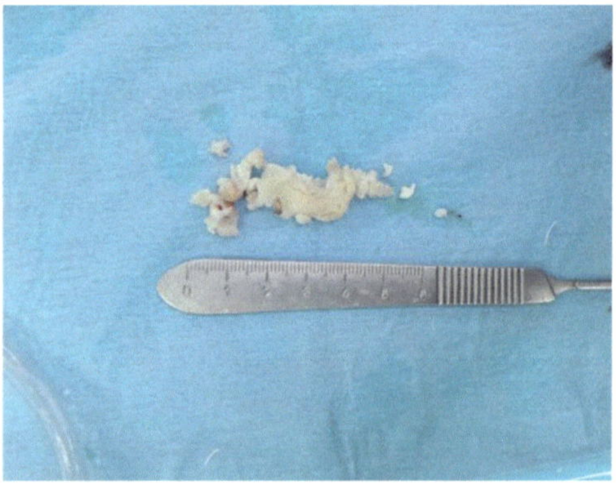

Figure 6.
The endoscopic view in the transforaminal approach.

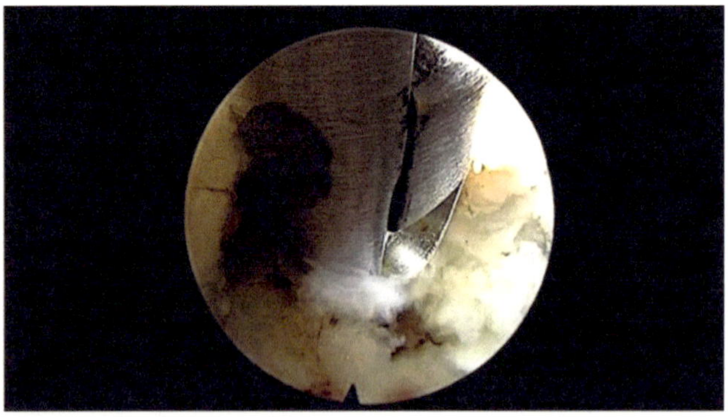

Figure 7.
Disc material after extraction by transforaminal approach.

3.1.2 Transforaminal lumbar foraminotomy/Transforaminal lateral recess decompression

Until recently, tubular microdiscectomy was the golden standard surgical option when it comes to dealing with degenerative stenotic pathological changes such as superior articulating process (SAP) or ligamentum flavum (LF) hypertrophy, osteophyte formation or associated dynamic or static instability [10], however, in recent years the endoscopic approach has risen to be a strong competitor.

A. Indications:

- lateral recess/foraminal stenosis

B. Contraindications:

- Similar to the aforementioned contraindications.

C. Technique [8]:

- docking the port at the lower foramen (caudal surface of the SAP).
- The tip of the SAP is excised by reaming. It is done blindly under fluoroscopic control with the medial pedicle line as the limit, and the giveaway feeling suggests the completeness of bony resection. It, though, appears risky for early endoscopy surgeons. However, there is a soft layer of capsule and ligamentum flavum that is still between the reamer and the traversing root.
- Visualized endoscopic burred foraminoplasty can also be done, which is apparently safe.
- exposed ligamentum flavum and capsule are removed
- For foraminal stenosis, the focus is on the cranial aspect of foramen and removal of the tip of SAP, capsule, and ligamentum flavum.
- For the lateral recess stenosis, the caudal foramen is focused.
- Visualization of the pulsatile exiting nerve root is the end point of decompression.

3.1.3 Interlaminar lumbar discectomy

A. Indications: (Soft LDHs that were technically inaccessible in the transforaminal approach) [8, 11–13]

- L5-S1 level with high iliac crest level.
- High-grade migrated disc herniation, either cranial or caudal direction.
- Calcified discs.

- The sufficient interlaminar window between the cranial and caudal lamina and the midline and mediodorsal borders of the inferior articular process (IAP) measuring at least 6 mm.
- Central canal stenosis
- Ligamentum flavum hypertrophy
- Lateral recess stenosis and Foraminal stenosis (shared with transforaminal approach)
- Synovial cysts.
- Hypertrophic facet.

B. Contraindications:

- General surgical contraindications.

C. Technique [9]:

- The patient is positioned in the prone position, on a radiolucent table, under general anesthesia (In this technique, general anesthesia is necessary because it is vital to move away from the neural root).
- The interlaminar window at the level is marked on the skin with the use of X-ray, and a 1-cm longitudinal access is made near the midline.
- dilator is put in the interlaminar space
- the endoscope is inserted.
- musculature is dissected to the ligamentum flavum, which is opened to expose the descending root and the epidural fat.
- The opening of the yellow ligament is a fundamental step during endoscopic surgery by the interlaminar approach, to access the nerve structures and the intervertebral disc.
- The nerve root is protected with a beveled cannula.
- The intervertebral disc is perforated and decompressed.
- At the end of the procedure, a thermal nucleoplasty is done.

3.2 Thoracic spinal endoscopy

A. Indications:

- Soft thoracic disc herniation in paracentral and lateral locations.

B. Contraindications [14]:

- Neurological deficits and significant myelopathy
- History of previous spine surgery
- Multi-level involvement.

C. Technique resembles that of the lumbar spine approach.

3.3 Cervical spinal endoscopy

A. Indications [8, 15–17]:

- cervical radiculopathy due to disc herniation or foraminal stenosis.
- Contraindications [8]:
- Calcified discs
- Severe compressive cervical myelopathy.
- Cervical segmental instability.
- Previous neck surgery.

B. Technique [9]:

Posterior approach:

- Prone positioning of the patient.
- The neck is extended and the head is fixed in place with tape.
- The arms are positioned towards the caudal on the body with gentle tension.
- The line of spinal joints is marked X-ray (2 cm lateral from the midline).
- Insertion of the sheath with the dilator beveled opening.
- The dilator is removed.
- operation is performed under visual control and continuous irrigation with saline solution.
- foraminotomy is done with resection of the lateral aspect of the ligamentum flavum, and identification of the lateral edge of the spinal cord and branching of the spinal nerves.
- Bipolar coagulation of the venous plexus.
- If disc herniation occurs, the nerves should be immobilized, and the herniated disc material should be resected.

- Depending on the pathology, the foraminotomy can be extended.

Anterior approach [18]:

- The patient is set in the supine position with her neck in slight extension.
- A 3 cm anterolateral incision, centered at C/6 as localized using a radiographic image intensifier, allowed exposure of the anterior spine medial to the carotid sheath.
- Under lateral fluoroscopic guidance, needle is inserted obliquely into each affected disc.
- After guide-wire insertion, guiding rods and a dilating tube are then passed, followed by a working cannula with an outer diameter of 4.8 mm.
- After resection of the margin of the uncinate process, the endoscope is then used to visualize the disc.
- The posterior part of the nucleus pulposus is first partially removed with grasping forceps for preliminary decompression.
- The endoscope is then advanced to the posterior annular margin of the disc to identify the target fragments, with particular care taken not to damage the nerve roots or the dura mater.

So, what about other indications, such as fusion? In other words, can spinal endoscopy expand its indications to fill the role of conventional open spine surgery? [19].

To answer that question, you must know that the development process of spinal endoscopic surgery can be divided mainly into four generations (**Table 1**) [20].

- The first generation: the transforaminal approach
- The second generation is an interlaminar approach which was developed to tackle herniations that were difficult to access with a transforaminal approach.

	1st generation	**2nd generation**	**3rd generation**	**4th generation**
Endoscopy systems	Uniportal	Uniportal	Uniportal/Biportal	Uniportal/ Biportal
Indication	Disc herniation	Disc herniation	Disc herniation Central stenosis Foraminal stenosis	Stenosis Instability
Lesion	Lumbar	Lumbar	Lumbar Thoracic Cervical	Lumbar Lumbar interbody fusion
Approach	Transforaminal	Interlaminar	Posterior interlaminar Transforaminal	Trans-Kambin Posterolateral

Table 1.
The advancing generation of endoscopic spine surgery.

- The third generation, spinal stenosis could be approached. Moreover, endoscopic treatment was possible the cervical and thoracic spine as well.

- The fourth generation endoscopic lumbar interbody fusion can be attempted.

Image-guided assistance is feasible and applicable in endoscopic spinal approach. It will provide several advantages over conventional C-arm fluoroscopy.

On the other hand, the method is still heavy, time consuming, and might be improved according to the radiological facilities [21].

4. Learning curve

It comes as no surprise that the field of endoscopic spine surgery, like any other novel field in surgery, requires the surgeon to overcome the barriers that come along the transition from open or microscopic spine surgery to more minimally invasive yet technically demanding approaches, Therefore, to guarantee a successful transition from conventional open spine surgery to an endoscopic spine practice surgeons should aim to [22, 23].

- Have a good fundamental grasp the pathophysiology of neurogenic pain

- Correlate surgical anatomy with symptomatic pain generators.

- Employ a staged management approach going from least invasive to most invasive.

- Avoid doing fusions for pain management unless there is gross instability or deformity.

When it comes to data entailing the number of cases in a learning curve, Hsu et al. showed that the plateauing of the learning curve for the transforaminal approach occurred around the 10th case [9, 24], Lee et al. reached a similar finding by observing a significant reduction in the operative time after the17th patient was treated by percutaneous endoscopic lumbar discectomy [9, 25]. At the same time, Choi et al. recommended supervision by an experienced surgeon in the initial 10 cases to overcome the learning curve for the interlaminar procedure at L5-S1 [9, 26] and the approximate cutoff point of the learning curve of biportal endoscopy surgery was around 54 cases [27].

Therefore, certain considerations must be put in mind to tackle this learning curve [22]:

- Define the patient target group.

- Identify endoscopic surgeries to learn.

- Attend professional and society meetings and courses.

- Practice in cadaver workshops.

- Identify mentors and observe live surgeries.

- Employ reliable diagnostic prognosticators.
- Start with selective blocks.
- Then start with simple far lateral soft disc herniations.
- Expand to paracentral and central disc herniations.
- Expand to foraminal and lateral recess stenosis.
- Analyze outcomes and contribute.
- Present and publish your outcomes.
- Teach others and become a mentor.

And always remember that a learning curve is not an achievement curve, proper guidelines and goal setting for education and training are more important than ever, and it is necessary to discuss creating a consensus between endoscopic academic societies and experts [28].

5. Complications and limitations

5.1 Dural tear

Dura tear rate is approximately 3% in endoscopic spine surgery [29, 30]. The rate is higher in decompression and fusion than in discectomy.

To give a general estimation of the magnitude of such complications, let us look at the study conducted by Lewandrowski et al. covering more than 64,000 cases of spinal endoscopy; where the durotomy incidence was that of 1.07% [31].

Medium-sized dural tears (1–10 mm) were the most common (52.2%; 48/93). Small pinhole durotomies (less than 1 mm) were the second most common type (46.7%; 43/93). Rootlet herniations were seen by 46.2% (43/93) of responding surgeons.

The posterior dural sac injury during the interlaminar approach (57%; 53/93) occurred more frequently than traversing nerve-root injuries (31.2%) or anterior dural sac (23.7%; 22/93).

Exiting nerve-root injuries (10.8%;10/93) were less common.

The majority of participating surgeons (64%; 57/89) reported that the long-term outcome was unaffected. Only 18% of surgeons reported having seen the development of a postoperative cerebrospinal fluid (CSF)-fistula (18%;16/89). However, the absolute incidence of CSF fistula was only 0.025% (16/64 470).

Severe radiculopathy with dysesthesia; sensory loss; and motor weakness in association with an incidental durotomy were reported by 12.4% (11/89), 3.4% (3/89), and 2.2% (2/89) of surgeons, respectively [31].

5.2 Vascular injury

Injuries to the segmental artery are the main concern.

Segmental artery injury mainly occurs during transforaminal work, especially when decompressing the exiting nerve root; because the segmental artery passes under the exiting nerve root, this segmental artery injury may induce serious retroperitoneal hematoma [32, 33].

5.3 Infections

Discitis or any other SSI after lumbar endoscopic surgery is very rare.

One study reported an infection rate of 0.11% [32, 34].

5.4 Water irrigation-related neck and head pain

Postoperative raised ICP can occur secondary to high endoscopic saline inflow and it can lead to cerebral edema and seizure, which can also be intraoperatively [35]. Prevention is key.

The ideal water pressure used is said to be around 30 mmHg (25–50 mmHg) [29, 35, 36].

5.5 Hematoma

Kim et al. showed approximately 25% hematoma rate in biportal endoscopic spine surgery, with only 1.2% requiring revision due to the hematoma.

Careful hemostasis is key to preventing postoperative hematoma formation. In the presence of an increase in the neurological deficit of bilateral limbs postoperatively, a low threshold for revision decompression and hematoma drainage is necessary [29, 37].

5.6 Postoperative dysesthesia

Postoperative dysesthesia is a common complaint.

Minimal dorsal root ganglion retraction is essential for preventing postoperative dysesthesia. Kim et al. showed interlaminar contralateral approach has less postoperative dysesthesia rate than transforaminal endoscopic lumbar discectomy [29, 38].

5.7 Missed fragments

Even in experienced hands, some herniations remain technically difficult. In literature, huge central disc herniations and highly migrated disc herniations have high failure rates [30, 39, 40].

The success of the procedure is attributed to proper preoperative planning based on the MRI.

Avoidance of complications is enhanced by the ability to visualize normal and pathoanatomy clearly, and use of local anesthesia and conscious sedation rather than general or spinal anesthesia [41].

6. The future of endoscopic spine surgery

With advancements in implant and instrument technology and the incorporation of robotic technology, surgical indications may be expanded into motion-preserving scoliosis surgeries, tumor resections, and more complex surgical procedures. As we move towards a patient-centered and cost-effective healthcare model, we may see endoscopic spine surgery become increasingly relevant to the future of spine surgical practice with improved patient outcomes and decreased medical costs [42].

The reasons behind the hindered widespread acceptance and uptake could, in part be the parallel explosions in other potentially more lucrative fields within spinal surgery, such as instrumentation, expandable technologies, biologics, navigation, and robotics [43] along with the unfamiliarity with the equipment and approach.

Over the few years, increasing recognition of the physiological footprint imparted upon the patient by traditional open surgery, combined with a historically nihilistic approach to operating upon the elderly and infirm, a population that often needs our help the most, and traditionally negative public perceptions of spinal surgery, have led to the rise of enhanced recovery after surgery (ERAS) programs, with endpoints of reducing pain and narcotic consumption, hastening postoperative mobility and recovery, improving patient satisfaction, and reducing the length of stay and costs [44, 45].

So all data suggests that there will be a decisive shift towards such techniques in the upcoming years once we set up plans to overcome the difficulties, tackle the learning curve, and set up systemized training programs.

7. Conclusion

Spinal endoscopy is a minimally invasive procedure used to diagnose and treat spinal disorders. It involves inserting a small camera and specialized instruments into the spinal canal through a small incision in the skin. Spinal endoscopy is less invasive than traditional open surgery, which can result in less blood loss, less pain, and faster recovery times.

Recent advances in technology and surgical techniques have made spinal endoscopy a safe and effective option for many spinal conditions. Spinal endoscopy is being used to treat conditions such as spinal stenosis, herniated discs, and spinal tumors. It has also been used in spinal fusion procedures and to address failed back surgery syndrome.

While spinal endoscopy has shown promising results, it is not always the best option for every patient or condition. The decision to use spinal endoscopy should be made by a skilled and experienced surgeon who can evaluate each patient's unique needs and medical history.

The learning curve for spinal endoscopy can be steep, as the procedure requires a high level of technical skill and expertise. The surgeon must be able to navigate the instruments and camera through the narrow spinal canal while avoiding damage to the delicate spinal structures.

Training in spinal endoscopy typically involves a combination of didactic instruction, observation of experienced surgeons, and hands-on practice in cadaveric and animal models. Surgeons may also participate in live surgery courses and attend conferences to develop their skills further.

In addition to technical skills, surgeons must thoroughly understand spinal anatomy and pathology to perform spinal endoscopy safely and effectively. They must also be able to recognize and manage potential complications, such as nerve damage or cerebrospinal fluid leaks.

While the learning curve for spinal endoscopy is steep, many surgeons can perform the procedure safely and effectively with appropriate training and practice.

As with any surgical procedure, patient outcomes depend on the surgeon's skill and experience, as well as the patient's medical history and condition.

The future for spinal endoscopy is bright, and it is a trend that every spine surgeon should seek and a skill that each acquires.

Author details

Ghazwan Abdulla Hasan[1*] and Mustafa Hayder Qatran[2]

1 Al-Kindy Teaching Hospital, Baghdad, Iraq

2 Mustansiriyah University College of Medicine - Department of Orthopedics, Baghdad, Iraq

*Address all correspondence to: dr.bayaty@gmail.com

References

[1] Michael Mayer H. A history of endoscopic lumbar spine surgery: What have we learnt? BioMed Research International. 2019, Article ID 4583943;**2019**:8. DOI: 10.1155/2019/4583943

[2] Hijikata S, S. A. A method of percutaneous nuclear extraction. Journal of Toden Hospital. 1975;**5**(5):39

[3] Forst R, Hausmann B. Nucleoscopy--a new examination technique. Archives of Orthopaedic and Trauma Surgery. 1978). 1983;**101**(3):219-221. DOI: 10.1007/BF00436774

[4] Kambin P, Nixon JE, Chait A, Schaffer JL. Annular protrusion: Pathophysiology and roentgenographic appearance. Spine (Phila Pa 1976). 1988;**13**(6):671-675

[5] Simpson AK. Spinal endoscopy: Evidence, techniques, global trends, and future projections. The Spine Journal. 2022;**22**(1):64-74

[6] Hofstetter CP, Ahn Y, Choi G, et al. AOSpine consensus paper on nomenclature for Working-Channel endoscopic spinal procedures. Global. Spine Journal. 2020;**10**(Suppl. 2):111S-121S. DOI: 10.1177/2192568219887364

[7] Ahn Y. Current techniques of endoscopic decompression in spine surgery. Annals of Translational Medicine. 2019;7(S5):S169-S169. DOI: 10.21037/atm.2019.07.98

[8] Krishnan A, Kim HS, Raj A. Bharat R Dave: Expanded indications of full endoscopic spine. Journal of Minimally Invasive Spine Surgery and Technique. 2020;**6**(Suppl. 1):S130-S156. DOI: 10.21182/jmisst.2021.00129

[9] Larocca Kulcheski Á, Graells SIX, Luís Sebben A. Spine Endoscopy. In: Endoscopy - Novel Techniques and Recent Advancements. London, UK, London, UK: IntechOpen; 2019. DOI: 10.5772/intechopen.79298

[10] Englund J. Lumbar spinal stenosis. Current Sports Medicine Reports. 2007;**6**:50-55. DOI: 10.1007/s11932-007-0012-0

[11] Ahn Y. Endoscopic spine discectomy: Indications and outcomes. International Orthopaedics. 2019;**43**(4):909-916. DOI: 10.1007/s00264-018-04283-w Epub 2019 Jan 5

[12] Wagner R, Haefner M. Indications and contraindications of full-endoscopic Interlaminar lumbar decompression. World Neurosurgery. 2021;**145**:657-662. DOI: 10.1016/j.wneu.2020.08.042 Epub 2020 Aug 15

[13] Yue JJ, Long W. Full endoscopic spinal surgery techniques: Advancements, indications, and outcomes. International Journal of Spine Surgery. 2015;**9**:17. DOI: 10.14444/2017

[14] Choi G, Munoz-Suarez D. Transforaminal endoscopic thoracic discectomy: Technical review to prevent complications. Neurospine. 2020;**17**(Suppl. 1):S58-S65. DOI: 10.14245/ns.2040250.125 Epub 2020 Jul 31

[15] Ruetten S, Komp M, Merk H, Godolias G. Full-endoscopic cervical posterior foraminotomy for the operation of lateral disc herniations using 5.9-mm endoscopes: A prospective, randomized, controlled study. Spine (Phila Pa 1976). 2008;**33**(9):940-948. DOI: 10.1097/BRS.0b013e31816c8b67

[16] Ahn Y. Percutaneous endoscopic cervical discectomy using working

channel endoscopes. Expert Review of Medical Devices. 2016;**13**(6):601-610. DOI: 10.1080/17434440.2016.1180245 Epub 2016 Apr 27

[17] Ruetten S, Komp M, Merk H, Godolias G. Full-endoscopic anterior decompression versus conventional anterior decompression and fusion in cervical disc herniations. International Orthopaedics. 2009;**33**(6):1677-1682. DOI: 10.1007/s00264-008-0684-y Epub 2008 Nov 18

[18] Middleton SD, Wagner R, Gibson JNA. Multi-level spine endoscopy: A review of available evidence and case report. EFORT Open Reviews. 2017;**2**(7):317-323 Retrieved Feb 28, 2023, from https://eor.bioscientifica.com/view/journals/eor/2/7/2058-5241.2.160087.xml

[19] Kim HS, Wu PH, Raorane HD, Jang IT. Generation change of practice in spinal surgery: Can endoscopic spine surgery expand its indications to fill in the role of conventional open spine surgery in Most of degenerative spinal diseases and disc Herniations: A study of 616 spinal cases 3 years. Neurology India. 2020;**68**(5):1157-1165. DOI: 10.4103/0028-3886.299145

[20] Dong H, Dong L, Hyeun-Sung K, Hungtae C. Recent trends and changes in the endoscopic spinal surgery. Journal of Minimally Invasive Spine Surgery and Technique. 2021;**6**:S81-S83. DOI: 10.21182/jmisst.2021.00136

[21] Assaker R, Reyns N, Pertruzon B, Lejeune JP. Image-guided endoscopic spine surgery: Part II: Clinical applications. Spine (Phila Pa 1976). 2001;**26**(15):1711-1718. DOI: 10.1097/00007632-200108010-00016

[22] Ransom NA, Gollogly S, Lewandrowski KU, Yeung A. Navigating the learning curve of spinal endoscopy as an established traditionally trained spine surgeon. Journal of Spine Surgery. 2020;**6**(Suppl. 1):S197-S207. DOI: 10.21037/jss.2019.10.03

[23] Hasan GA. How to Go Further with My Clinical Practice on Unilateral Biportal Endoscopy. In Springer eBooks. 2022. pp. 125-135. DOI: 10.1007/978-3-031-14736-4_10

[24] Hsu HT, Chang SJ, Yang SS, Chai CL. Learning curve of full-endoscopic lumbar discectomy. European Spine Journal. 2013;**22**(4):727-733. DOI: 10.1007/s00586-012-2540-4 Epub 2012 Oct 17

[25] Lee DY, Lee SH. Learning curve for percutaneous endoscopic lumbar discectomy. Neurologia Medico-Chirurgica (Tokyo). 2008;**48**(9):383-388; discussion 388-9. DOI: 10.2176/nmc.48.383

[26] Choi G, Lee SH, Raiturker PP, Lee S, Chae YS. Percutaneous endoscopic interlaminar discectomy for intracanalicular disc herniations at L5-S1 using a rigid working channel endoscope. Neurosurgery. 2006;**58**(Suppl. 1):ONS59-ONS68; discussion ONS59-68. DOI: 10.1227/01.neu.0000192713.95921.4a

[27] Xu J, Wang D, Liu J, Zhu C, Bao J, Gao W, et al. Learning curve and complications of unilateral Biportal endoscopy: Cumulative sum and risk-adjusted cumulative sum analysis. Neurospine. 2022;**19**(3):792-804. DOI: 10.14245/ns.2143116.558 Epub 2022 Aug 15

[28] Bae J, Kim JS. Building a successful practice of endoscopic spine surgery: Learning, setting the goal, and expanding the border. Neurospine. 2022;**19**(3):571-573. DOI: 10.14245/ns.2244712.356 Epub 2022 Sep 30

[29] Wu PH, Kim HS, Choi DJ, Gamaliel Y-HT. Overview of tips in overcoming learning curve in Uniportal and Biportal endoscopic spine surgery. Journal of Minimally Invasive Spine Surgery & Technique. 2021;**6**(Suppl. 1):S84-S96. DOI: 10.21182/jmisst.2020.00024

[30] Kim HS, Sharma SB, Wu PH, Raorane HD, Adsul NM, Singh R, et al. Complications and limitations of endoscopic spine surgery and percutaneous instrumentation. Indian Spine Journal. 2020;**3**:78-85

[31] Lewandrowski KU, Hellinger S, De Carvalho PST, Freitas Ramos MR, Soriano-SáNchez JA, Xifeng Z, et al. Dural tears during lumbar spinal endoscopy: Surgeon skill, training, incidence, risk factors, and management. International Journal of Spine Surgery. 2021;**15**(2):280-294. DOI: 10.14444/8038 Epub 2021 Apr 1

[32] Lewandrowski K-U, Telfeian AE, Hellinger S, León JFR, Teixeira PS, de Carvalho MRF, et al. Anthony Yeung: Difficulties, challenges, and the learning curve of avoiding complications in lumbar endoscopic spine surgery, international journal of spine. Surgery. 2021;**15**(suppl. 3):S21-S37. DOI: 10.14444/8161

[33] Zhou C, Zhang G, Panchal RR, Ren X, Xiang H, Xuexiao M, et al. Unique complications of percutaneous endoscopic lumbar discectomy and percutaneous endoscopic Interlaminar discectomy. Pain Physician. 2018;**21**(2):E105-E112

[34] Lewandrowski KU. Incidence, management, and cost of complications after transforaminal endoscopic decompression surgery for lumbar foraminal and lateral recess stenosis: A value proposition for outpatient ambulatory surgery. International Journal of Spine Surgery. 2019;**13**(1):53-67. DOI: 10.14444/6008

[35] Parpaley Y, Urbach H, Kovacs A, Klehr M, Kristof RA. Pseudohypoxic brain swelling (postoperative intracranial hypotension-associated venous congestion) after spinal surgery: Report of 2 cases. Neurosurgery. 2011;**68**(1):E277-E283. DOI: 10.1227/NEU.0b013e3181fead14

[36] Choi G, Kang HY, Modi HN, Prada N, Nicolau RJ, Joh JY, et al. Risk of developing seizure after percutaneous endoscopic lumbar discectomy. Journal of Spinal Disorders & Techniques. 2011;**24**(2):83-92. DOI: 10.1097/BSD.0b013e3181ddf124

[37] Kim JE, Choi DJ, Park EJ. Evaluation of postoperative spinal epidural hematoma after Biportal endoscopic spine surgery for single-level lumbar spinal stenosis: Clinical and magnetic resonance imaging study. World Neurosurgery. 2019;**126**:e786-e792. DOI: 10.1016/j.wneu.2019.02.150 Epub 2019 Mar 14

[38] Kim HS, Kim JY, Wu PH, Jang IT. Effect of dorsal root ganglion retraction in endoscopic lumbar Decompressive surgery for Foraminal pathology: A retrospective cohort study of Interlaminar contralateral endoscopic lumbar Foraminotomy and discectomy versus Transforaminal endoscopic lumbar Foraminotomy and discectomy. World Neurosurgery. 2021;**148**:e101-e114. DOI: 10.1016/j.wneu.2020.12.176 Epub 2021 Jan 11

[39] Choi KC, Lee JH, Kim JS, Sabal LA, Lee S, Kim H, et al. Unsuccessful percutaneous endoscopic lumbar discectomy: A single-center experience of 10,228 cases. Neurosurgery. 2015;**76**(4):372-380; discussion 380-1; quiz 381. DOI: 10.1227/NEU.0000000000000628

[40] Lee SH, Kang BU, Ahn Y, Choi G, Choi YG, Ahn KU, et al. Operative failure of percutaneous endoscopic lumbar discectomy: A radiologic analysis of 55 cases. Spine (Phila Pa 1976). 2006;**31**(10):E285-E290

[41] Percutaneous Endoscopic Spine Surgery (History, Indications and Complications) [internet]. Available from: http://www.axis-hospital-croatia.com/percutaneous-endoscopic-spine-surgery-history-indications-and-complications/

[42] Moon ASM, Rajaram Manoharan SR. Endoscopic spine surgery: Current state of art and the future perspective. Asian Spine Journal. 2018;**12**(1):1-2. DOI: 10.4184/asj.2018.12.1.1 Epub 2018 Feb 7

[43] Yoon J, Wang M. The evolution of minimally invasive spine surgery. Journal of Neurosurgery: Spine. 2019;**30**:149-158. DOI: 10.3171/2018.11.SPINE181215

[44] Dietz N, Sharma M, Adams S, Alhourani A, Ugiliweneza B, Wang D, et al. Enhanced recovery after surgery (ERAS) for spine surgery: A systematic review. World Neurosurgery. 2019;**130**:415-426. DOI: 10.1016/j.wneu.2019.06.181 Epub 2019 Jul 2

[45] Is There a Bright Future for Endoscopic Spinal Surgery?[internet]. Available at: https://spinalnewsinternational.com/is-there-a-bright-future-for-endoscopic-spinal-surgery/

Chapter 2

Endoscopic Technique for Multilevel Spine Degeneration Based on 3 Column Theory: Do We Need Fusion?

Aloysius Bambang Darwono and Volodymyr Radchenko

Abstract

Multilevel spine degeneration with deformity should be described in 3 column theory of lumbar degeneration cascade to detect completely the degenerative damages or deformers. Theory of degenerative spine deformity is a combination between 2 factors: 1. spine stabilizer (disc, 2 facet joints, anterior and posterior longitudinal ligament, supra-spinatus ligament, multifidus muscle) and 2. spine deformer (degenerative injury). The common gold standard is to remove the deformer by open surgery, but this open surgery will sacrifice the stabilizer, so it requires artificial stabilizer or fusion device. The concept of minimally invasive endoscopic spine surgery is simply to remove the deformer while retaining the stabilizer. After deformer are removed, the stabilizers will be reapplied, and the deformity can be corrected naturally.

Keywords: endoscopy, spine degeneration, deformity, fusion, 3 column theory

1. Introduction

Surgery for treatment of multilevel spine degeneration with deformity, where are we now: open surgery, minimally invasive spine surgery, fusion or non-fusion. In fusion technique related to the nature of illness, the degenerative cascade will go to the adjacent level [1–7]. In non-fusion technique or decompression, the degenerative damages should be removed completely related to the nature of illness [8–10].

The theory of nature of illness in spine degeneration and deformity, including the nature of healing after surgery, will be discussed.

2. Three columns theory of lumbar degenerative

2.1 Cascade and classification

The axial stability is maintained along a vertical column system, three columns from C2 to the sacrum. The anterior column is formed by the vertebral bodies and discs, and the two posterior columns by posterior joints. Anterior column consist of vertebral bodies, discs, anterior, and posterior ligament. The articular facet joint and flavum ligament are middle column, while the posterior column consist of spinous process, inter- and supraspinatus ligament include multifidus muscle [11–14].

Three joint complex theory of lumbar degenerative cascade by Kirkaldy-Willis et al. described the detail of pathologic changes of the disc and two posterior joints, but this only describe the 2 vertical columns, anterior and middle column [15]. Christian Ingerslev Baastrup a Danish radiologist Copenhagen [16] described degenerative cascade of the posterior vertical column, pathologic changes on the spinous processes in the lumbar vertebrae including the soft tissues between them which was mentioned as kissing spine. His publication was supported by studies by Auckland and Bristol study group (2010), described a breakdown of the inter-spinous ligament and leading to a development of neo-arthrosis between adjacent spinous processes, characterized by abutment, enlargement, sclerosis and bursa [12, 14, 16–18].

The new three columns theory of Lumbar degenerative cascade related to the nature of illness of lumbar degeneration is built combining both theory to give a clear understanding about lumbar degenerative process: that may start from either one of the three columns, alone or together, starting from inflammatory to a compressive reactions, change the bio-mechanic construct of the lumbar spine, single or multi-levels and leading to a deformity or de novo scoliosis (**Figure 1**) [12, 14].

The new classification based on three columns theory of lumbar degenerative cascade could give a complete description about the various individual cascade of lumbar degeneration, and has the consequence in the clinical application of evidence-based treatment related to this theory: the justification of treatment for various individual cases will be different. The classification should describe a complete assessment of the bio-mechanic construct changes due to degenerative damages involving the three columns using the radiologic parameters of dynamic lumbosacral x-rays and MRI studies and could show the different cascade of each column. The grading classification consist of:

Grade 1, involve either one of the columns, each level in different cascade,

Grade 2, involve either 2 columns, each column or level in different cascade,

Grade3, involve 3 columns, each column or level in different cascade (**Figure 2**).

Purpose of this classification is to describe completely the bio-mechanic construct changes due to degenerative damages, involving all column of mobile segment, each column in different level and different cascade. It can be used as a guideline to fix and

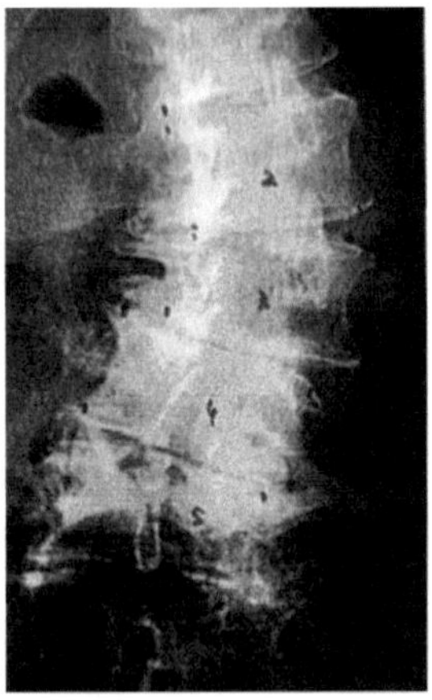

Figure 1.
De novo scoliosis.

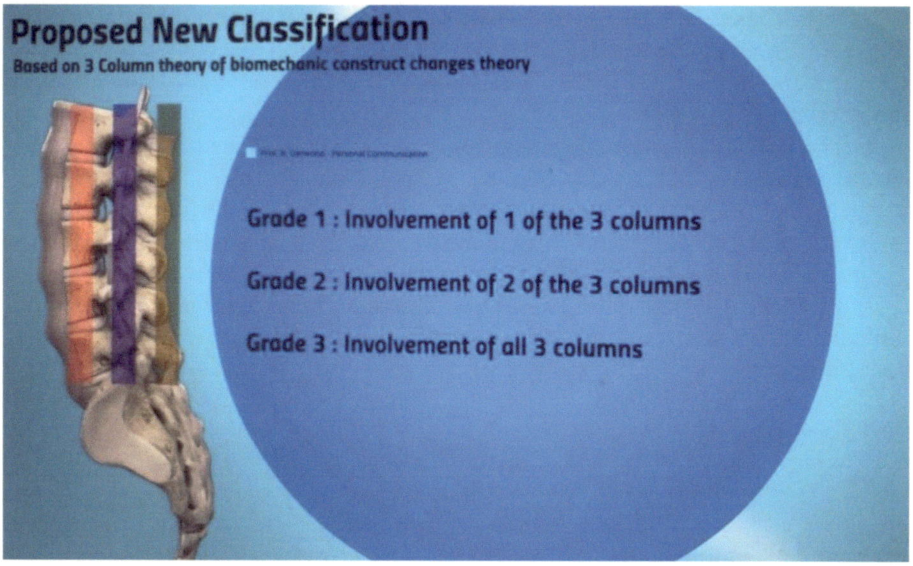

Figure 2.
Proposed new classification.

reconstruct all the degenerative damages, specially in preserving the spine motion, as an evidence-based consideration to justify the different methods of treatment for the various cases of lumbar degeneration [14].

3. Degenerative spine deformity

Lumbar spine stability during the dynamic movement is supported by disc, facet joint and strong ligament: anterior longitudinal, posterior longitudinal, and

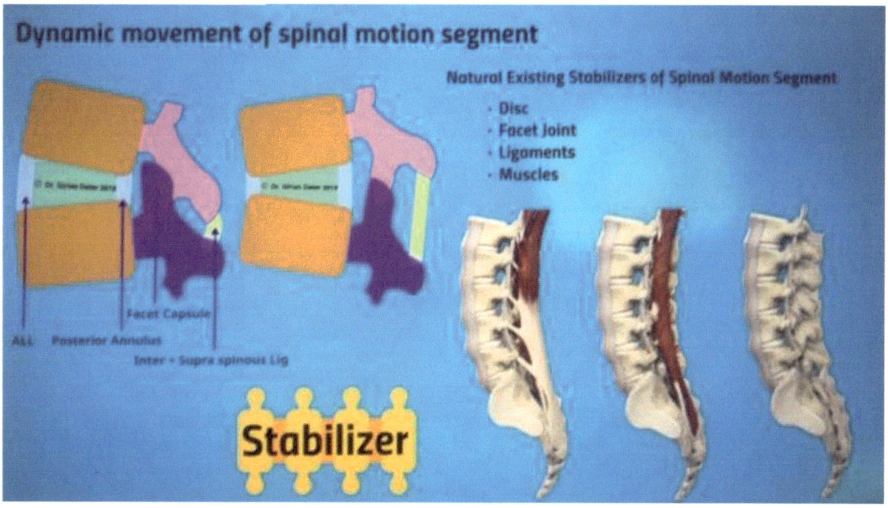

Figure 3.
Spine stabilizer.

supraspinatus ligament complex. According to Wolfgang Rauschning the supraspinatus ligament complex is not a ligament, but multiple tendon insertion of multifidus muscle [10, 13, 14, 19–25]. All the above anatomy including the muscle are known as spine stabilizer (**Figure 3**).

Anatomical changes due to degenerative damage occur in three columns: osteophyte, hypertrophy facet, lamina, spinous process, canal stenosis, disc herniation, disc narrowing, flavum in-folding and hypertrophy, kissing spine, kissing lamina, all of these are known as deformer in degenerative cascade because it will dysfunction the spine stabilizer (**Figure 4**) [14].

The degenerative spine deformity is a combination between two factors: spine stabilizer and spine deformer, creating instability and deformity in the three columns (**Figure 5**).

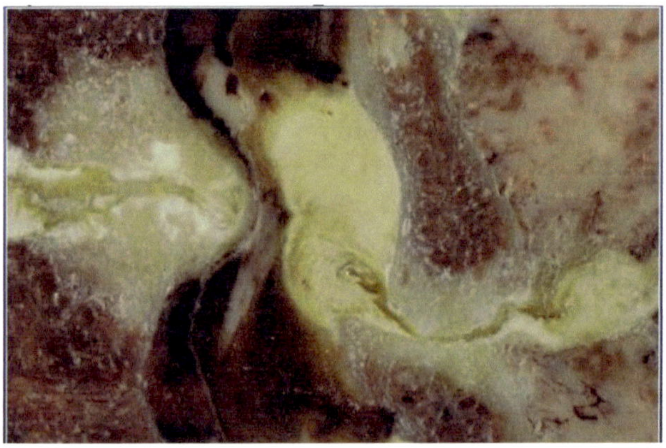

Figure 4.
Kissing lamina as deformer (courtesy of Rauschning).

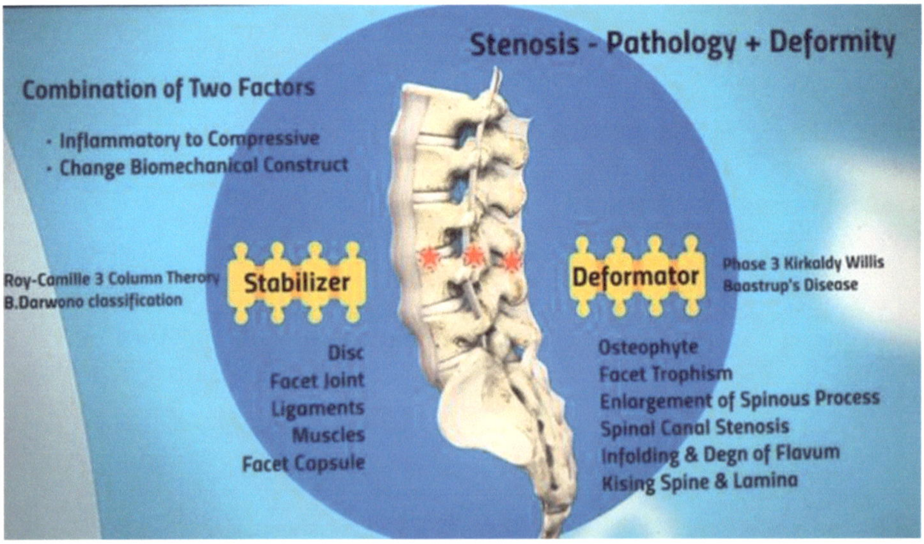

Figure 5.
Deformity as combination of two factors.

4. Option of treatment

The gold standard of treatment is open surgery or decompression to remove the deformer, but anyway this technique will sacrifice some of the stabilizer and as a consequence need to use artificial stabilizer or fusion to restabilize (**Figure 6**) [19, 20, 26, 27].

The question is, if the technique of surgery could preserve the stabilizer, does the artificial stabilizer is needed. Minimally invasive spine surgery using endoscope was developed to answer the question. A long evolution in developing this technology starting from Hijikata 1970s, Parviz Kambin 1980s, Screiber, Suezawa, Leu using discoscopy late 1980, Anthony Yeung transforaminal under continuous irrigation 1990s, Sebastian Rutten interlaminar and application of arthroscopic technique 2000s.

The disruptive surgical technology of spine endoscope is from dry environment in simple endoscopy to arthroscopic surgical dissection performed in the spine underwater with continuous irrigation and suction. Advantages of disruptive technology are:

- docking system and closed system irrigation, the water irrigation and suction could be controlled better,

- the continuous water irrigation will create a better visibility in the surgical area, reduce intra and postop bleeding and infection rate significantly,

- the range of approaches increased from pure transforaminal or posterolateral to interlaminar, because rongeur, high-speed drills, other instruments could be used and has a wider horizon of view.

- The current indication spectrum for lumbar, thoracic, and cervical applications become wide and covers all types of degenerative (and other) pathologies, which have been the domain of microsurgical techniques in the past.

The new concept of endoscopic surgical technique based on three columns theory is:

- Preserve the three columns spine stabilizers.

- Decompression to remove spine de-formators due to degenerative damage constricting the spinal canal in three columns.

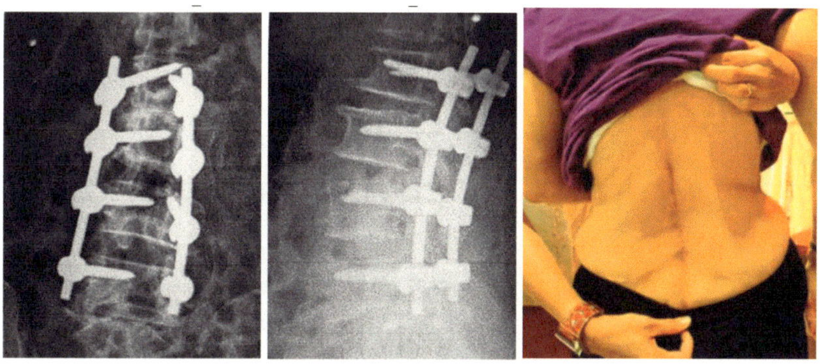

Figure 6.
Artificial stabilizer.

- Decompression will naturally refunction the spine stabilizers and could reduce the deformity without using artificial stabilizers.

- Deformity reduction is similar as the second decompression, because the best decompression is deformity correction.

5. Cases

Case 1: Lady 83, Low back pain and sciatica, spine deformity, wheelchair case. MRI show lumbar spondylosis with severe stenosis on L 3-4 and L 4-5. Treatment by endoscopic decompression from interlaminar and deformity was corrected well (**Figures** 7 and **8**).

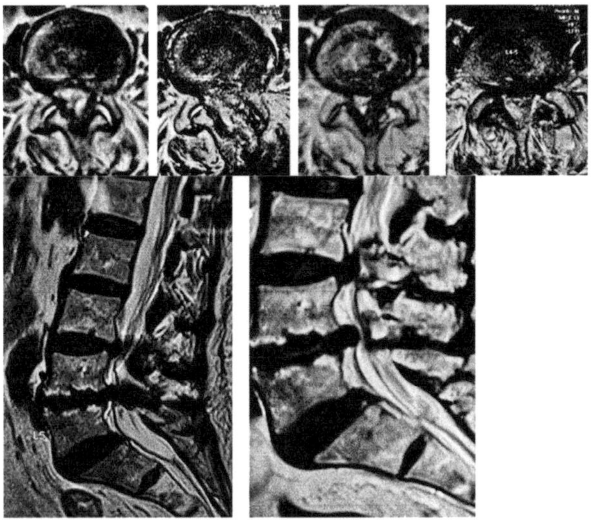

Figure 7.
MRI L 3-4, L 4-5, before and after endoscopic treatment.

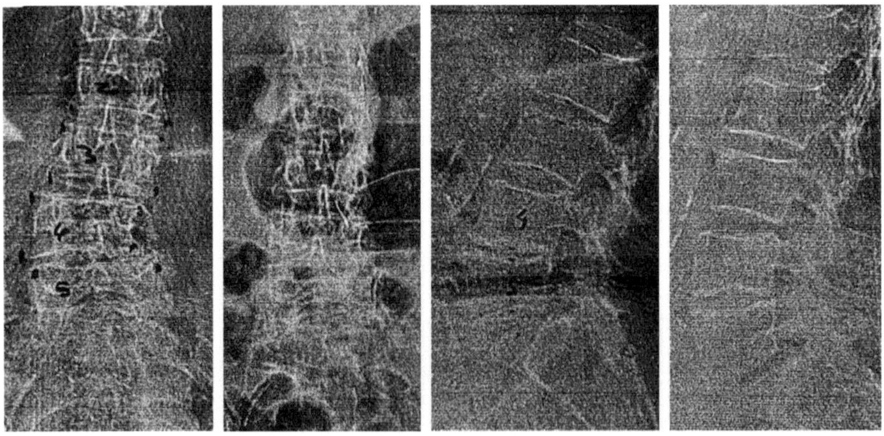

Figure 8.
Deformity corrected.

Case 2: Lady 62, Low back pain and sciatica with deformity, on MRI lumbar spondylosis L 2-3, 3-4, 4-5. Deformity was corrected after decompression by endoscopic interlaminar (**Figures 9** and **10**).

Case 3: Lady 55, low back pain and sciatica with deformity, claudication, wheelchair case. On MRI lumbar spondylosis and severe stenosis L 4-5. Deformity correction after endoscopic decompression interlaminar (**Figures 11** and **12**).

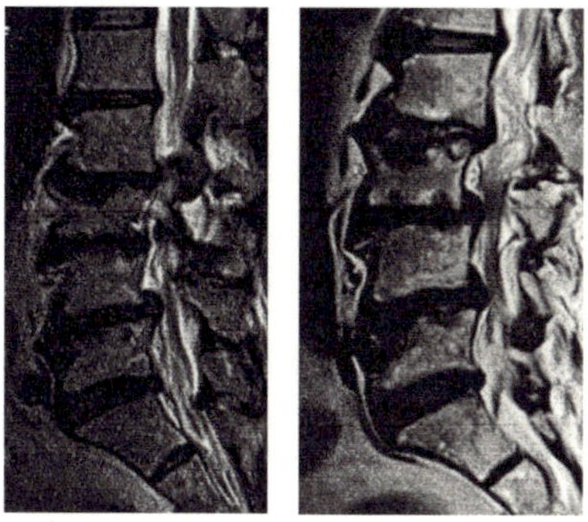

Figure 9.
MRI L2-3, 3-4, 4-5 before and after surgery.

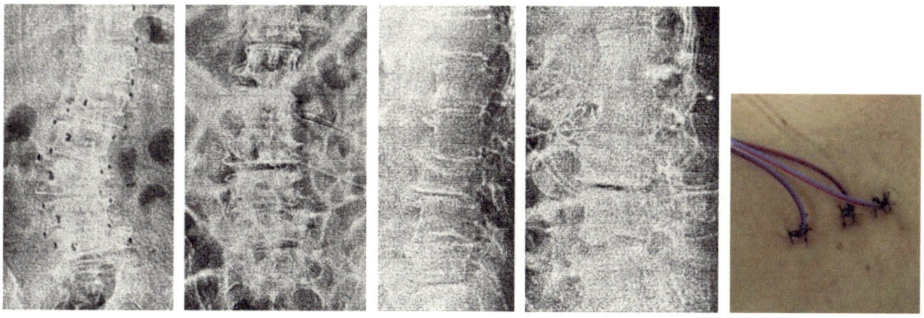

Figure 10.
Deformity corrected.

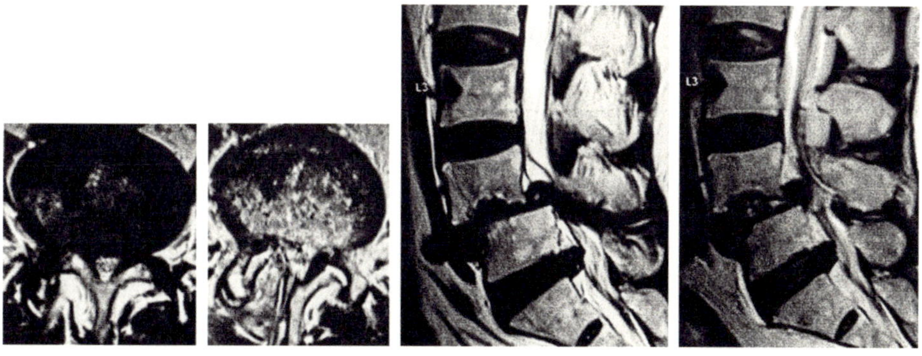

Figure 11.
MRI before and after surgery L 4-5.

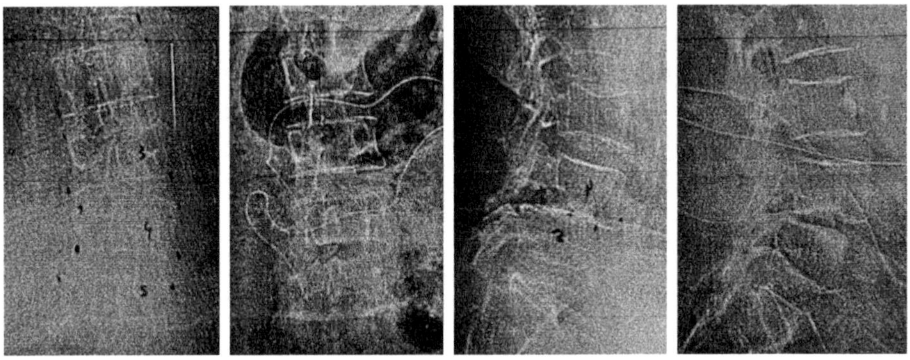

Figure 12.
Deformity corrected.

6. Conclusion

Spine is a life tissue and has the nature of healing after surgery that should be well supported. The new classification of spine degeneration describe all deformer of spine degeneration in three columns. Degenerative spine deformity is a combination of 2 factors: spine stabilizer and deformer. Removing all deformer could support the function of spine stabilizer to reduce the deformity. The disruptive technology of endoscopy using arthroscopic concept for the spine could remove all deformer while retaining the spine stabilizer. After deformer is removed, the stabilizer will be reapplied and the deformity can be corrected naturally.

Author details

Aloysius Bambang Darwono[1*] and Volodymyr Radchenko[2]

1 Gading Pluit Hospital, Medical Faculty of Tarumanagara University, Jakarta, Indonesia

2 Sytenko Institute of Spine and Joint Pathology, Kharkiv, Ukraine

*Address all correspondence to: bdarwono@yahoo.com.au

References

[1] Eck JC, Humphreys SC, Hodges SD. Adjacent-segment degeneration after lumbar fusion. A review of clinical, biochemical, and radiologic studies. The American Journal of Orthopedics. 1999;**28**:336-340

[2] Etebar S, Cahill DW. Risk factors for adjacent-segment failure following lumbar fixation with rigid instrumentation for degenerative instability. Journal of Neurosurgery. 1999;**90**:163-169

[3] Lee CK. Accelerated degeneration of the segment adjacent to a lumbar fusion. Spine. 1988;**13**(3):375-377

[4] Lindsey DP, Swanson KE, Fuchs P, et al. The effects of an interspinous implant on the kinematics of the instrumental and adjacent levels in the lumbar spine. Spine. 2003;**28**(19):2192-2197

[5] Molz F, Partin J, Kirkpatrick J. The acute effect of L3/L4 fusion on the motion of vertebrae in whole lumbar cadaveric spine. In: Presented at the Annual Meeting of the International Society for the Study of the Lumbar Spine; Vancouver, BC. 2003

[6] Patel C, Truumees E, Gittlin J, et al. Symptomatic spinal stenosis adjacent to a previous lumbar fusion. The Spine Journal. 2002;**2**:54S-55S

[7] Weinhoffer SL, Guyer RD, Herbert M, et al. Intradiscal pressure measurements above an instrumented fusion. A cadaver study. Spine. 1995;**20**(5):526-531

[8] Kanayama M, Hashimoto T, Shigenubu K, et al. Adjacent-segment morbidity after graft ligamentoplasty compared with posterolateral lumbar fusion. Journal of Neurosurgery. 2001;**95**(1 Suppl):5-10

[9] Kanayama M, Hashimoto T, Shigenubu K, et al. Non-fusion surgery for degenerative spondylolisthesis using artificial ligament stabilization: Surgical indication and clinical results. Spine. 2005;**30**(5):588-592

[10] Stoll TM, Dubois G, Schwarzenbach O. The dynamic neutralization system for the spine: A multi-center study of a novel non-fusion system. European Spine Journal. 2002;**11**(Suppl. 2):170-178

[11] Roy-Camille R. Traitement des fractures du rachis dorsolumbaire par la method de Bohler. Revue de Chirurgie Orthopédique et Réparatrice de l'Appareil Moteur. 1989;**75**(7):E109-E114

[12] Darwono B, Radchenko V. New classification 3 columns theory of lumbar degenerative cascade (literature review). Orthopaedics, Traumatology and Prosthetics. 2018;**610**(1):96-104. DOI: 10.15674/0030-59872018196-104

[13] Louis R. Spinal stability as defined by the three-column spine concept. Anatomica Clinica. 1985;7:33-42

[14] Darwono B. MISS Concept based on theory of three columns-lumbae degenerative cascade. In: Bambang Darwono: Presented at SICOT 42th Annual Meeting, Kuala Lumpur, Malaysia. 2022

[15] Kirkaldy-Willis WH, Wedge JH, Yong-Hing K, et al. Pathology and pathogenesis of lumbar spondylosis and stenosis. Spine. 1978;**3**:319-328

[16] Baastrup C. On the spinous processes of the lumbar vertebrae and the soft tissue between them, and on pathological changes in that region. Acta Radiologica. 1933;**14**:52-54

[17] Aylott CE, Puna R, Robertson PA, Walker C. Spinous process morphology: The effect of ageing through adulthood on spinous process size and relationship to sagittal alignment. European Spine Journal. 2012;**21**(5):1007-1012. DOI: 10.1007/s00586-011-2029-6

[18] Kwong Y, Rao N, Latief K. MDCT findings in Baastrup disease: Disease or normal features of the aging spine? AJR. American Journal of Roentgenology. 2011;**196**(5):1156-1159. DOI: 10.2214/AJR.10.5719

[19] Frymoyer JW, Krag MH. Spinal stability and instability: Definitions, classification, and general principles of management. In: Kahn A, editor. The Unstable Spine. New York: Grune & Startton; 1986

[20] Frymoyer JW, Sellby DK. Segmental instability. Rationale for treatment. Spine. 1985;**10**:280-286

[21] Fujiwara A, Lim TH, An HS, et al. The effect of disc degeneration and facet joint osteoarthritis on segmental flexibility of the lumbar spine. Spine. 2000;**25**(23):3036-3044

[22] Fujiwara A, Tamai K, An HS, et al. The relationship between disc degeneration, facet joint osteoarthritis, and stability of the degenerative lumbar spine. Journal of Spinal Disorders. 2000;**13**:444-450

[23] Okawa A, Shinomiya K, Komori H, et al. Dynamic motion study of the whole lumbar spine by video-fluoroscopy. Spine. 1998;**23**(916):1743-1749

[24] Paajanen H, Tertti M. Association of incipient disc degeneration and instability in spondylolisthesis. A magnetic resonance and flexion-extension radiographic study of 20-year-old low back pain patients. Archives of Orthopaedic and Trauma Surgery. 1991;**111**:16-19

[25] Pearcy MD, Tibrewal SB. Lumbar intervertebral disc and ligament deformations measured in vivo. Clinical Orthopaedics;**184, 191**:281-286

[26] DePalma AF, Rothman RH. Surgery of the lumbar spine. Clinical Orthopaedics. 1969;**63**:162-170

[27] Keller TS, Hanson TH, Abram AC, et al. Regional variations in the compressive properties of lumbar vertebral trabeculae. Effect of disc degeneration. Spine. 1989;**14**:1012-1019

Chapter 3

Endoscopic Transforaminal Lumbar Interbody Fusion

Jincai Yang, Yong Hai, Peng Yin, Bo Han, Honghao Yang and Jixuan Huang

Abstract

One of the most common surgical cures for lumbar degenerative illnesses is lumbar fusion. Traditional open lumbar fusion is often used in clinical settings and has positive clinical results. However, there are some disadvantages of the traditional open approach, such as tremendous surgical invasiveness and a high risk of complications in the perioperative period. The gold standard for minimally invasive surgical techniques in recent years has been minimally invasive transforaminal lumbar interbody fusion (MIS-TLIF). With the advancement of full-endoscopic spine surgical techniques, endoscopic lumbar surgery has rapidly developed from simple discectomy to decompression of spinal stenosis. Currently, the endoscopic lumbar interbody fusion procedure has been performed. On the basis of adequate spinal canal decompression and dependable interbody fusion, endoscopic lumbar interbody fusion could reduce surgical invasiveness and improve patient recovery. In this chapter, we will give a brief introduction to the advance in endoscopic transforaminal lumbar interbody fusion, focusing on the indication, technical aspects, clinical effectiveness, safety, fusion devices, and novel techniques that could be applied in the near future.

Keywords: endoscopic, transforaminal lumbar interbody fusion, percutaneous, minimally invasive, biportal

1. Introduction

Since the first description of endoscopic transforaminal lumbar interbody fusion (TLIF) by Leu et al. in 1997 [1], this technique has undergone more than 20 years of evolution. Concerns have centered on the efficacy and safety of endoscopic TLIF for neural decompression and solid interbody fusion. Numerous studies have demonstrated the efficacy of endoscopic TLIF in relieving low back and leg pain and enhancing the quality of life [2, 3]. Some research has also reported a high incidence of surgical complications, such as nerve root injury, cage migration, and pseudarthrosis, which have been the obstacles to the further development of endoscopic TLIF [4].

Surgeons from all over the world have conducted valuable explorations, including the innovations of endoscopic instruments and improvements in surgical technique. These advancements have increased the effectiveness and safety of endoscopic TLIF, allowing it to be applied as a routine procedure of minimally invasive spine surgery.

IntechOpen

In this chapter, we will give a brief introduction to the advance in endoscopic TLIF, focusing on the indication, technical aspects, clinical effectiveness, safety, fusion devices, and novel techniques that could be applied in the near future.

2. Surgical Indications and Stepwise selection

2.1 Surgical indications

Discogenic low back pain, lumbar foraminal or lateral recess stenosis with segmental instability, and Meyerding Grade I-II degenerative/isthmic spondylolisthesis should be the indications for endoscopic TLIF.

2.2 Stepwise selection of indications

According to the technical demanding level, the risks of complications, the controllability of operating time, and the surgeon's proficiency in endoscopic techniques, a stepwise selection of indications for endoscopic TLIF should be considered.

Single-level and unilateral diseases that do not require radical nerve decompression, such as discogenic low back pain, lumbar segmental instability, Meyerding Grade I lumbar spondylolisthesis, and unilateral symptomatic lumbar lateral recess stenosis, should be selected in the early stages of implementing endoscopic TLIF.

Surgeons with sufficient experience in endoscopic decompression and fusion techniques could choose to treat lumbar disc herniation or lumbar spinal stenosis requiring unilateral decompression at double segments or bilateral decompression at single segment, as well as Meyerding grade II lumbar spondylolisthesis.

After proficiently mastering endoscopic fusion techniques, surgeons could choose more challenging lumbar diseases, such as revision surgery for postendoscopic decompression.

For lumbar ossification-related disorders with cauda equina syndrome or revision surgery for postoperative segmental instability, endoscopic TLIF should be performed with caution. However, as endoscopic techniques and instruments continue to advance, the indications for endoscopic TLIF may be expanded.

3. Technical aspects

3.1 Percutaneous endoscopic transforaminal lumbar interbody fusion

Percutaneous endoscopic transforaminal lumbar interbody fusion (PE-TLIF) is performed while the patient is prone under general anesthesia or low-dose epidural anesthesia combined with local anesthesia. Using C-arm fluoroscopy, the lumbar segment is validated. After placing the functional conduit through Kambin's triangle, the endoscope system is connected. Under endoscopic observation, the ligament flavum is dissected, and the superior articular process (SAP) is excised with micro scissors or a burr drill. Then, the lateral spinal canal is decompressed, and the nerve root that traverses the canal is released. Endoscopic confirmation that the traversing and exiting nerve roots are protected from the working channel is followed by the discectomy and removal of the cartilaginous endplates. After the endplates have been sufficiently prepared, the endoscope is removed and the 7 mm PEEK or titanium expandable fusion cage is inserted through the working channel under radiography. The endoscope is used to examine the spinal canal and foramina to ensure that the nerve root is relieved. Using the radioscopic device, four pedicle screws are percutaneously implanted into the predetermined locations. Inserting two rods and tightening the screw-rod attachment. The epidermis is sutured, and the position of the fasteners and cage is re-evaluated using a C-arm fluoroscope.

3.2 Surgical innovations in PE-TLIF contributed by the authors

3.2.1 Safe removal of the superior articular process

The authors innovated in the safe removal of the SAP, as an innovative concept [5, 6]. In brief, syringe needles are used to identify the pedicle positions. Four incisions (5 mm) are made and then 4 primary guide pins are inserted. The depth is determined by fluoroscopy. The inferior primary guide on the hypothetically symptomatic side is confirmed as the first guide pin. At the end of the first guide pin, the specially designed oriented SAP resection device is installed. With the aid of this device, a secondary guide pin is percutaneously inserted into the SAP (**Figure 1**). After removing the guide, a 12-mm skin incision is made along the secondary guide pin. Dilating and protection cannulas are inserted progressively with the help of a secondary guide pin. While soft tissues and nerves are protected by the protection cannula, the part of the SAP is excised and taken out using a ring saw (**Figure 2**).

The primary benefit of this method is its ability to safely and effectively resect SAP. The design of the oriented SAP resection device is based on the relatively constant anatomical relationship between SAP and pedicles in the lumbar spine, allowing the removal of a portion of SAP without nerve damage when the standard procedure is followed.

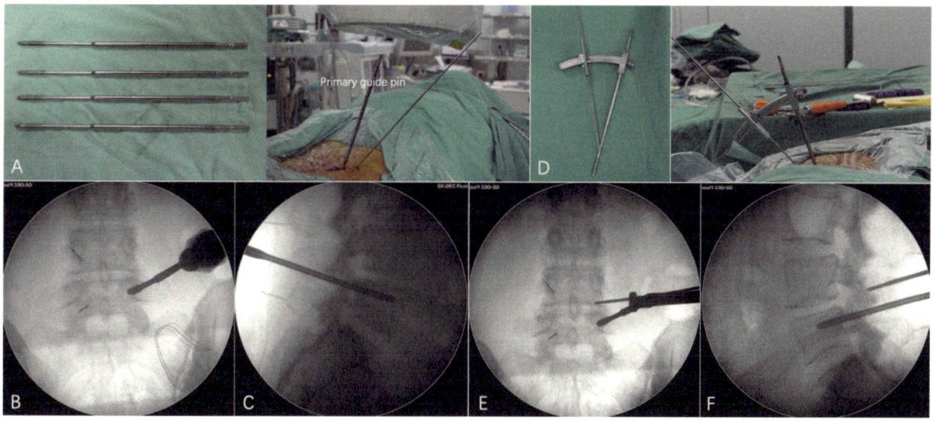

Figure 1.
Guide pin insertion under fluoroscopy. (A) The primary guide pin (left), whose front end is threaded and can be firmly fixed in the pedicle, and its position are readily identifiable under fluoroscopy; the primary guide pin is percutaneously inserted into the vertebral pedicle and rotated to fix (right). (B–C) C-arm anteroposterior and lateral fluoroscopy confirms that the primary guide pin penetrates the pedicle and that the upper thread edge is below the dorsal lateral level of the superior articular process. (D) Physical view of the specially designed SAP guider; the first and second guide pins are connected by a connecting arch, and the angle and depth of the second guide pin's perforation can be adjusted on the connecting arch. (E–F) C-arm anteroposterior and lateral fluoroscopy confirms that the second guide pin is attached to the superior articular process's posterior aspect. Reproduction permission was acquired from Yin et al. [5]. Originally published by and used with permission from Dove Medical Press Ltd.

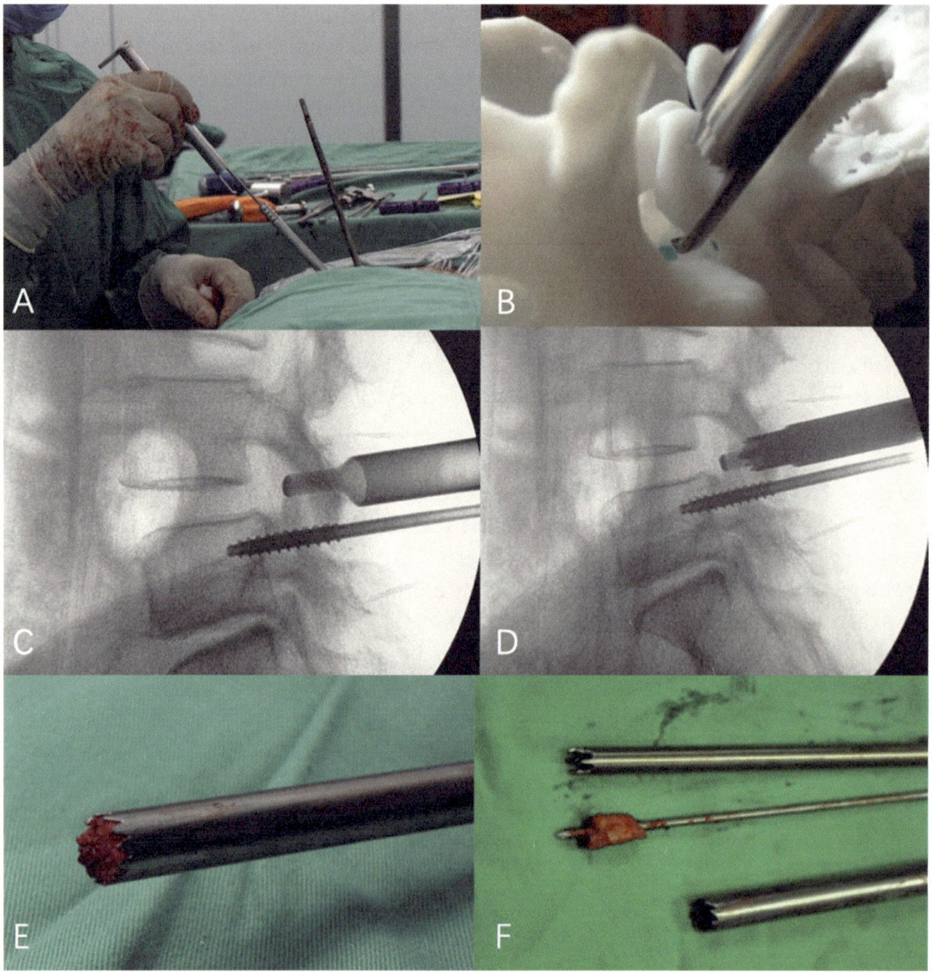

Figure 2.
A-F: Resection method of the superior articular process: the hook-shaped protective sleeve clings to the lateral cortex of the superior articular process, reaches the ventral side of the articular process, protects the exiting nerve root and can control the cutting depth of the trephine at the same time, protects the dura mater and nerve root, and rotates the trephine to remove the superior articular process.

In the meantime, the hook-shaped device in front of the cannula for SAP resection could limit the depth of incision, thereby preventing trepan-cutting of the nerve root and dura mater.

3.2.2 Innovative surgical instruments for intervertebral space handling

The authors developed a set of innovative surgical instruments for intervertebral space handling, including a width-adjustable intervertebral chisel and various nerve-protecting sheaths. These tools could assist the surgeon in precisely placing surgical instruments and endoscopes into the intervertebral space, facilitating safer and more precise operations (**Figure 3**).

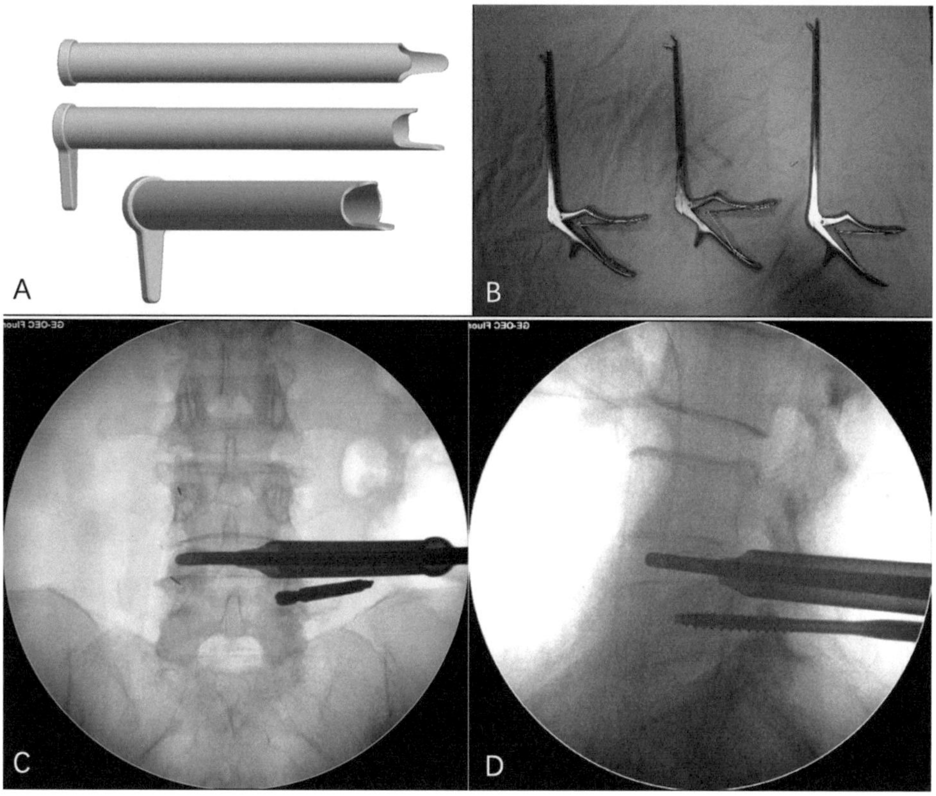

Figure 3.
Intervertebral space handling by the working sleeve. (A) Bone grafting channel with double tongue-shaped nerve-protecting sheaths. The tongue flaps are at the front end, one is long and the other is short; the tongue flap is designed according to the working sleeve tilted at 45°; the long tongue flap is used to protect the dura and nerve root in the spinal canal; and the short tongue flap is used to protect the exit nerve roots; they could simultaneously protect the traversing nerve root and the exiting nerve root outside the bone grafting channel. (B) The 4.5 mm straight and elbow rongeur are used to remove disc tissue. (C–D) Rongeur is used to remove the intervertebral disc tissue and confirm the position of the rongeur to ensure adequate resection of the disc.

3.2.3 Height-adjustable interbody fusion cage

The authors designed a height-adjustable interbody fusion cage, which could withstand greater motion and compressive loads, with its functionality remaining normal even under a 3000N compressive force [5]. Although its implantation channel requires an 8 mm working channel, larger than the B-Twin intervertebral fusion cage's minimum 5 mm channel, the round front end of the adjustable intervertebral fusion cage is more prone to be implanted. The maximal height of 13 mm after expansion could enhance the tension of the longitudinal ligament and annulus fibrosus while decreasing the risk of vertebral body fracture due to excessive expansion. The adjustable intervertebral fusion cage is designed with the characteristics of parallel expansion and a 3°~8° lordosis angle, which could not only consist with the stability of the superior/inferior endplates but also meet the sagittal lordosis requirement of lumbar spine. Moreover, its tapered sawtooth cross-section can reduce the risk of fusion cage migration (**Figure 4**).

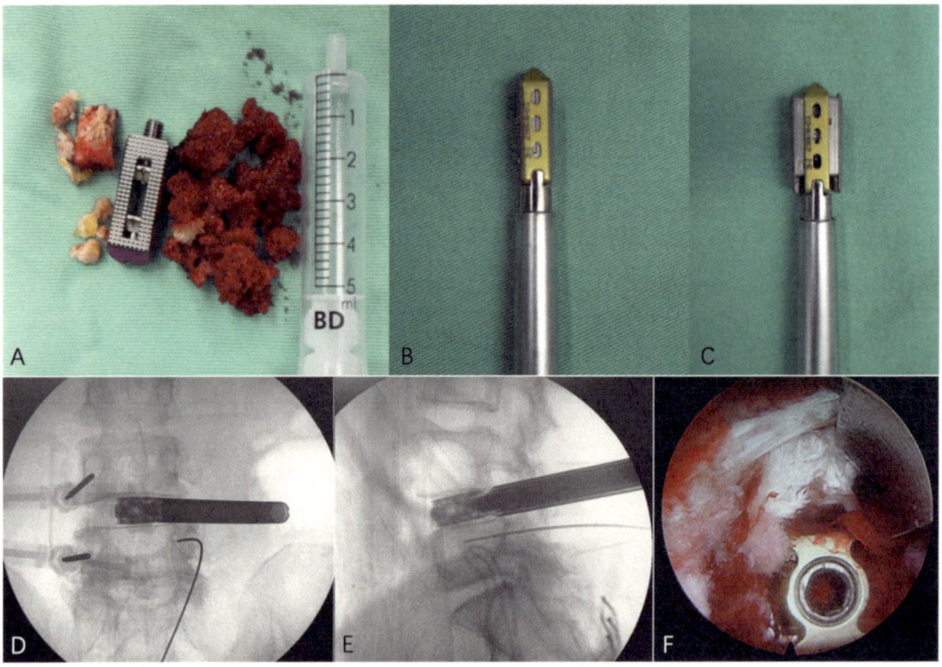

Figure 4.
Bone graft and interbody fusion cage implantation. (A–C) Height-adjustable cage, the autogenous bone, and allogenic bone are prepared for implantation. (D–E) The height-adjustable fusion cage is positioned at the center of the interbody space in the anteroposterior radiograph, and the leading edge reaches the position of the iliac crest. (F) The height-adjustable cage is confirmed in a satisfactory position under endoscopy. Nerves are not compressed by bone graft. Reproduced with permission from Yin et al. [5]. Originally published by and used with permission from Dove Medical Press Ltd.

3.3 Unilateral biportal endoscopic transforaminal lumbar interbody fusion

UBE-TLIF combines the benefits of open and endoscopic surgery. UBE-TLIF is performed while the patient is prone under general or epidural anesthesia. All decompression and interbody fusion procedures are carried out utilizing a biportal endoscopic system. Briefly, the installation of watertight draperies and the establishment of portal sites under fluoroscopic guidance. Two ipsilateral skin incisions are made in the paramedian region, one centimeter above and one centimeter below the midpoint of the intervertebral space, as well as on the ipsilateral medial border of the pedicle. In the left-sided approach, the upper orifice serves as the endoscopic portal, whereas the lower hole is the functional portal. After making two small incisions in the epidermis and fascia, adequate portals are created using serial dilators. Using a specialized lamina dissector inserted through the working portal, the lamina is then dissected. During the procedure, an endoscopic irrigation system is utilized, and irrigation fluid is drained from the endoscopic portal to the working portal. If the irrigation flow is inadequate, a small endoscopic retractor can be utilized to enhance the flow, ensure adequate visibility, and reduce soft tissue edema. Using a radiofrequency coagulator, further osseous dissection and control of hemorrhage are performed. Using a tubular retractor and a microscope, the UBE-TLIF technique is comparable to the MIS-TLIF technique. Endoscopic burrs and Kerrison punches are used to conduct ipsilateral hemilaminectomy. After adequate ipsilateral decompression, the ligamentum flavum is removed by decompressing the contralateral sublaminar portion with sublaminar drilling. Using endoscopic burrs and osteotomes, a unilateral facetectomy is then conducted to harvest autograft bone. Complete exposure of the ipsilateral and contralateral nerve roots should be confirmed. Using pituitary forceps and reamers, the disc is radically removed after complete dorsal decompression. Under endoscopic observation, the cartilaginous endplate is removed completely using curettes. Under fluoroscopic guidance, bone fragments from the lamina and facet are impacted into the disc space, and an interbody fusion cage containing bone grafts and fusion material is inserted. The procedure concludes with the insertion of additional percutaneous pedicle screws and a drain catheter to prevent epidural hematoma.

4. Clinical effectiveness and safety

The main criteria for evaluating endoscopic TLIF remain clinical outcomes, complications, operating time, and surgical invasiveness. Compared to the conventional MIS-TLIF, a well-established endoscopic TLIF should present comparable clinical outcomes, complication rate, and operating time. In addition, it should result in less invasiveness, less estimated blood loss, and improved postoperative recovery.

4.1 Clinical outcomes

A large amount of research has confirmed that PE-TLIF, UBE-TLIF, and MIS-TLIF all have the capacity to achieve satisfactory clinical effects, with no significant differences in mid- to long-term outcomes. Several meta-analyses have reported that both PE-TLIF and UBE-TLIF are superior to MIS-TLIF in early relief of low back pain, especially within three months after surgery; however, there is no significant difference between the alleviation of leg discomfort and the enhancement of the Oswestry Disability Index [7, 8]. These results suggest that endoscopic TLIF could achieve adequate nerve decompression, with less ischemic damage to paraspinal muscles, ligaments, and posterior soft tissue.

4.2 Complications

In the early stages of application, the complication rate of endoscopic TLIF procedures was relatively high. In 2013, Jacquot et al. reported a complication rate of 36.8% in 57 cases of PE-TLIF surgery, mainly including nerve root injury and cage migration, and 13 cases (22.8%) required revision of surgery [9]. With advancements in endoscopic instruments and surgical techniques, the incidence of complications in endoscopic TLIF has decreased dramatically in recent years. A recent meta-analysis showed that the incidence of complications in PE-TLIF was 10.1%, which is close to that of MIS-TLIF (12.7%); the incidence of complications in UBE-TLIF (7.8%) was also similar to that of MIS-TLIF (7.1%) [8, 10]. The most common complications are dura tear, nerve injury, endplate injury, and screw misplacement. Most of the complications are mild in symptoms, which can be improved with conservative treatment.

4.2.1 Dural tear and nerve injury

Dural tear and nerve injuries are the most common complications of endoscopic TLIF surgery. In the literature, the incidence of these complications is 0.1-8% for

PE-TLIF and 3-10% for UBE-TLIF, which is slightly higher than that in MIS-TLIF [11]. Endoscopic TLIF surgery may have a high risk of exiting nerve root irritation; however, the majority of these complications occurred during the initial phases of the learning curve and diminished as proficiency increased. Local anesthesia or general anesthesia with neuromonitoring may be an effective measure to reduce the risks of nerve injury.

4.2.2 Cage subsidence/migration

Cage subsidence or migration is a common complication in endoscopic TLIF surgery, with a slightly higher incidence than MIS-TLIF. Apart from osteoporosis, endplate injury is the culprit for cage subsidence. Intraoperatively, if the cage could not be implanted parallel to the endplate, the risk of endplate injury may increase. It is also important to note the bleeding from cancellous bone, which indicates injury to the bony endplate. Literature reports that in the early stages of PE-TLIF, the incidence of cage migration is 2 to 4%, while it is less common in UBE-TLIF [12, 13]. This may be due to the limited size of the instruments used, resulting in lower efficiency and insufficient handling of the intervertebral space.

4.2.3 Hematoma

According to previous studies, the incidence of postoperative hematoma in UBE-TLIF is higher than that of PE-TLIF, with an incidence of about 4% [14]. This may be due to the need to dissect more soft tissue and remove more bony structures in UBE-TLIF. The continuous fluid irrigation in the water-based endoscopic system may also impact the operation of hemostasis, causing an increased rate of postoperative hematoma. Active bleeding during the operation could be controlled by bipolar radio-frequency ablation, and hemostatic materials could be used to reduce the hemorrhage associated with epidural veins and bone surfaces.

4.2.4 Systemic complications

Research shows that the incidence of infection in endoscopic TLIF procedures is lower than that in MIS-TLIF, which may be attributed to the less invasiveness of endoscopic lumbar fusion surgery [15]. In terms of other systemic complications such as urinary retention, pneumonia, pulmonary embolism, and deep vein thrombosis, the endoscopic TLIF also presents a significantly lower incidence than MIS-TLIF. This may be related to enhanced recovery and early ambulation after endoscopic lumbar fusion surgery.

4.3 Operating time

Most literature reports a longer operating time in endoscopic TLIF procedures than that in MIS-TLIF [8]. The most time-consuming aspect of endoscopic lumbar fusion surgery is the handling of intervertebral space and endplate preparation. Although the improvement of endoscopic instruments has significantly increased the efficiency of these procedures, intraoperative evaluation of the endplate preparation status still requires a considerable amount of time. Unlike MIS-TLIF, which only requires palpation to assess the status of endplate preparation, endoscopic surgery needs additional visual observation or fluoroscopy to clearly ensure it.

4.4 Surgical invasiveness

MIS-TLIF necessitates extensive paraspinal muscle dissection and removal of the facet joint, partial lamina, and ligamentum flavum, whereas endoscopic TLIF aims to preserve these structures while ensuring adequate operative space, thereby significantly reducing surgical invasiveness. Both PE-TLIF and UBE-TLIF were shown by meta-analysis to substantially reduce intraoperative estimated blood loss compared to MIS-TLIF [8, 10]. In patients undergoing endoscopic TLIF, postoperative drainage, blood loss, and inflammatory indicators (e.g., C-reactive protein) were all reduced, and they also experienced a significantly shorter duration of ambulation and discharge from hospital. These effects of enhanced recovery after surgery are attributed to less invasiveness by endoscopic lumbar fusion surgery.

5. Learning curve

The learning curve for endoscopic TLIF is relatively long, and surgeons are required to have proficient endoscopic decompression experience before performing endoscopic lumbar fusion. In 2019, Kolcun et al. reported a case series of 100 consecutive patients undergoing PE-TLIF [16]. Complications occurred in four cases but three of which were developed in the initial stage of applying this procedure. Xu et al. suggested that at least 54 cases of endoscopic decompression were needed before performing UBE-TLIF [17]. Based on our experience, it is necessary to perform 20-30 endoscopic decompression procedures before the transition to more complex cases requiring lumbar interbody fusion.

6. Selection of fusion cages

In the early stages of endoscopic TLIF, the fusion process involved only interbody bone grafting, which resulted in a high incidence of postoperative bone graft absorption, displacement, and pseudarthrosis. As of now, fusion cages combined with autologous or synthetic bone implants are regarded as the gold standard. Based on the categories of materials used for fusion cages, they can be classified into metallic materials, polymer materials, and biomaterials.

The main types of metallic materials applied in endoscopic spine fusion cages are titanium alloys, which exhibit good mechanical properties and stability, making them suitable for the 3D printing of personalized and expandable fusion cages. However, metallic fusion cages have several disadvantages, such as a high elastic modulus, a high risk of subsidence, and metal artifacts, which can impact fusion status assessment. Polymer materials, such as polyetheretherketone (PEEK) and carbon fiber reinforced polymer (CFRP), are characterized by bone tissue-matched elastic modulus, low-stress shielding, and no artifacts. Additionally, fusion cages made of polymers can be designed into different shapes, such as bullet- or kidney-shaped, which are appropriate for endoscopic lumbar fusion surgery. Degradable polymers, such as polycarbonates, have excellent biocompatibility; however, the clinical application is limited by their high brittleness, long bone healing time, and adverse reactions caused by degradation products. Biomaterials, such as allogeneic bone, can shorten the duration of fusion but their low mechanical stiffness is not conducive to maintaining intervertebral height. Currently, expandable fusion cages made of titanium alloys or nonexpandable fusion cages made of polymer materials are the main alternative for endoscopic lumbar fusion surgery, but clinical trials with large sample sizes and long-term follow-up are still required.

Although there are various types of fusion cages, the safety of implantation procedures should be ensured. Fusion cages could be implanted through expandable channels and in the guidance of wires or tracks. Among the fusion cages that are commonly used, the size of titanium alloy expandable devices is relatively small, and they can be directly implanted through an endoscopic protective sheath tube. When passing through the Kambin triangle, expandable fusion cages have the least impact on nearby nerves, thus presenting high neuro-safety.

7. Fusion rate

According to clinical research, the fusion rate of endoscopic TLIF is comparable to that of MIS-TLIF. The fusion rate was 95.0% (360/379) and 94.9% (451/457) for patients undergoing PE-TLIF and MIS-TLIF, respectively [10]. The fusion rate between UBE-TLIF and MIS-TLIF is also comparable. However, some studies have indicated that the endoscopic TLIF would require more time to achieve fusion status than MIS-TLIF, with a fusion rate of 85.3% at 12 months for PE-TLIF and 92.3% for MIS-TLIF [2]. This discrepancy may be due to the continuous irrigation of bone surfaces with saline during endoscopic lumbar fusion procedures. Bone graft bed quality, bone graft material, fusion cage design, fusion status assessment criteria, and length of follow-up are all related to fusion success. Bone morphogenetic protein-2 has the potential to greatly increase the pace of fusion and decrease the time needed to achieve a fusion state.

8. Advanced techniques and future

Attributed to the development of imaging technologies and computer science, digital/intelligent surgery and implants would be the future of spine surgery. Robotic-assisted systems, mixed reality, and artificial intelligence (AI)–based surgical planning and implant design are expected to deeply integrate with endoscopic TLIF surgery. These techniques could further reduce surgical invasiveness, improve surgical efficiency, decrease the risks of neurological and vascular complications, and provide lower radiation to patients.

8.1 Robotic-assisted system

In the realm of spine surgery, a robot-assisted system is predominantly utilized for pedicle screw placement, presenting increased accuracy and diminished radiation exposure compared to traditional fluoroscopy [18]. Despite the similarities to O-arm navigations, a robot-assisted system could provide more precise physical guidance for surgeons to execute the surgical plan. Endoscopic lumbar fusion requires recurrent fluoroscopy for percutaneous pedicle screw insertion because the entry points of the pedicle screw are not visible. Therefore, the role of robotic-assisted surgery is more significant in endoscopic TLIF, and the safety and efficacy of the robot-assisted system in PE-TLIF have been well-validated by Chang et al. [19]. With the advent of an autonomous robotic system, decompression and facetectomy by a robot in endoscopic TLIF may be realized in the near future.

8.2 Mixed reality

Mixed reality (MR) technology is a combination of virtual reality and augmented reality, which anchors 3D hologram into the physical object and establishes an interactive feedback loop between the virtual and real world. In surgery, with the MR, a 3D anatomical model based on patients' imaging data could be seamlessly integrated into the real surgical site, enabling surgeons to have a 3D vitalization and get real-time interaction. MR has been applied in various spine surgery, mainly for pedicle screw fixation [20]. Although it is similar to conventional navigation, MR is more adequate to facilitate synchronization between the image and the surgical field. Butler et al. reported the first case series of 164 patients with percutaneous pedicle screw fixation under the MR system [21]. In this study, only 3 minutes and 54 seconds were required from registration to placement for each screw, and high accuracy was achieved. Therefore, with the development of display and wearable devices, MR has the potential to be routinely used in endoscopic TLIF in the future.

8.3 Artificial intelligence–based surgical planning and implants design

A variety of AI automatic surgical planning and implant design systems for spine surgery have been reported. Caprara et al. employed an AI preoperative planning system to find the optimized pedicle screw trajectories by maximizing the CT-derived bone mechanical properties [22]. Recently, Ma et al. developed an innovative CT image-based AI technique for screw trajectory planning, including components of automatic vertebral detection, auto-simulation of pedicle screw placement, bone mineral density estimation, and screw pull-out simulations [23]. The optimized trajectories demonstrated significantly higher bone mineral density and pull-out force than the conventional trajectories, which would especially benefit patients with osteoporosis. Similarly, AI automatic design system for fusion cages was also developed. In addition to morphological matching, the fusion cages designed by this system have personalized biomechanical adaptability. Compared to titanium alloys or PEEK fusion cages, it possesses a more gradual stepwise elastic modulus, which matches the bone strength of patients. It is no doubt that the AI-based surgical planning and implant design system would provide more appropriate and personalized surgical planning for each patient, and it would have an important role in endoscopic TLIF surgery to further improve clinical outcomes.

9. Conclusion

Endoscopic TLIF requires proficiency in endoscopic decompression techniques as a foundation, coupled with a deep understanding of open fusion surgery or the MIS-TLIF technique. Surgeons should strictly select appropriate indications and choose suitable endoscopic lumbar fusion procedures based on their technique level and case characteristics, with an emphasis on surgical safety, effectiveness, and long-term clinical outcomes. Although the current limitations of endoscopic TLIF include a long learning curve, a lack of long-term interbody fusion outcomes, and the absence of standardized surgical procedures, the future prospects for endoscopic TLIF will be better with the improvement of endoscopic instruments, bone graft materials, imaging technologies, and AI system.

Conflict of interest

The authors declare no conflict of interest. This work was supported by Shoufa grant [2020-2-2038].

Author details

Jincai Yang, Yong Hai*, Peng Yin, Bo Han, Honghao Yang and Jixuan Huang
Department of Orthopedic Surgery, Beijing Chaoyang Hospital, Capital Medical University, Beijing, China

*Address all correspondence to: prof.haiyong@yahoo.com

References

[1] Leu HF, Hauser RK, Schreiber A. Lumbar percutaneous endoscopic interbody fusion. Clinical Orthopaedics and Related Research. 1997;**337**:58-63

[2] Ao S, Zheng W, Wu J, Tang Y, Zhang C, Zhou Y, et al. Comparison of preliminary clinical outcomes between percutaneous endoscopic and minimally invasive transforaminal lumbar interbody fusion for lumbar degenerative diseases in a tertiary hospital: Is percutaneous endoscopic procedure superior to MIS-TLIF? A prospective cohort study. International Journal of Surgery. 2020;**76**:136-143

[3] Wang JC, Cao Z, Li ZZ, Zhao HL, Hou SX. Full-endoscopic lumbar interbody fusion versus minimally invasive transforaminal lumbar interbody fusion with a tubular retractor system: A retrospective controlled study. World Neurosurgery. 2022;**165**:e457-ee68

[4] Kolcun JPG, Brusko GD, Wang MY. Endoscopic transforaminal lumbar interbody fusion without general anesthesia: Technical innovations and outcomes. Annals of Translational Medicine. 2019;7(Suppl 5):S167

[5] Yin P, Ding Y, Zhou L, Xu C, Gao H, Pang D, et al. Innovative percutaneous endoscopic transforaminal lumbar interbody fusion of lumbar spinal stenosis with degenerative instability: A non-randomized clinical trial. Journal of Pain Research. 2021;**14**:3685-3693

[6] Yin P, Gao H, Zhou L, Pang D, Hai Y, Yang J. Enhanced recovery after an innovative percutaneous endoscopic transforaminal lumbar interbody fusion for the treatment of lumbar spinal stenosis: A prospective observational study. Pain Research & Management. 2021;**2021**:7921662

[7] Guo H, Song Y, Weng R, Tian H, Yuan J, Li Y. Comparison of clinical outcomes and complications between endoscopic and minimally invasive transforaminal lumbar interbody fusion for lumbar degenerative diseases: A systematic review and meta-analysis. Global Spine Journal. 2022:21925682221142545

[8] Yang H, Cheng F, Hai Y, Liu Y, Pan A. Unilateral biportal endoscopic lumbar interbody fusion enhanced the recovery of patients with the lumbar degenerative disease compared with the conventional posterior procedures: A systematic review and meta-analysis. Frontiers in Neurology. 2022;**13**:1089981

[9] Jacquot F, Gastambide D. Percutaneous endoscopic transforaminal lumbar interbody fusion: Is it worth it? International Orthopaedics. 2013;**37**(8):1507-1510

[10] Zhu L, Cai T, Shan Y, Zhang W, Zhang L, Feng X. Comparison of clinical outcomes and complications between percutaneous endoscopic and minimally invasive transforaminal lumbar interbody fusion for degenerative lumbar disease: A systematic review and meta-analysis. Pain Physician. 2021;**24**(6):441-452

[11] Ahn Y, Youn MS, Heo DH. Endoscopic transforaminal lumbar interbody fusion: A comprehensive review. Expert Review of Medical Devices. 2019;**16**(5):373-380

[12] Nagahama K, Ito M, Abe Y, Murota E, Hiratsuka S, Takahata M. Early clinical results of percutaneous endoscopic

Transforaminal lumbar interbody fusion: A new modified technique for treating degenerative lumbar spondylolisthesis. Spine Surgery and Related Research. 2019;**3**(4):327-334

[13] Butler AJ, Brusko GD, Wang MY. Awake endoscopic Transforaminal lumbar interbody fusion: A technical note. HSS Journal. 2020;**16**(2):200-204

[14] Youn MS, Shin JK, Goh TS, Lee JS. Full endoscopic lumbar interbody fusion (FELIF): Technical note. European Spine Journal. 2018;**27**(8):1949-1955

[15] Zhao XB, Ma HJ, Geng B, Zhou HG, Xia YY. Early clinical evaluation of percutaneous full-endoscopic transforaminal lumbar interbody fusion with pedicle screw insertion for treating degenerative lumbar spinal stenosis. Orthopaedic Surgery. 2021;**13**(1):328-337

[16] Kolcun JPG, Brusko GD, Basil GW, Epstein R, Wang MY. Endoscopic transforaminal lumbar interbody fusion without general anesthesia: Operative and clinical outcomes in 100 consecutive patients with a minimum 1-year follow-up. Neurosurgical Focus. 2019;**46**(4):E14

[17] Xu J, Wang D, Liu J, Zhu C, Bao J, Gao W, et al. Learning curve and complications of unilateral Biportal endoscopy: Cumulative sum and risk-adjusted cumulative sum analysis. Neurospine. 2022;**19**(3):792-804

[18] Li HM, Zhang RJ, Shen CL. Accuracy of pedicle screw placement and clinical outcomes of robot-assisted technique versus conventional freehand technique in spine surgery from nine randomized controlled trials: A meta-analysis. Spine (Phila Pa 1976). 2020;**45**(2):E111-E1e9

[19] Chang M, Wang L, Yuan S, Tian Y, Zhao Y, Liu X. Percutaneous endoscopic robot-assisted transforaminal lumbar interbody fusion (PE RA-TLIF) for lumbar spondylolisthesis: A technical note and two years clinical results. Pain Physician. 2022;**25**(1):E73-e86

[20] Lu L, Wang H, Liu P, Liu R, Zhang J, Xie Y, et al. Applications of mixed reality Technology in Orthopedics Surgery: A pilot study. Frontiers in Bioengineering and Biotechnology. 2022;**10**:740507

[21] Butler AJ, Colman MW, Lynch J, Phillips FM. Augmented reality in minimally invasive spine surgery: Early efficiency and complications of percutaneous pedicle screw instrumentation. The Spine Journal. 2023;**23**(1):27-33

[22] Caprara S, Fasser MR, Spirig JM, Widmer J, Snedeker JG, Farshad M, et al. Bone density optimized pedicle screw instrumentation improves screw pull-out force in lumbar vertebrae. Computer Methods in Biomechanics and Biomedical Engineering. 2022;**25**(4):464-474

[23] Ma C, Zou D, Qi H, Li C, Zhang C, Yang K, et al. A novel surgical planning system using an AI model to optimize planning of pedicle screw trajectories with highest bone mineral density and strongest pull-out force. Neurosurgical Focus. 2022;**52**(4):E10

Chapter 4

Foraminoplasty

Pablo Pazmiño

Abstract

The lumbar foraminoplasty is a novel surgical option for appropriately indicated patients, and high success rates have been reported in the literature. Complications and failures are often associated with patient indications or technical variables, and the goal of this chapter is to assist surgeons in understanding these factors.

Keywords: lumbar foraminoplasty, foraminoplasty, radiculopathy, stenosis, foraminal stenosis, foraminotomy lumbar degenerative disc disease, lumbar disc herniation, herniated disc

1. Introduction

Spine surgeons are confronted with several surgical approaches when managing lumbar stenosis and radicular pains which have not responded to conservative treatment options. There are several conventional approaches to addressing foraminal stenosis, each facing specific challenges in the operative setting. Often in order to perform a sufficient foraminal decompression surgeons must balance the resection of a considerable amount of the overlying facet joints, with the need to preserve and maximize their bony architecture in order to ensure postoperative spinal stability. In fact residual foraminal stenosis has been shown to be a leading cause of failed back surgery syndrome [1]. Moreover, there are other potential long term drawbacks with the standard decompression ranging from the development of instability, postlaminectomy syndrome, neuropathic pain, residual disc, persistent pain, and the degeneration of adjacent segments [1–3]. During a standard foraminotomy instruments can only reach a specified distance within the neuroforamina, and this often leads to an incomplete decompression Video 1a, https://drive.google.com/file/d/1b9-zjYYhP_EsOkEB_Qmo-HsWe-p037TvS/view. In efforts to reach far lateral pathology standard instruments could potentially excise more of the facet joint than required, which could inadvertently lead to long term segmental instability. Ahuja et al. have demonstrated that a resection of 30% of the facet joint led to an increase in mediolateral spinal mobility [4, 5]. The same study found that an excision of 45% of the facet joints resulted in an increase of segmental instability in both anteroposterior and mediolateral planes, which was compounded with bilateral resections [4, 5].

In patients with symptomatic lumbar neuroforaminal stenosis, there has been a growing enthusiasm towards definitive management in the form of a foraminoplasty with a microblade shaver [6–10]. In essence the lumbar foraminoplasty is a reshaping and restructuring of the neuroforaminal arch using a flexible microblade shaver

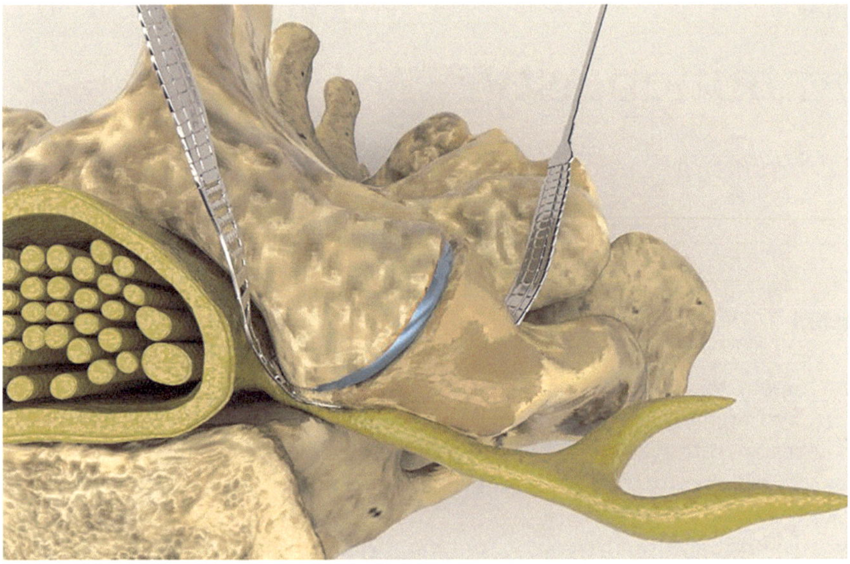

Figure 1.
The lumbar foramina prior to reciprocations with neuroforaminal stenosis and the microblade shaver in place.

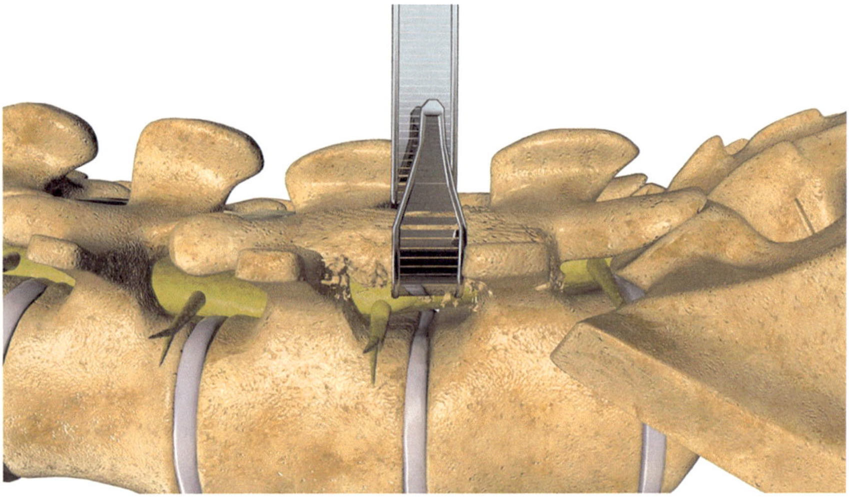

Figure 2.
The foraminoplasty involves a foraminal decompression through a remodeling of the neuroforaminal arch with a thin microblade shaver.

(Spinal Elements, Carlsbad, California) **Figures 1** and **2** and Video 1b, https://drive.google.com/file/d/1VnbEUGuI0eyiYCglgFkSAxwF9MKH1UNV/view; https://drive.google.com/file/d/1474vZSCOC3gRnhcICipt1fYkH8o_OH6p/view; https://drive.google.com/file/d/1nremJQLLeceyb15qJLozVvOtAVyvKksz/view and Video 1c, https://drive.google.com/file/d/1sFq3vwLhxOoUXF1QV3qJwE3sG_HAfFvQ/view. This is performed in conjunction with neuromonitoring and fluoroscopy, which maximizes neural safety while providing live onscreen visualization as the neural arch is expanded and remodeled. Foraminoplasty with a microblade shaver provides the unique opportunity to perform a full foraminal decompression along the entire length and width of the superior articular process. Lauryssen et al. compared traditional decompression techniques with the microblade shaver in order to discover any iatrogenic insults which could later lead towards the development of segmental instability [9]. Using quantitative image CT scan analysis they determined the microblade shaver excised less laminar bone, less bone from the central canal, and less bone from the structural pars compared with traditional decompression methods. Moreover they found the foraminoplasty decompressed and reshaped the foramina in an anteroposterior plane, as opposed to the traditional medial to lateral plane, while simultaneously increasing the neuro foraminal volume. Compared to traditional instrumentation the microblade shaver was also found to have resected less facet width, facet cross sectional and facet surface area from both nondiseased and stenotic spines [9, 10]. This procedure has been demonstrated to be a safe and effective means of treating single or multiple level lumbar neuroforaminal stenosis by several studies as well as from the United States Food and Drug Administration [6, 8–10].

1.1 Facet joint biomechanics and degeneration

Morphologically the spinal facets are paired diarthrodial joints with opposing articular cartilaginous surfaces that provide a low friction environment which are designed to guide and constrain motion while dispersing loads [11–14]. Anatomical studies have demonstrated that contact is not uniform across the lumbar facet articular surfaces [15–18]. Specifically the regions being contacted vary in accordance to the given loading scenario and activity. This in turn influences the overall architecture and creates unique distortions along the surface of the individual facet joints [15, 19]. In addition to mitigating compressive loads along the spine, spinal facet joints also provide torsional constraint, and impedance to shear. The orientation of the facet bony articular pillars serve to resist vertebral translation. Peripherally the capsular ligaments and synovial lining help limit joint distraction. Ultimately spinal degeneration fundamentally leads to an alteration along the avascular layer of hyaline cartilage and the development of osteoarthritis. Initially this is marked by the development of microtears along the superficial cartilaginous surface, which leads to fibrillation along the periphery and the evolution of ulcers spanning the superficial and transitional zones. Exposure of the deep cartilaginous zone threatens the underlying subchondral bone and in direct response there is a development of cysts, osteophytic bone spurs and a calcification of the facet joint capsule [20–22]. The ensuing ligamentum flavum and facet joint bony hypertrophy gradually begins to compromise the neuroforaminal volume, leading to varying degrees of stenosis.

2. Methodology

2.1 Indications

Surgeons interpret the severity of neuroforaminal stenosis through the lens of their own training, expertise, and experience. For surgeons addressing the foramina begins with developing an awareness of the locus of the pathology and then deploying various tactics either percutaneous, or open to decompress the foraminal obstruction. While indications for foraminoplasty and foraminal decompression are always in a state of flux certain considerations can be made to this point.

Foraminoplasty Inclusion Criteria:

- Lumbar foraminal pathology at one or more levels (from L1 to S1) requiring surgical treatment and involving intractable radiculopathy, and/or back pain.

- Lumbar disc pathology at one or more levels (from L1 to S1) requiring surgical treatment and involving intractable radiculopathy, and/or back pain.

- Herniated disc and/or osteophyte formation that is producing symptomatic nerve root and/or thecal sac compression. The pathology correlates directly with documented findings on patient history and exam (e.g., back pain with concordant leg pain, functional deficit and/or neurological deficit), and the requirement for surgical treatment is confirmed by imaging studies (e.g., MRI, CT, x-rays, etc.).

- Subadjacent facet cyst pathology at one or more levels (from L1 to S1) requiring surgical treatment and involving intractable radiculopathy, and/or back pain.

- Must be at least 18 years of age and be skeletally mature at the time of surgery;

- Advanced degeneration and/or enlargement of the facet joints on the back of the spine.

2.2 Contraindications

Often with lumbar foraminal pathology a simultaneous fusion based implant may be warranted, so for the purpose of this chapter we will set our focus on contraindications specific to the foraminoplasty.

- Advanced abnormal changes such as bony collapse at the proposed surgery level.

- Pars defect and/or fracture such that foraminoplasty can lead to further instability

- An active systemic infection or infection at the surgical site.

- An unnatural shape (e.g. hyperkyphosis deformity, hyperlordosis deformity) of the back.

- Documented or diagnosed lumbar instability relative to adjacent segments at either level, defined by dynamic (flexion/extension) radiographs showing:

- Sagittal plane translation >3.5 mm

- Previously diagnosed with osteopenia or osteomalacia.

- Previously diagnosed with diagnosis of osteoporosis

- If the level of bone mineral density is a T score of −1.5 or lower

- Presence of spinal metastases and/or primary tumors along the spinal column.

- Overt or active bacterial infection, either local or systemic.

- Chronic or acute renal failure or prior history of renal disease.
- Received drugs or therapies that may interfere with bone metabolism within 2 weeks prior to the planned date of spinal surgery (e.g., chemotherapy, radiation, steroids or methotrexate), excluding routine perioperative anti-inflammatory drugs.
- History of an endocrine or metabolic disorder known to affect osteogenesis (e.g., Paget's Disease, renal osteodystrophy, Ehlers-Danlos Syndrome, or osteogenesis imperfecta).
- A condition that requires postoperative medications that could interfere with postoperative healing/stability such as steroids, chemotherapy, or radiation. (This does not include low-dose aspirin for prophylactic anticoagulation and routine perioperative anti-inflammatory drugs).
- A history of heterotopic ossification
- Abnormal anatomy which could necessitate supplemental procedures i.e. Conjoined nerve root, Tarlov Cysts
- History of a prior failed or attempted foraminoplasty at the proposed arthroplasty level.

3. Implants

3.1 Microblade shaver implants

The disposable microblade shaver comes in a variety of widths (5.5 mm, 7.5 mm, 10 mm, 12 mm) which can allow for a customized decompression of the given neuroforamina **Figure 3** and Video 2, https://drive.google.com/file/d/1BJVSFnid_oXpfKfXyy06VLNRHvoGskZC/view?usp=sharing. Along the entire length of the microblade is a flattened bezeled surface designed to run safely against the ventral

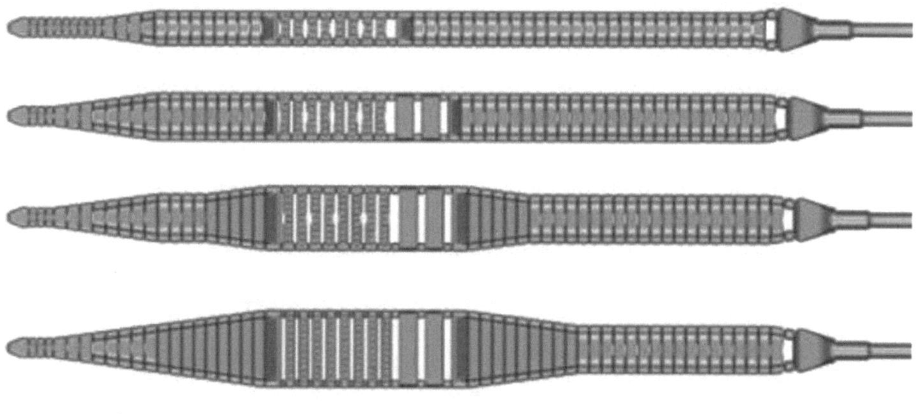

Figure 3.
The disposable microblade shaver comes in a variety of widths (5.5, 7.5, 10, and 12 mm) which can allow for a customized decompression of the given neuroforamina.

aspect of the neuroforamina inclusive of any neurovascular structures. Each stainless steel shaver has a narrow distal tapered section, to allow for a gradual foraminal entry. The mid aspect of the microblade contains a chamfered surface with both bone and ligament cutting teeth designed to manually grind away any deterrent pathology. While performing sequential reciprocations the transition from smooth to barbed cutting teeth is tangible and as such allows the surgeon to confine the working zone to a distinct intended area.

4. Surgical rationale and decision making

4.1 Implant placement and rationale

The sequence of implantation should be considered well in advance in order to limit unnecessary complications. Based on the imaging, pathology, and the patient's symptoms the decision should be made to either proceed with a laminotomy or a full laminectomy. It should be noted that a foraminoplasty with a microblade shaver provides the unique opportunity where through one laminotomy aperture the surgeon can address the exiting and traversing nerve roots of both the ipsilateral and contralateral sides **Figure 4** and Video 3, https://drive.google.com/file/d/1a7EkR4T-y4xpJ9o979evwACiGhxMJWRW/view?usp=sharing. However, if used in conjunction with a full laminectomy then the microblade shaver should be sequentially placed ipsilaterally within each individual neuroforamina to perform each foraminoplasty.

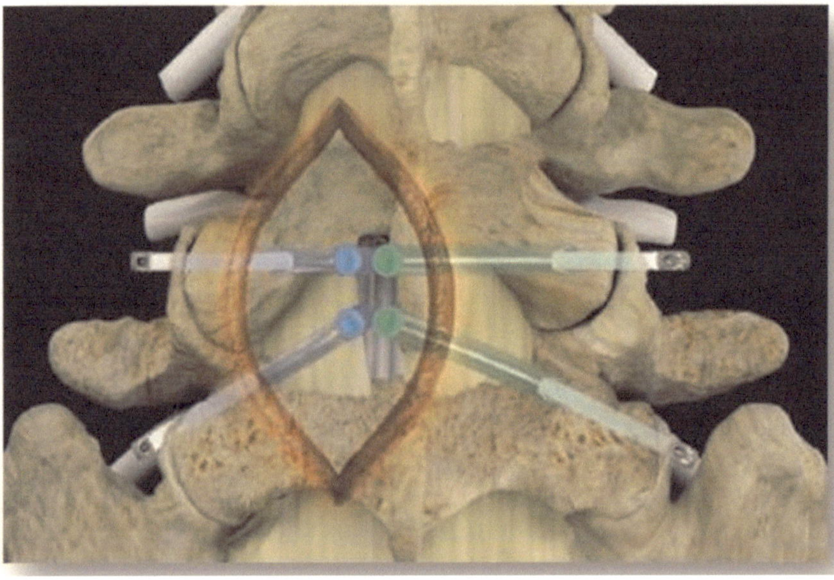

Figure 4.
It should be noted that a foraminoplasty with a microblade shaver provides the unique opportunity where through one laminotomy aperture the surgeon can address the exiting and traversing nerve roots of both the ipsilateral and contralateral sides.

5. Surgical technique and pearls

5.1 Patient positioning

The patient should be positioned prone on the operative frame, with the abdomen slightly elevated off the bed to allow for decreased intra abdominal and epidural venous pressure. The shoulders and arms should be abducted 90 degrees and raised overhead to allow for intraoperative fluoroscopic visualization. Once all bony prominences are padded, a wider than normal surgical prep and drape should be performed to allow sufficient room for potential guidewire egress **Figure 5**.

5.2 Surgical approach and foraminoplasty

5.2.1 Sequence of implantation

A standard laminotomy or laminectomy is performed to provide initial access to the neuroforamina. If a microdiscectomy is needed at the index level, it should be performed prior to foraminoplasty as the procedure will result in bleeding bony surfaces which may later serve to obstruct visualization. Prior to implant insertion in the laminotomy, it is first necessary to confirm adequate clearance for the intended

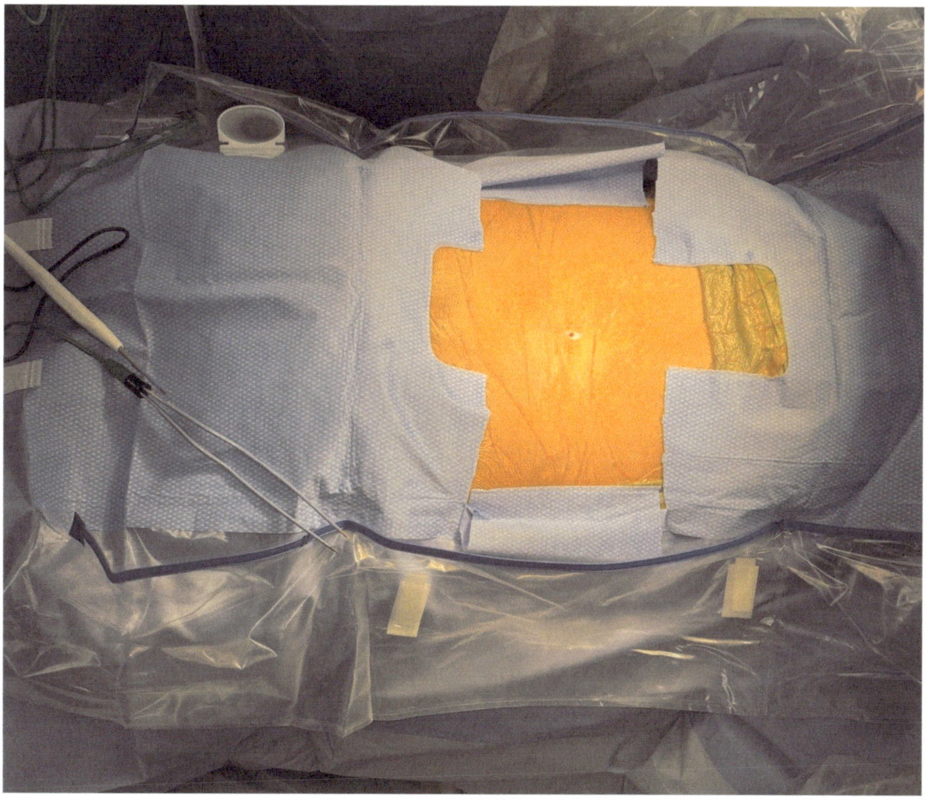

Figure 5.
A wider than normal surgical prep and drape should be performed to allow sufficient room for potential guidewire egress. Here the surgical drape is cut and folded backwards. Later in the procedure this will allow for sufficient room to visualize the guidewire as it exits the skin laterally.

shaver. This can be ascertained by placing a Woodson dental within the laminotomy defect and confirming a 360 degree clearance around the perpendicular post of the instrument handle **Figure 6** and Video 4, https://drive.google.com/file/d/1f6_55Ohf WI0GSbYsELtEniVgTmmzMP6r/view?usp=sharing. If there are still aspects of the hemilaminae abutting the post of the instrument then, prior to microblade insertion, a wider laminotomy should first be performed. Once sufficient clearance has been obtained the ipsilateral or contralateral probe is placed through the laminotomy and into the neuroforamina. During entry the probe should make direct contact against the bone, as if scraping the undersurface of the facet joints as it is being inserted into the neuroforamina. This maneuver provides tactile confirmation the probe was kept in a dorsal plane upon foraminal entry which provides an initial safeguard against any potential ventral nerve entrapment. Fluoroscopic imaging confirms exact placement of the probe within the neuroforamina at the intended position. Placement of the probe within the inferior third of the neuroforamina is recommended to avoid the more cephalad neural elements, while maximizing decompression of the superior articular process. A guidewire is placed through the hollow probe and exits the skins laterally. The hollow probe is subsequently removed leaving the guidewire in place, which will serve to establish the eventual trajectory of the microblade shaver. Next the guidewire is connected to the neurocheck device which will be used to localize the position of the nerve within the foramina. The banded neurocheck is a radiopaque flexible flat 2 sided channel bipolar array with an active central region bordered by proximal and distal markers visible under fluoroscopy. Once in the neuroforamina the banded neurocheck device resembles a parabola under fluoroscopy. Its ideal position is with the proximal marker at the nadir of the curve, thus ensuring the active region is securely centered within the neuroforamina **Figure 7**. Once in position the neurocheck device is designed to provide distinct dorsal and ventral measurements in

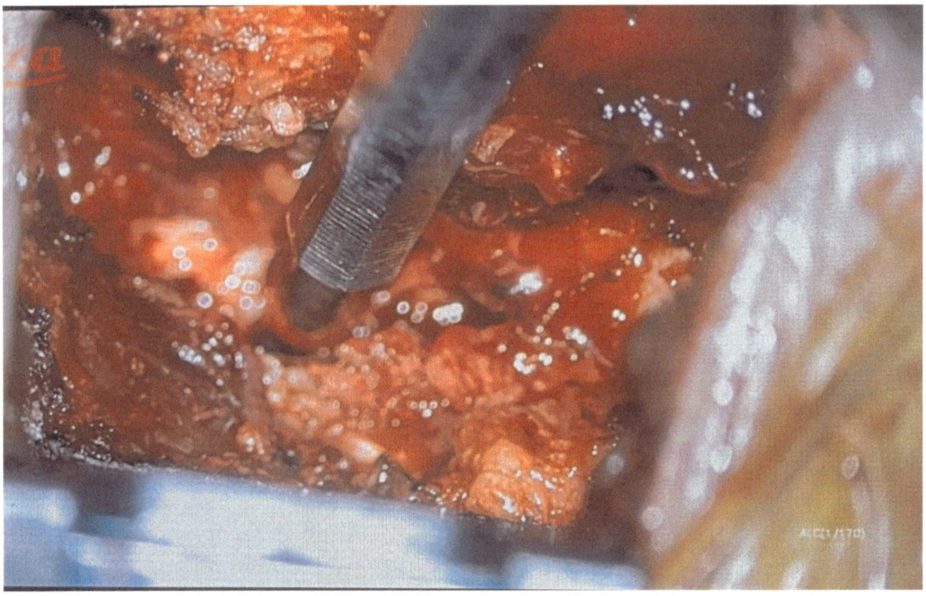

Figure 6.
Prior to insertion of the microblade shaver, sufficient clearance can be confirmed by first placing a Woodson dental probe within the laminotomy defect inside the neuroforamina. If there is a 360 degree clearance around the perpendicular post of the instrument handle then there will be sufficient clearance for the microblade shaver.

order to help pinpoint the exact location of the nerve. These readings are then compared in relation to each other in order to confirm the neural elements lie safely in a plane ventral to the shaver's intended path. The microblade should only be inserted once the dorsal neurocheck reading measures a difference of 3 mA (milliamperes) greater than the corresponding ventral measurement. If the reading is equal to or less than 3 mA then the guidewire should be completely removed and the entire process should be repeated in a new position within the foramina to ensure neurovascular safety.

5.2.2 Measuring intraoperative width

Fluoroscopic imaging can be used to determine the expected width of the microblade shaver. The neurocheck device is 4.1 mm wide and can be easily visualized within the neuroforamina on the lateral fluoroscopic image **Figure** 7. The width of the microblade shaver is selected based on which size can sufficiently reach and therefore decompress the most cephalad tip of the superior articular process. Therefore an extrapolation of neurocheck's size can be applied towards determining which size microblade shaver (5 mm, 7.5 mm, 10 mm and 12 mm) the neuroforamina can most comfortably accommodate.

5.2.3 Microblade placement

The neurocheck device is removed and the guidewire is then attached to the microblade shaver, which is slowly introduced into the neuroforamina. As the device

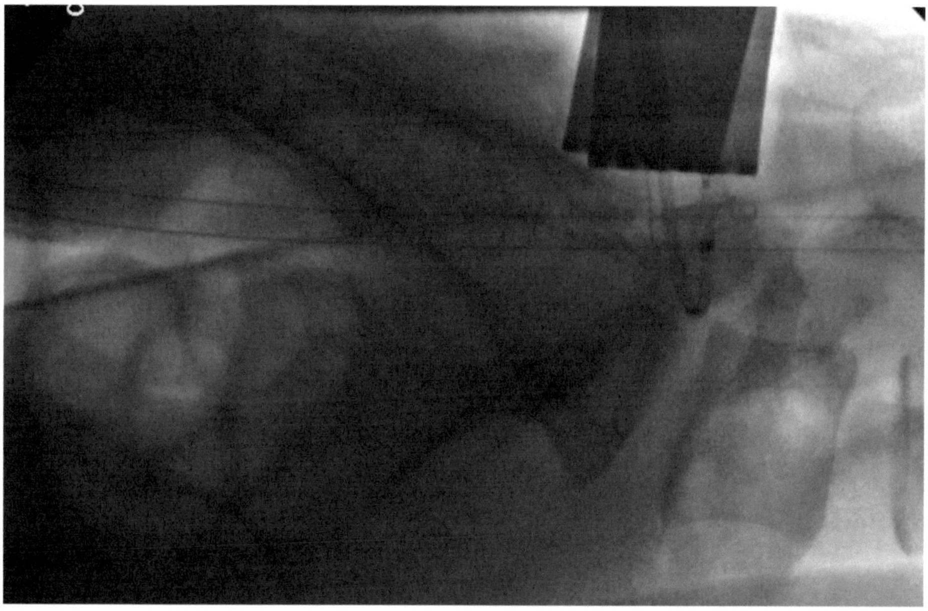

Figure 7.
Once in the neuroforamina the neurocheck device bends into a parabolic shape and is visible under fluoroscopy. The ideal neurocheck position is with the proximal marker at the bottom of the parabola's curve, as this ensures the active bipolar region is securely centered within the neuroforamina. Dorsal and ventral readings are obtained and compared with each other. If the dorsal reading is 3 mA (milliamperes) greater than the ventral reading then this confirms the neural elements are ventral to the intended path of the microblade shaver. The reference guideline of 3 mA is based on data compiled from the initial successful treatment of over 8000 neuroforamina. Fluoroscopic imaging can be used to determine the expected width of the microblade shaver. The neurocheck device is 4.1 mm wide and its size can be applied towards determining which size microblade shaver (5, 7.5, 10, and 12 mm) can be inserted.

is guided into position within the neuroforamina attention is placed towards any potential neural activity or irritation. A pre reciprocation fluoroscopic image is obtained and saved for later comparison. The microblade shaver is then pulled dorsally against the neuroforamina, and if there is no neural activity, gentle reciprocations are performed. During consecutive oscillations a tactile feeling of where the cutting teeth are centered within the device can help control bony resection and ultimately limit blood loss.

5.2.4 Measuring the amount of facet resection

During the foraminoplasty the goal is to maximize the overall neuroforaminal volume by maximizing the ligament and bony resection while in essence recreating the neuroforaminal arch. The neuroforaminal arch spans the inferior third of the neuroforamina and is comprised of the curvature formed by the superior border of the pedicle and the ventral cortical limb of the superior articular process. The neuroforaminal arch is biomechanically designed to tolerate multiaxial, translational, compressive and torsional forces **Figure 8**. Bony outgrowth in the form of facet hypertrophy can inadvertently compress the neuroforamina and lead to differing grades of neuroforaminal stenosis. In order to limit bony resection, prior to reciprocations the original contour of the neuroforaminal arch can be estimated, and the foraminoplasty should conclude as the shaver nears this boundary **Figures 9–11**. The pre reciprocation fluoroscopic image is saved and compared to imaging obtained from sequential reciprocations until the neuroforaminal arch, and therefore a sufficient volume of the neuroforamina, has been restored Video 5, https://drive.google.com/file/d/1k8wFSAWeuPBwc4ArN8YsqrFgVPRZbRpK/view and Video 1b, https://drive.google.com/file/d/1VnbEUGuI0eyiYCglgFkSAxwF9MKH1UNV/view; https://drive.google.com/file/d/1474vZSCOC3gRnhcICipt1fYkH8o_OH6p/view; https://drive.google.com/file/d/1nremJQLLeceyb15qJLozVvOtAVyvKksz/view.

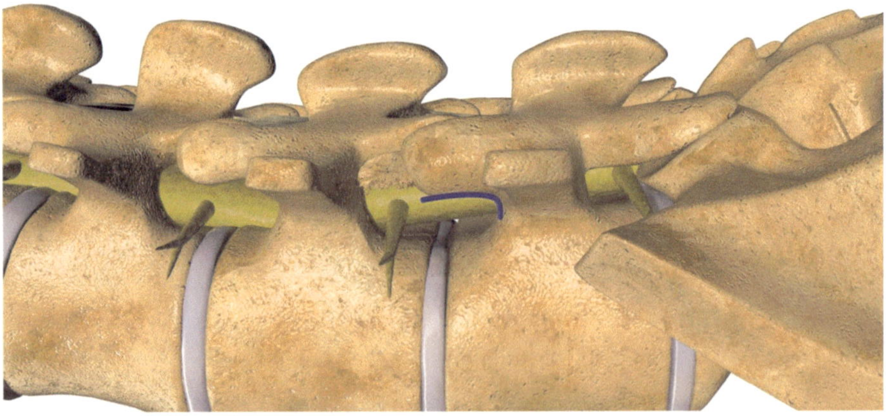

Figure 8.
The neuroforaminal arch spans the inferior third of the neuroforamina and is comprised of the curvature formed by the superior border of the pedicle and the ventral cortical limb of the superior articular process. The neuroforaminal arch is biomechanically designed to tolerate multiaxial, translational, compressive and torsional forces.

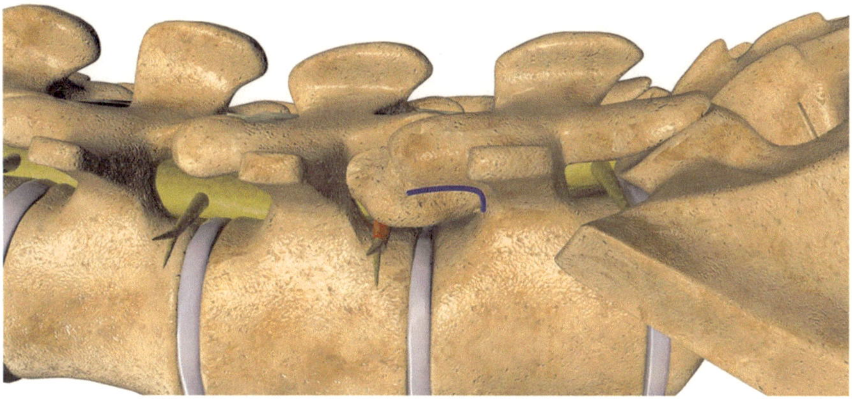

Figure 9.
In order to limit excessive bony resection, prior to reciprocations the original contour of the neuroforaminal arch can be estimated.

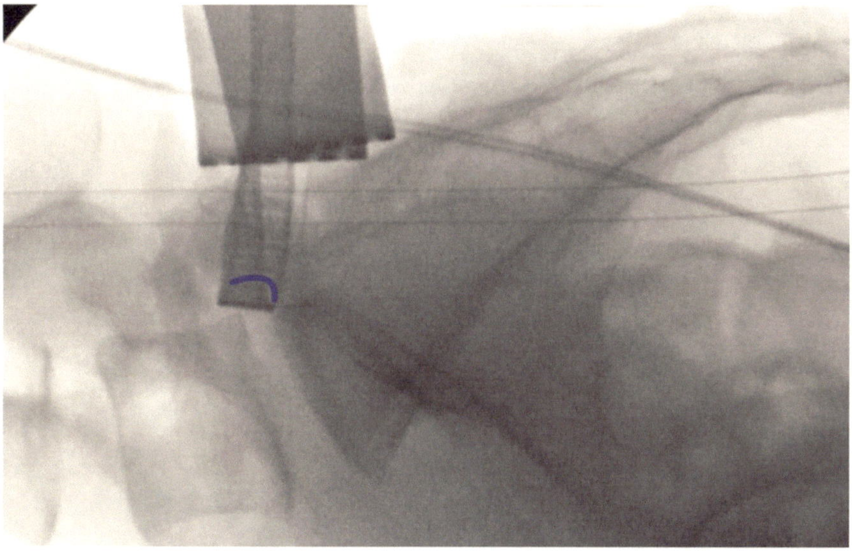

Figure 10.
Prior to any reciprocations an initial image is saved and will be used to compare against with sequential images. Mentally the surgeon makes an approximation of the neuroforaminal arch (Blue curved line) on the fluroscopic image.

5.2.5 Complications

As the microblade shaver has been incorporated into mainstream clinical practices, the literature remains somewhat limited in regards to its long term results, efficacy and complications. Overall the incidence of neural and vascular complications compare favorably to the rates seen with standard means of decompression [23, 24]. The incidence of surgery-related complications in the initial 59 patients treated was found to be 5.1% [6]. Dickinson et al. described a 3.4% incidence of nerve complications ranging from transient "paresthetic" foot pain (n = 59, 1.7%), worsening of sciatic pain, and a postoperative weakness of the decompressed nerve (n = 59, 1.7%) [7].

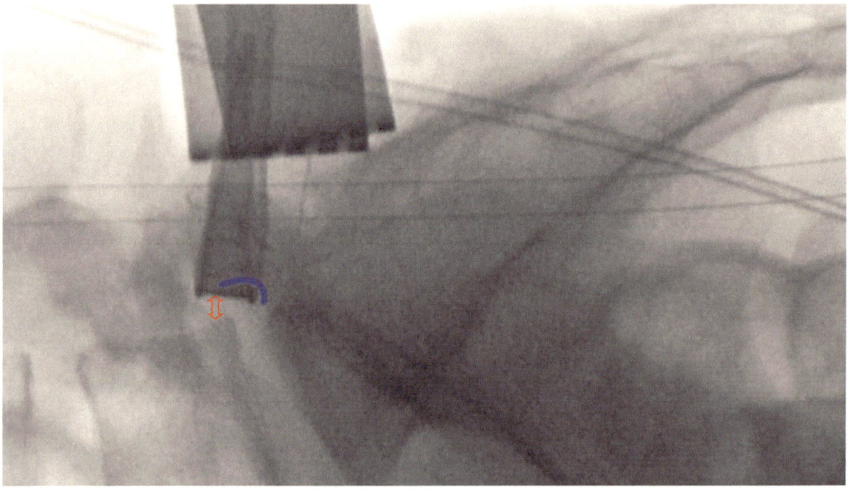

Figure 11.
The pre reciprocation fluoroscopic image is compared to sequential images until the neuroforaminal arch and therefore a sufficient volume of the neuroforamina has been restored (Double headed red arrow). Several images should be obtained throughout the surgery and the foraminoplasty should conclude as the shaver nears this boundary. If the shaver touches the arched boundary line then an inadvertent facetectomy could be performed.

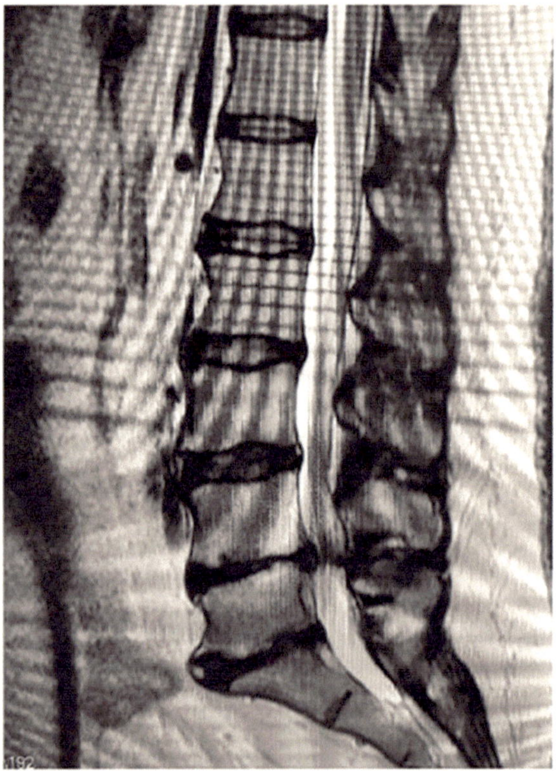

Figure 12.
Preoperative Lumbar Sagittal MRI Demonstrating some decreased height and signal intensity at the L4-L5 and L5-S1Disc concomitant disc herniation.

When poor neurocheck signals were obtained the flexible shaver system was abandoned in favor of a traditional decompression [6]. A recent series evaluated 31 consecutive patients with a mean age of 54.6 years and the procedure was performed with a neural mapping SentioMMG system. Buraimoh et al. detailed a 9.7% rate of transient numbness postoperatively, with 3.2% complaining of transient hypersensitivity pain and no postoperative motor deficits [25]. The composite nerve complication rate was 12.9%.With widespread use reports of complications have ranged from dural tears, post-surgical hematomas, infections, neural complications, paresthesias, foot drop, and fractures of the articular process [26, 27].

5.3 Case study

61 year old female presents with lumbar complaints which are 80% bilateral leg pain and 20% low back pain. The radiculopathy is rated 6 to 8 out of 10. The radicular pains are more severe in the right leg. The patient has tried and failed a course of conservative measures inclusive of transforaminal epidural injections, physical therapy, bracing, acupuncture, and Nonsteroidal anti inflammatories. Lumbar MRI demonstrated a considerable amount of Central stenosis, Right and Left sided Foraminal Stenosis **Figures 12–14**. Her diagnosis for neuroforaminal encroachment leading to radiculopathy was confirmed by three separate L4–5 transforaminal epidural steroid injections performed a minimum of 2 months apart. L4–5 central decompression and foraminoplasty was performed bilaterally through L4–5 laminotomies without complication **Figures 15** and **16**. Postoperatively the patient noted a resolution of both back pain and radiculopathy and returned to regular activities including work within 3 months. She remained asymptomatic at her 1 year postoperative appointment.

6. Case study

51 year old male presents with lumbar complaints which are 70% Right leg pain and 30% low back pain. The radiculopathy and back pains are both rated 8 out of 10. The patient has tried and failed a course of conservative measures inclusive of physical therapy, bracing, acupuncture, and Nonsteroidal anti inflammatories. Lumbar MRI

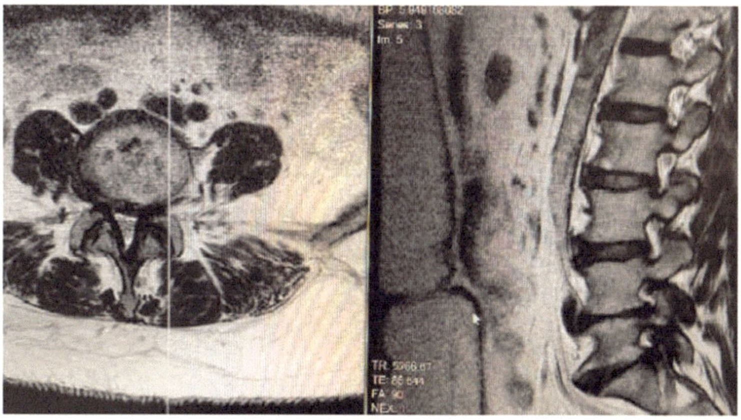

Figure 13.
Left Parasagittal Lumbar MRI of Lumbar 45 demonstrates Severe neuroforaminal stenosis and central stenosis as a result of ligamentum flavum hypertrophy and facet joint hypertrophy.

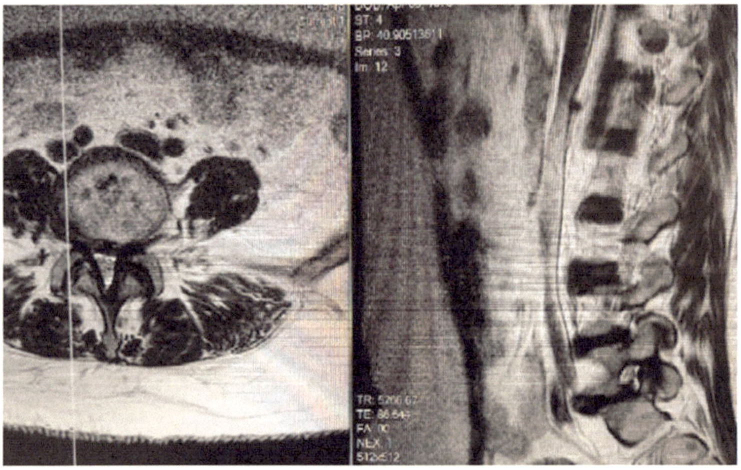

Figure 14.
Right Parasagittal Lumbar MRI of Lumbar 45 demonstrates Severe neuroforaminal stenosis and central stenosis as a result of ligamentum flavum hypertrophy and facet joint hypertrophy.

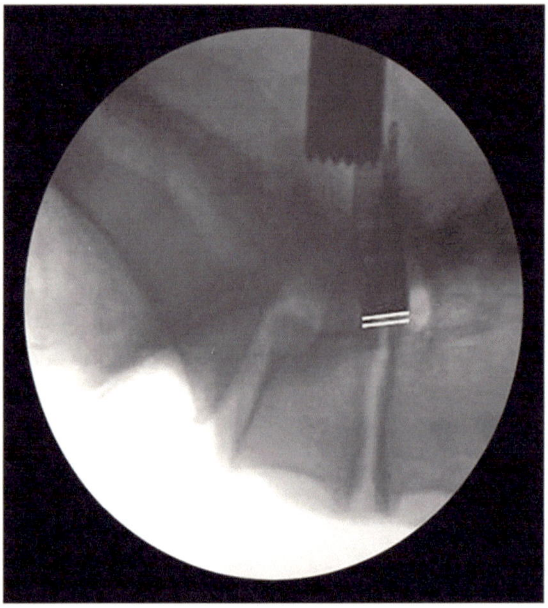

Figure 15.
PreReciprocation Lateral Fluoroscopy: The microblade shaver is slowly inserted into the neuroforamina and a lateral radiograph is obtained. The baseline anteroposterior foraminal depth is delineated by the white reference lines depicting the anterior aspect of the microblade shaver in relation to the posterior margin of the vertebral body. Note the decreased neuroforaminal volume present.

demonstrated a considerable amount of Right sided Foraminal Stenosis and a large disc herniation **Figures 17–19**. His diagnosis for right sided neuroforaminal encroachment leading to radiculopathy was confirmed by three separate transforaminal epidural steroid injections performed a minimum of 3 months apart. First a microdiscectomy was performed at L5-S1. Then a foraminoplasty was performed on the right side through the same laminotomy without complication **Figures 20** and **21**.

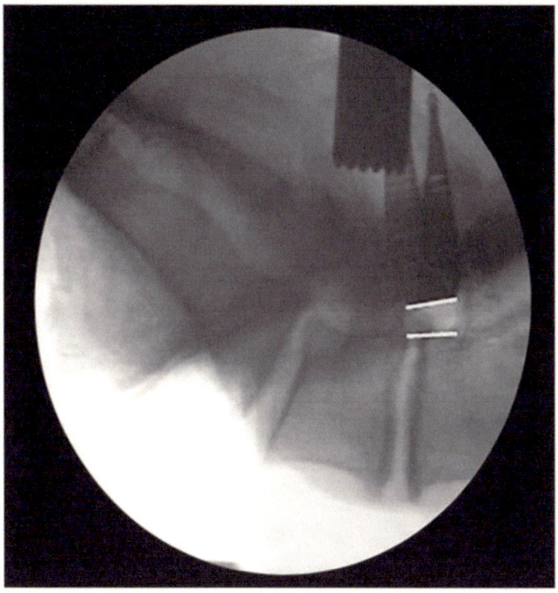

Figure 16.
PostReciprocation Lateral Fluoroscopy: The foraminoplasty is performed under live fluoroscopy or with sequential lateral imaging. There is a notable increase in the anteroposterior neuroforaminal depth and volume.

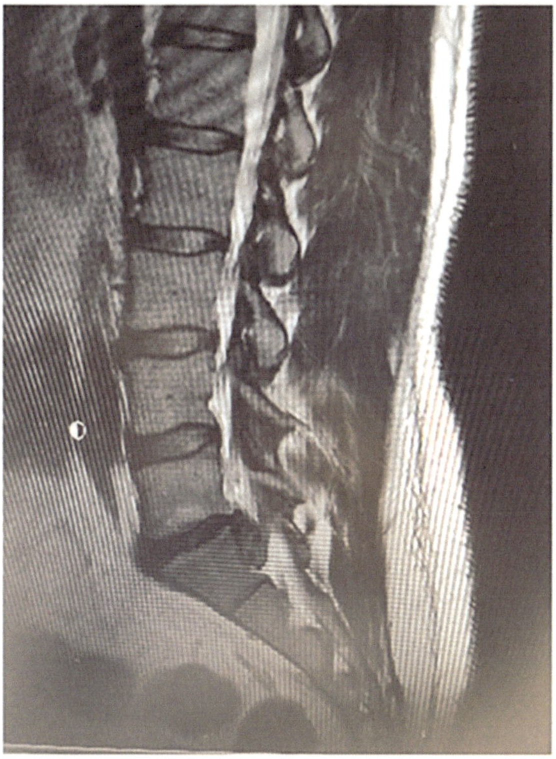

Figure 17.
Sagittal MRI of L5S1 demonstrating decreased signal intensity with a large extruded fragment lodged posterior to the sacral one vertebral body.

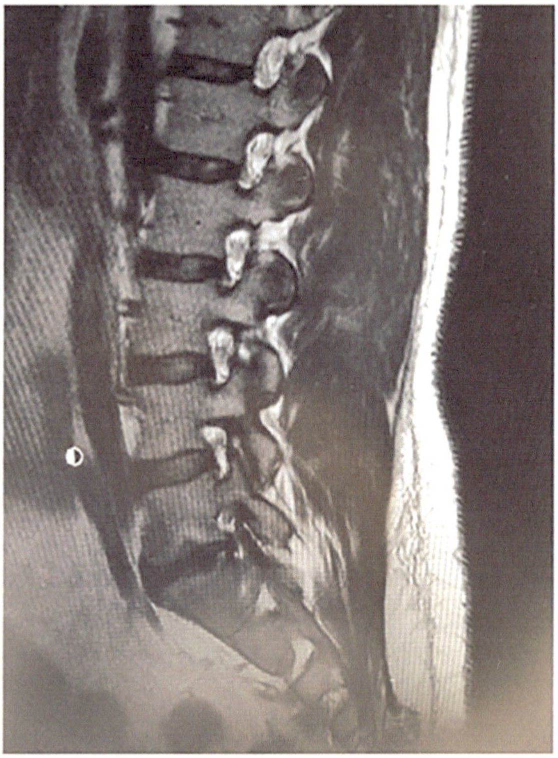

Figure 18.
Right Parasagittal Lumbar MRI demonstrates Severe Lumbar 5-S1 neuroforaminal stenosis.

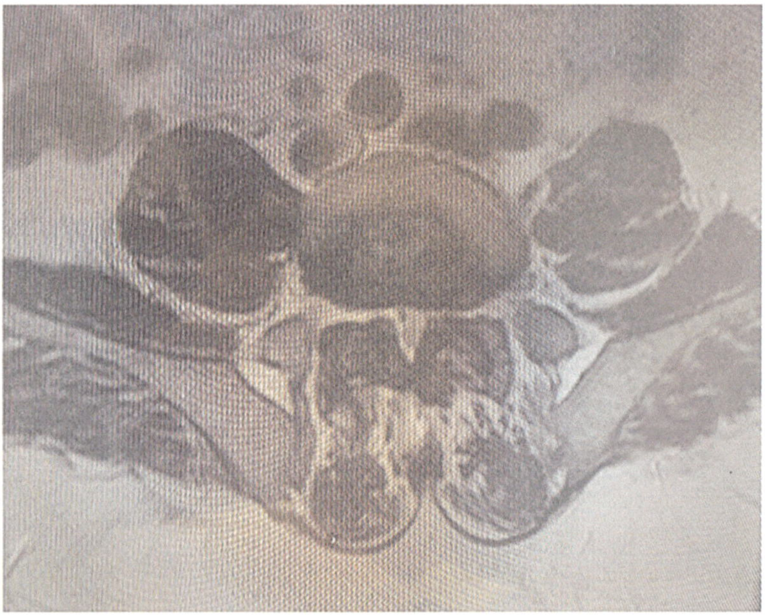

Figure 19.
Axial MRI demonstrating central stenosis and severe facet joint hypertrophy causing neuroforaminal stenosis along the lateral recess with extension into the foraminal zone.

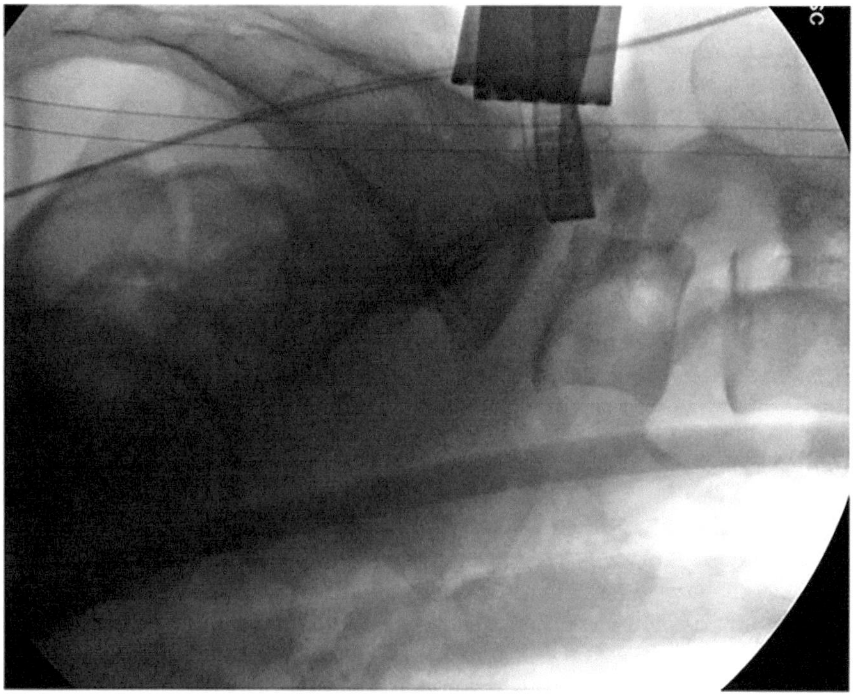

Figure 20.
PreReciprocation Lateral Fluoroscopy: Following the microdiscectomy, the microblade shaver was slowly inserted into the neuroforamina and a lateral radiograph is obtained. The baseline anteroposterior foraminal depth is delineated by the anterior aspect of the microblade shaver in relation to the posterior margin of the vertebral body. Note the decreased neuroforaminal volume present.

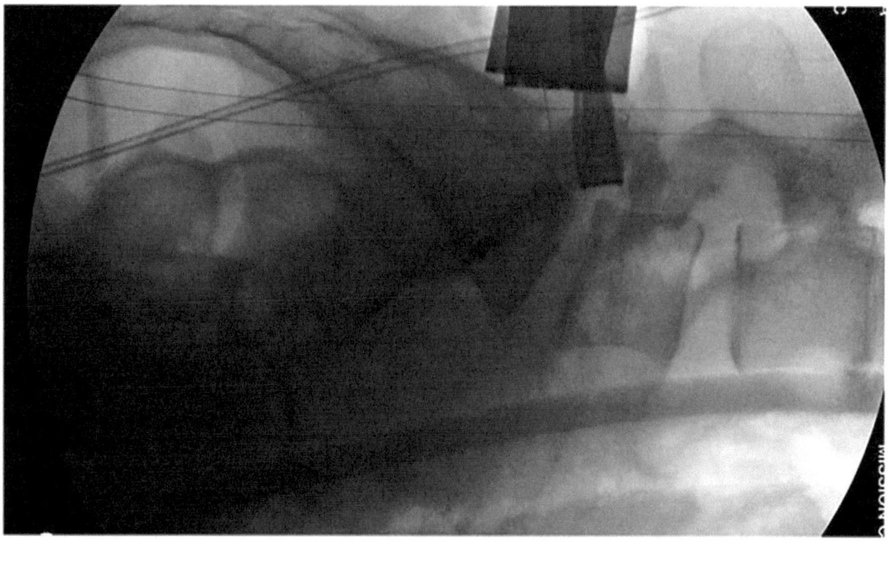

Figure 21.
PostReciprocation Lateral Fluoroscopy: The foraminoplasty is performed under live fluoroscopy or with sequential lateral imaging. There is a notable increase in the anteroposterior neuroforaminal depth and volume.

Postoperatively the patient noted a resolution of both back pain and radiculopathy and returned to regular activities including work within 6 weeks. He remained asymptomatic at his 1 year postoperative appointment and the final flexion and extension plain films demonstrated no segmental instability.

7. Conclusions

There has been an association of decreased lower back pains in the majority of patients who have undergone the microblade foraminoplasty and this may represent important areas for further study [25, 28–30]. The statistically significant improvement in VAS and ODI scores postoperatively may be attributed towards the removal of painful bony architecture, or an incidental disruption of the medial branch fibers of the posterior ramus which can occur during the foraminoplasty.

In clinical practice the progression of radiculopathy from foraminal stenosis is of great concern. With properly indicated patients, meticulous preoperative planning, and sound surgical technique, lumbar foraminoplasty offers an excellent surgical option for many patients with symptomatic foraminal stenosis. Foraminoplasty performed in conjunction with fluoroscopy provides an effective means of definitively controlling the extent of the foraminal decompression while directly visualizing the foraminoplasty as it occurs under live fluoroscopy. Moreover the decompression can be performed in concert with neuromonitoring in order to maximize neural safety while maintaining the overall strength and integrity of the newly reconstructed neuroforaminal arch.

Conflict of interest

The author declares no current conflict of interest. From 2011 to 2013 Dr. Pazmiño worked as a surgeon clinical instructor for Baxano.

Author details

Pablo Pazmiño
SpineCal, Santa Monica, CA, USA

*Address all correspondence to: doctor@spinecal.com

References

[1] Schofferman J, Reynolds J, Herzog R, Covington E, Dreyfuss P, O'Neill C. Failed back surgery: Etiology and diagnostic evaluation. The Spine Journal. 2003;**3**(5):400-403. DOI: 10.1016/s1529-9430(03)00122-0

[2] Carroll SE, Wiesel SW. Neurologic complications and lumbar laminectomy. A standardized approach to the multiply-operated lumbar spine. Clinical Orthopaedics and Related Research. 1992;**284**:14-23

[3] McLain RF, Bell GR, Kalfas I, Tetzlaff JE, Yoon HJ. Complications associated with lumbar laminectomy: A comparison of spinal versus general anesthesia. Spine. 2004;**29**(22):2542-2547. DOI: 10.1097/01.brs.0000144834.43115.38

[4] Ahuja S, Moideen AN, Dudhniwala AG, Karatsis E, Papadakis L, Varitis E. Lumbar stability following graded unilateral and bilateral facetectomy: A finite element model study. Clinical Biomechanics. 2020;**75**:105011. DOI: 10.1016/j.clinbiomech.2020.105011

[5] Ahuja S, Dudhniwala AG, Tsouknidas A, Sarrigiannidis S, Michailidis N. Lumbar stability following graded unilateral and bilateral graded facetectomy - A finite element model study. The Spine Journal. 2016;**16**:S46-S47. DOI: 10.1016/j.spinee.2016.01.030

[6] Dickinson LD, Phelps J, Summa CD, Vanichkachorn JS, Jeshuran WR, Randall JB, et al. Facet-sparing decompression with a minimally invasive flexible microblade shaver. Journal of Spinal Disorders & Techniques. 2013;**26**:427-436. DOI: 10.1097/bsd.0b013e318290fc62

[7] Dickinson LD, Phelps J, Summa CD, Vanichkachorn JS, Jeshuran WR, Randall JB, et al. Facet-sparing decompression with a minimally invasive flexible microblade shaver: A prospective operative analysis. Journal of Spinal Disorders & Techniques. 2013;**26**(8):427-436

[8] Lauryssen C. Technical advances in minimally invasive surgery: Direct decompression for lumbar spinal stenosis. Spine. 2010;**35**(26 Suppl):S287-S293

[9] Lauryssen C, Berven S, Mimran R, Summa C, Sheinberg M, Miller LE, et al. Facet-sparing lumbar decompression with a minimally invasive flexible MicroBlade Shaver® versus traditional decompression: Quantitative radiographic assessment. Clinical Interventions in Aging. 2012;**7**:257-266

[10] Block J, Miller L, Berven M, Summa, et al. Facet-sparing lumbar decompression with a minimally invasive flexible MicroBlade Shaver® versus traditional decompression: Quantitative radiographic assessment. Clinical Interventions in Aging. 2012;**7**:257. DOI: 10.2147/cia.s32536

[11] Sharma L, Kapoor D, Issa S. Epidemiology of osteoarthritis: An update. Current Opinion in Rheumatology. 2006;**18**:147-156. DOI: 10.1097/01.bor.0000209426.84775.f8

[12] Côté P, Cassidy JD, Carroll L, Frank JW, Bombardier C. A systematic review of the prognosis of acute whiplash and a new conceptual framework to synthesize the literature. Spine. 2001;**26**(19):E445-E458. DOI: 10.1097/00007632-200110010-00020

[13] White AA. Clinical biomechanics of cervical spine implants. Spine. 1989;

14(10):1040-1045. DOI: 10.1097/00007632-198910000-00002

[14] Adams MA, Hutton WC. The effect of posture on the role of the apophysial joints in resisting intervertebral compressive forces. Journal of Bone and Joint Surgery. British Volume (London). 1980;**62**(3):358-362. DOI: 10.1302/0301-620X.62B3.6447702

[15] Dunlop RB, Adams MA, Hutton WC. Disc space narrowing and the lumbar facet joints. Journal of Bone and Joint Surgery. British Volume (London). 1984; **66**(5):706-710. DOI: 10.1302/0301-620X.66B5.6501365

[16] Zhu QA, Park YB, Sjovold SG, Niosi CA, Wilson DC, Cripton PA, et al. Can extra-articular strains be used to measure facet contact forces in the lumbar spine? An in-vitro biomechanical study. Proceedings of the Institution of Mechanical Engineers. Part H. 2008; **222**(2):171-184. DOI: 10.1243/09544119JEIM290

[17] Wilson DC, Niosi CA, Zhu QA, Oxland TR, Wilson DR. Accuracy and repeatability of a new method for measuring facet loads in the lumbar spine. Journal of Biomechanics. 2006; **39**(2):348-353. DOI: 10.1016/j.jbiomech.2004.12.011

[18] Kim K, Lee S-K, Kim YH. The biomechanical effects of variation in the maximum forces exerted by trunk muscles on the joint forces and moments in the lumbar spine: A finite element analysis. Proceedings of the Institution of Mechanical Engineers, Part H: Journal of Engineering in Medicine. 2010;**224**: 1165-1174. DOI: 10.1243/09544119jeim765

[19] Rousseau M-A, Bradford DS, Bertagnoli R, Hu SS, Lotz JC. Disc arthroplasty design influences intervertebral kinematics and facet forces. The Spine Journal. 2006;**6**(3): 258-266. DOI: 10.1016/j.spinee.2005.07.004

[20] Jeffrey JE, Gregory DW, Aspden RM. Matrix damage and chondrocyte viability following a single impact load on articular cartilage. Archives of Biochemistry and Biophysics. 1995;**322**(1):87-96. DOI: 10.1006/abbi.1995.1439

[21] Whiteside RA, Jakob RP, Wyss UP, Mainil-Varlet P. Impact loading of articular cartilage during transplantation of osteochondral autograft. The Journal of Bone and Joint Surgery. 2005;**87**(9): 1285-1291. DOI: 10.1302/0301-620X.87B9.15710. Erratum in: Journal of Bone and Joint Surgery. British Volume (London) 2005;87(11): 1583

[22] Morel V, Merçay A, Quinn TM. Prestrain decreases cartilage susceptibility to injury by ramp compression in vitro. Osteoarthritis and Cartilage. 2005;**13**:964-970. DOI: 10.1016/j.joca.2005.06.016

[23] Desai A, Ball PA, Bekelis K, Lurie J, Mirza SK, Tosteson TD, et al. SPORT: Does incidental durotomy affect long-term outcomes in cases of spinal stenosis? Neurosurgery. 2011;**69**(1): 38-44

[24] Weinstein JN, Tosteson TD, Lurie JD, Tosteson A, Blood E, Herkowitz H, et al. Surgical versus nonoperative treatment for lumbar spinal stenosis four-year results of the Spine Patient Outcomes Research Trial. Spine. 2010;**35**(14):1329-1338

[25] Buraimoh M, Ansok C, Pawloski J, Jung EK, Bartol S. Facet sparing foraminal decompression using the flexible shaver foraminotomy system:

Nerve safety, pain relief, and patient satisfaction. International Journal of Spine Surgery. 2018;**12**(2):92-97

[26] Pazmino PR. Conversations and Lectures Baxano Faculty Meeting. California: Napa; 2013

[27] Pazmino PR, Verma RB. Conversations With Rohit Binod Verma. New York: NY; 2018

[28] Pazmino PR, Lauryssen CL. Lifestyle Outcomes Analysis After Minimally Invasive Microscopic Decompression for Lumbar Spinal Stenosis. Orlando, Florida: Presented at The Annual Meeting of The AANS/CNS Section on Disorders of the Spine and Peripheral Nerves; 2008

[29] Pazmino Lauryssen CL. Lifestyle Outcomes Analysis After Minimally Invasive Microscopic Decompression For Lumbar Spinal Stenosis. London: Presented at sAS 9 Spine Arthroplasty Society Annual Meeting, England; 2009

[30] Pazmino PR. IoFlex Baxano Neuroforaminal Decompression Following Traumatic Radiculopathy. Paris France: Annual Meeting of The World Congress on Minimally Invasive Spine Surgery and Techniques Association; 2014

Chapter 5

Perspectives of Endoscopic Spine Surgery in Athletes and Practitioners of Physical Activity

João Paulo Machado Bergamaschi,
Marcelo Botelho Soares de Brito, Ariel Falbel Lugão,
Thiago Queiroz Soares, Gustavo Vitelli Depieri,
Edgar Takao Utino, Fábio da Silva Forti,
Kai-Uwe Lewandrowski and Fernanda Wirth

Abstract

Spinal degenerative diseases are common in physical activity practitioners and even athletes and may require surgical intervention. A great training routine, especially at young ages may lead to raised chances of spine degeneration and back pain. However, endoscopic spine surgery (ESS) seems to be a viable alternative, especially in the case of athletes, as recovery time and time away from the play are much shorter than in open surgery. Open surgery requires longer hospitalization time, has higher rates of infection, and, consequently, longer recovery time. Athletes and practitioners of physical activity can benefit from ESS as it is a minimally invasive procedure, with less tissue damage and shorter recovery time, which in many cases has the same benefits as open procedures for spinal disorders, but often with a shorter return to play (RTP) time.

Keywords: athletes, physical activity, spine degeneration, endoscopic spine surgery, back pain

1. Introduction

Physical activity has been seen as beneficial in spinal health, but spinal overuse has been associated with degenerative pathologies in the athletes and practitioners of some types of physical activity populations [1]. Degenerative pathology of the spine may be associated mainly with competitive sports activities [2] probably because of the placement of heavy loads on the intervertebral discs involved in some sports modalities. Due to this fact, athletes and practitioners of physical activity in some sports modalities have an increased predisposition to disc herniations because these heavy loads may predispose them to a raised risk for degenerative disc disease [3].

The treatment for symptomatic disc herniations in athletes is the same as in the non-athletic population [3]. Treatment of lumbar spine problems usually starts with conservative treatment, when there is no red flag sign or symptom, such as reduced anal sphincter tone, hyperreflexia, hyporeflexia or areflexia, lower extremity muscle weakness, and saddle anesthesia [4]. Conservative treatment can be composed of treatments such as physiotherapy, acupuncture, and pharmacological treatment. Medications usually involve nonsteroidal anti-inflammatory drugs and may include muscle relaxants if the athlete is undergoing muscle spasms [5]. In case of failure of conservative treatment and sufficient patient morbidity, surgery may be required [5, 6].

However, postoperative rehabilitation after spine surgery is another challenge. Some authors suggest that for the athlete over the age of 60 who underwent spine surgery, it is possible but not probable to RTP (return to play) in the previous level of athletic activity. Those under the age of 60, they should be able to RTP at a moderate level of sports participation [6]. This may be due to the damage to the back muscle [7]. For this reason, defining the ideal surgical approach is fundamental for the athletes' livelihood [8]. In this population, the minimally invasive spine procedures (MISP) may be welcome because they have been suffering rapid development because they confer less muscle crush injuries; pain; prevent soft tissue stripping, including muscles and ligamentous structures; confer decreased blood loss, bony resection, and hospitalization; besides they can promote high patient satisfaction and absence of arthrogenic inhibition due to the small incision and tissue adhesion due to scarring [9, 10]. Regarding the advantages of these procedures, the literature confirms the efficiency and efficacy of MISP concerning morbidity and safer complication profiles [9].

The RTP capability is frequently measured as a success factor in the athlete and practitioners of physical activity populations [3]. RTP is progressive according to the improvement of symptoms [5, 11, 12]. Some authors recommend that individuals are able to RTP if they have a full painless range of movement, the capability to preserve a neural spine position during specific exercises, control, endurance, and return of muscle strength [5, 11].

There are just a few case reports about ESS in athletes and no study or case report about ESS in practitioners of physical activity and for this reason, the aim of this chapter is to discuss the role of ESS in athletes and practitioners of physical activity through a literature review about the application of ESS in athletes and the role of physical activity in the context of ESS.

2. Advantages, indications, and techniques in the context of ESS

The increasing improvements in spine surgery over the last decades progressively reduced the size of skin incisions and gave rise to spine minimally invasive surgery [13, 14]. Yeung gave rise to ESS by developing microdiscectomy, percutaneous nucleotomy, and tubular discectomy with the use of tubular dilators. Finally, he introduced a multichannel endoscope with saline irrigation and a camera [13, 15].

The new surgical intervention methods aim to produce better functional preservation and faster recovery [16]. Endoscopic techniques provide a minimal approach while maximizing functional visualization and correction of pathological tissues [17]. In this context, the main method for the treatment of diseases such as lumbar disc herniations (LDH), cervical stenosis, thoracic disc herniations, and revision surgeries in different vertebral segments is ESS [8, 10, 18]. ESS may offer many advantages over other surgical approaches [19]. It involves minimal muscle dissection and a small incision [7, 20] while effectively treating spinal stenosis and/or disc herniation [8, 21, 22] and due to this fact, it can be performed under sedation and local anesthesia, which facilitates communication between the patient and the surgeon, so the surgeon can have the intraoperative feedback and improve safety during spinal surgery, besides the shorter recovery time and fewer side effects [23, 24].

Some of the benefits of the endoscopic approach are: decreased blood loss, shorter hospitalization, reduced postoperative pain, improved functional status, lower infection rates, improved biomechanical stability, absence of arthrogenic inhibition, reduced collateral damage, preservation of facet joint, better cost-effectiveness, and low risk of surgery-related morbidity [8, 10]. As a result of a great decrease in approach-related tissue damage, ESS is also related to low rates of perioperative complications [8, 25], with current estimates ranging from around 3% to 9.76% [8, 18, 26]. These features lead to faster rehabilitation for patients [27]. Regarding all these benefits, the ESS approach for spinal canal decompression is becoming a good option for athletes and practitioners of physical activity instead of traditional open surgical approaches [8] because biomechanical stability and postoperative time to recovery are critical points for the athletic population and all these benefits make this surgical approach adequate to athletes and practitioners of physical activity [8]. Biomechanical stability contributes to the control of postural and core stability and consequently to more effective functional movements specific to some particular sports [28]. The postoperative recovery time is a critical situation in terms of athletes' performance and financial terms since this population in general has sponsors. The result in general needs to be quick to meet the expectations of the athlete, the club, the sponsor, the family, and the fans. Furthermore, when compared with open discectomy and microdiscectomy, the ESS outcomes are similar to open spine surgery in terms of symptomatic relief [8] but with lower overall complications according to recent publications [13, 29]. Concerning professional athletes, ESS could be considered the ideal surgical intervention because of the minimum damage to the back muscles due to the use of small tubular retractors [7]. Previous studies on this topic appear to confirm the premise that minimization of approach-related tissue damage may help rehabilitation and increase functional recovery [8, 30–34]. Non-surgical treatments may improve RTP rates, but there is no consensus about this topic and more studies are necessary to better guide the treatment [35]. Another factor to be considered is that athletes have differentiated muscle conditioning, which can help in the recovery of the individual. Because of this differentiated muscle conditioning, the athlete will RTP much faster than the general population. It is worth bearing in mind that injured athlete usually receives care from various providers during rehabilitation and generally have a better commitment to their rehabilitation, due to the factors mentioned above [36]. Due to the development of better endoscopic equipment, new endoscopic approaches were developed, and the number of indications also increased during the last two decades [10], so this minimally invasive treatment is possible. Nowadays, endoscopes can provide optimal visualization, reducing the necessity for large incisions and changes in the biomechanics of the affected vertebral segment [8].

The indications for ESS expanded considerably during the last decade and they continue to evolve. They can involve degenerative pathology in all parts of the spine from low-complexity procedures like lumbar microdiscectomy to high-complexity procedures (for example, cervical stenosis and thoracic herniations) [8, 10, 18]. The lumbar ESS may include interbody fusion, spinal stenosis, disc herniations, infections, medial branch rhizotomy [17], dural injury [37], and osteoid osteoma [38]. Nevertheless, the viability of ESS and its approach should be determined according to the anatomical and clinical conditions of the patient [39]. In addition, the understanding of the various types of the disc prolapses pathology related to the neuroforamen often results in better surgical outcomes [17].

Owing to the continued evolution of these surgical techniques, the approaches for the cervical and thoracic spine gained wider appeal [18, 40, 41]. Endoscopic techniques have been used to treat many pathological conditions in terms of degenerative, and even cancer [42]. Several full-endoscopic spinal approaches have been reported and performed over the past three decades. The main approaches used in the context of ESS are transforaminal (TF) and interlaminar (IL) approaches. TF approaches were developed after the description of the medial aspect of the foraminal annular window as a safe area for disc space access, known as the Kambin triangle [43, 44]. This approach utilizes endoscopic visualization, and high-speed burrs [13]. A recent study demonstrated that ESS is superior to open discectomy regarding the rate of adverse events and total length of hospital stay [45]. It is possible to perform foraminoplasty and decompression of structures that may participate in the genesis of the degenerative disease of the segment approached (**Figure 1**) [46]. TF techniques can be separated into inside-out and outside-in techniques considering the surgical method. The inside-out is the technique that requires access to the intervertebral disc through an annulotomy and moves to the outside of the intervertebral disc to protect the epidural space. The outside-in technique starts from the outside of the intervertebral disc, protecting the epidural space and entering the disc space. Yet, the approach technique is based on the type of disc herniation [47]. **Figure 2A** shows a complete set of instruments from ESS. **Figure 2B** shows a surgical team performing a transforaminal approach in an ESS.

In more recent years, with the development of camera technology and better instruments, it has become possible the direct approaches to the spine by IL techniques thus facilitating the treatment of degenerative spinal pathology and resecting yellow ligament (ligamentum flavum) [43, 48]. This technique was developed to treat mainly disc herniations at the L5-S1 level. With the development of IL endoscopic techniques, the indications for ESS have further broadened. The entrance to the vertebral canal through the posterior approach is called the IL window. Regarding anatomy, the width at the bottom of the lower back increases, but its height decreases. Even though the IL window reduces in the lower lumbar segments, it will usually be about >10 mm at the L4-L5 and L5-S1 levels, thereby allowing endoscopic instruments to access the canal. Furthermore, the flexion position can increase the height [49].

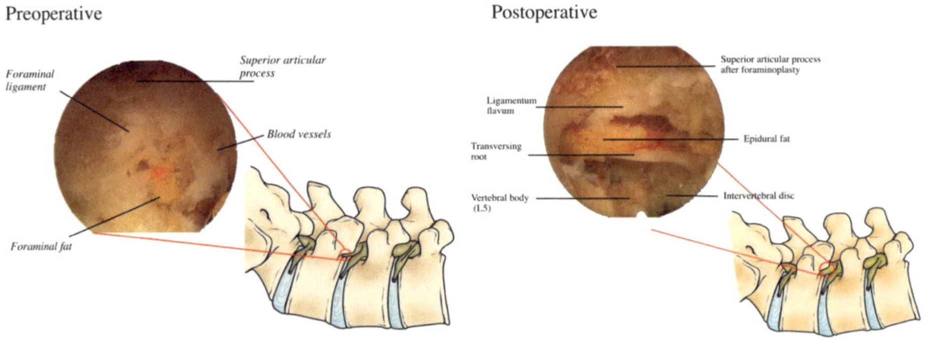

Figure 1.
Endoscopic view of the intervertebral foramen with stenosis (preoperative) and after foraminoplasty for root decompression (postoperative) using the full-endoscopic technique on the lumbar spine.

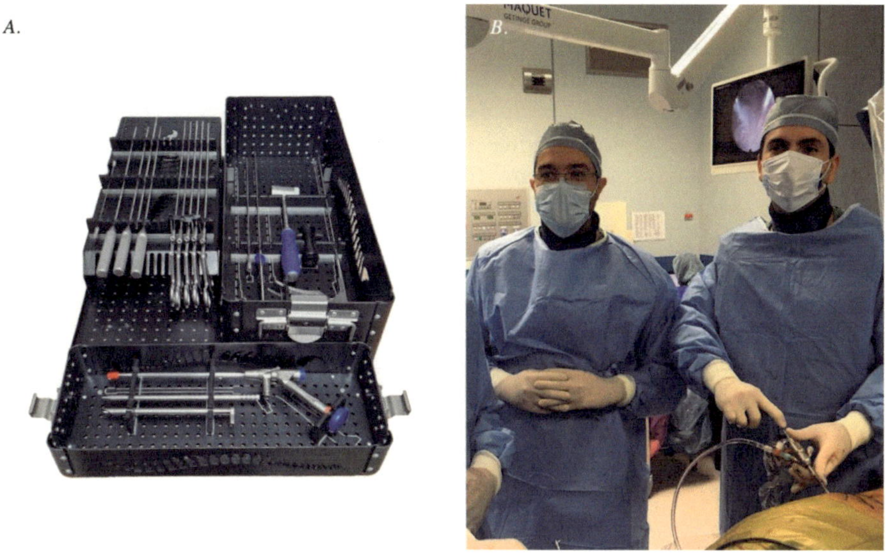

Figure 2.
A. Complete set of instruments from ESS. B. Surgical team performing a TF approach in an ESS.

3. ESS in athletes

Athletic activity has been seen as beneficial for spinal health, but spinal overuse has been associated with degradation in the athletic population [50]. A common type of overuse injury of the spine is stress fracture through pars interarticularis. These injuries are usual in all sports with high reclination load to the lumbar spine, early start of high training load, and year-round sports with insufficient time for recovery [51]. For this reason, athletes tend to have back pain (BP) more commonly than the general population, probably because of the repetitive physical exercises of their training, due to their training load and the overuse [8, 50, 52]. All this can result in repetitive traumatic discopathy (RTD), which is characterized by degeneration or herniation of the intervertebral discs. This happens mainly because of repeated traumatic movements, instability, and deterioration of the spine. RTD occurs more commonly at the spine level that is exposed to considerable mechanical stress [50]. Due to this mechanical stress, the intervertebral disc tissue loses volume and stability leading to a significantly higher prevalence of disc degeneration and RTD in athletes (75%) than in non-athletes (31%) [50, 53]. Some studies report that up to 75% of athletes that train and compete, experience one or more episodes of BP during their career [50, 54].

Spine injuries can be related to participation in sports that involve repetitive hyperextension, flexion, rotation, and axial loading. Mechanical loading of the spine during physical activity plays an important role in the etiology of BP and back injuries [5]. Gymnastics, ballet, rowing, football, swimming, wrestling, diving, dance, hockey, tennis, and soccer are examples of sports that are related to these repetitive movements and can consequently be related to spine problems [5, 55–58]. The main spine problem in the young athletic population is probably overuse injuries [57, 58]. These injuries can result from two types of force generation: acute macrotrauma or repetitive microtrauma, resulting in overuse injuries [59]. Overuse injuries often result in unsatisfactory performance or even incapability to perform, which may lead to a reduced career and financial loss because of absence from important championships [5].

Concerning professional athletes, ESS could be considered the ideal surgical intervention because of the minimum damage to the back muscles due to the use of tubular retractors [7]. Previous studies on this topic appear to confirm the premise that minimization of approach-related tissue damage may help rehabilitation and increase functional recovery [8, 30–34]. Yet, elite athletes are not usually considered in debates about spinal surgery [8]. Perhaps the main reason for that is the difficulty to apply to athletes the surgical outcomes from the general population to determine the success of the surgery because athletes are part of a special population in which the outcome must include factors such as the ability to RTP, endurance, flexibility, return to baseline strength, pain-free with a full range of motion [8, 58].

However, it is suggested that elite athletes may successfully RTP after ESS because this procedure has a favorable impact on the rehabilitation process, improving the outcome, especially on the subject of time to RTP. Still, there are no formal guidelines considering RTP aspects until now. The only pieces of evidence available in the literature include case series, case reports, and retrospective reviews. Although these data are narrow due to the lack of homogeneity and small sample size, they can support the idea that ESS provides advantages over traditional open surgery in terms of time and rate of RTP. Thus, ESS approaches to the spine may be the best choice for athletes that need to RTP as soon as possible because of the small tissue disruption and better and faster postoperative functional outcomes when compared to open approaches given the minimal approach applied [8].

Until this moment, there are only three randomized controlled trials compared ESS with traditional microdiscectomy published in the literature [60–62], and none of them include athletes or practitioners of physical activity. The first clinical trial was published in 2008 and found significantly lower postoperative opiate use, a shorter period of incapacity, and a similar reduction of leg pain when compared to traditional surgery [62]. The second clinical trial was published in 2017 by Gibson et al. This study found the advantage that at a 2-year follow-up the patients who underwent ESS improved leg pain better (decreased by 55 and 65% in the two groups) than the patients who underwent traditional discectomies [61]. The last clinical trial until this moment was published one year later, in 2018, by Chen et al. who did not find differences in outcomes between FESS and microendoscopic discectomy for LDH [60].

Considering the case reports and case series available in the literature, here we summarized them in **Table 1**. Current data available include various sports modalities, such as football, baseball, volleyball, tennis, basketball, bicycle race, boxing, soccer, golf, weightlift, etc., but something important to point out is that lumbar levels are the most frequent regarding injuries. Baseball and football seem to be the most frequent sports involved in spine injuries according to these case series and case reports. In ESS, there are low rates of complications in athletes reported in the literature, as well as high rates of rapid RTP. The spine level that is most often associated with injuries or herniations is the L4-L5 level. The cervical levels are infrequent, but there is one case report including full recovery after FESS in a weightlifter [65]. There are low rates of complications and the most common approach is a transforaminal endoscopic discectomy. The average time for rehabilitation varies from 1 to 3 months for training activities and most of the athletes return to their previous levels of sports activity and competitive level.

In summary, there is good evidence that ESS would be the ideal surgical intervention for athletes, but to confirm this hypothesis, more studies are necessary,

DOI: http://dx.doi.org/10.5772/intechopen.1001430

Reference	Study design	Technique	Number of patients	Sport	Complications	Spine level	RTP/considerations
[63]	Case series	Percutaneous endoscopic discectomy (TF)	21	Football, baseball, volleyball, tennis, track and field, basketball, bicycle race, boxing and ping-pong	No	L_4-L_5	• Return to sports activity 6 weeks after surgery • 95% (20/21) returned to the same level of sporting activity as before the procedure • RTP at an average of 9.2 weeks (ranging from 6 to 28 weeks) after PED
[30]	Case series	Endoscopic lumbar discectomy	25	"High-recreational" and competitive athletes	No	L_5-S_1, L_4-L_5 and L_3-L_4	• 19 patients (82.6%) returned to their original levels of sporting activity as before the procedure • 1 patient (4.4%) could not return to his pre-injury level of sporting activity because of residual pain • The mean period until complete RTP was 10.8 weeks (ranging from 5 to 16 weeks) • 3 patients (13.0%) could not return to sport activity because of residual pain
[64]	Case series	Endoscopic lumbar discectomy	4	Soccer, football, boat race, golf, discus thrower, baseball, handball	1 recurrence	L_2-L_3, L_3-L_4, and L_4-L_5	• All subjects (100%) were able to return to their original sport • 9 subjects were able to return to their original competitive level • RTP in 5–8 weeks
[31]	Case report	Percutaneous endoscopic discectomy (TF)	1	Hanball	Reherniation	L_4-L_5	• RTP in 2 months. • The patient developed reherniation at L_4-L_5 level • Returned to the original level of performance before the procedure
[32]	Case report	Endoscopic lumbar discectomy	1	Baseball	No	L_5-S_1	• The patient could return to light training at 4 weeks after surgery • RTP in 8 weeks after surgery
[34]	Case series	Endoscopic lumbar discectomy	12	Baseball, Keirin, Tennis, hammer throw, road bike	2 revision surgeries	L_4-L_5 and L_5-S_1	• All patients (100%) could return to the same level of play • RTP at 2.8 months after surgery except the two revision cases

Reference	Study design	Technique	Number of patients	Sport	Complications	Spine level	RTP/considerations
[65]	Case report	Anterior Full-endoscopic cervical discectomy, TF full-endoscopic lumbar discectomy	1	Weightlifter	No	C6-C7, L_4-L_5 and L_5-S_1	• He returned to normal training at 3 months after the procedure • 7 months after the procedure, the patient competed in the 2016 Rio Olympics
[7]	Case series	TF endoscopic lumbar discectomy	5	Baseball	No	L_4-L_5 and L_5-S_1	• 100% of patients returned to full-activity within 2 and 3 months after the surgery • 100% showed RTP at the professional level • 3 patients underwent surgery just after the season ended (around November) and they could play with no restrictions during the following season
[8]	Case series	IL endoscopic L_5/S_1 discectomy; TF endoscopic L_4/L_5 discectomy; and full-endoscopic unilateral approach for bilateral decompression	3	Soccer, football	No	L_4-L_5 and L_5-S_1	• Case 1: at 2 weeks postoperatively, the patient was cleared to return to light exercise. In the season after the surgery, the patient earned all-conference honors in one of the top collegiate divisions 1A conferences • Case 2: by 3 months after surgery, the patient returned to full play, earning all-conference honors • Case 3: RTP at 3 months and rejoined the active roster with playing time in one of the top division 1 collegiate conferences
[66]	Case series	TF endoscopic lumbar discectomy	55	Basketball, volleyball, weight lifting, wrestling	3.6% of patients expressed dysesthesia directly after surgery, but it was alleviated at the 6-week follow-up examination with conservative treatment	L_3-L_4, L_4-L_5 and L_5-S_1	• 100% of patients returned to their previous levels of sports activity at 6.7 weeks on average (ranging from 6 to 7 weeks) • RTP percentage was 100%

TF — transforaminal; IL — interlaminar.

Table 1.
Case series and case reports available in the literature.

preferentially clinical trials. Until now, there is no clinical trial in athletes published in the literature and all this information is based on case reports and case series.

4. ESS in practitioners of physical activity

BP seems to be the main cause of disability worldwide and its consequences are healthcare and loss of productivity costs [67]. BP does not seem to be directly related to physical activity, but to its intensity or sedentary lifestyle. In a recent prospective cohort study, the authors aimed to observe the association between total sitting time, low BP, LDH, and different levels of leisure physical activity. They found that 3.8% of all subjects reported BP and 1% had LDH. Moderate and vigorous physical activity were strongly associated with low BP compared to light physical activity [68]. In this context, another review concluded that continued heavy sports may increase the risk of low BP, however, a dose-response association regarding volume is unknown [69]. However, not all people with BP have a herniated disc. Considering only LDH, the study conducted by Balling and colleagues (2019) concluded that moderate physical activity had a positive relationship with LDH while no association was found for vigorous physical activity. The probable explanation for this finding could be that the individuals who practice vigorous physical activity may be practicing particular types of activity which are not connected to LDH [68].

There is a necessity to study the role of physical activity in the context of ESS [70, 71]. Some studies present a beneficial association between physical activity and improved outcomes after ESS because it improves physical and mental health in adults and children [72]. Besides that, physical activity has the collateral advantage of facilitating weight loss, which is beneficial for spinal health [72, 73]. Another point to remember is that after the treatment of LDH by a percutaneous transforaminal endoscopic discectomy, it is easier to recover the biomechanical balance of the spine in patients, even mainly due to less soft tissue injury [74, 75]. Furthermore, studies have demonstrated that it is required to conduct a functional exercise to promote early recovery and prevent relapses [76–78]. It occurs because muscles without functional exercises tend to have a worse capillary response, which produces an inadequate blood supply of muscles, and the consequences of that are: failure to guarantee a supply of nutritional components; makes muscle produce glycogen and accumulate a large amount of lactic acid under hypoxia conditions. This accumulation of lactic acid generates pain and leads to muscle edema [75–78].

In this context, Zhang and colleagues [75] conducted a study to evaluate the effects of postoperative functional exercise on patients who underwent percutaneous transforaminal endoscopic discectomy for LDH. They found that after 1 year after the procedure, patients who had functional exercise (intervention group) after surgery had a significantly more effective treatment than the control group (patients who did not have functional exercise after the procedure). After 3 years of follow-up, patients in the intervention group had a significantly more effective treatment than the control group. In summary, this study showed that postoperative functional exercise significantly improved short-term and long-term rehabilitation in patients with LDH [75].

For practitioners of physical activity, ESS may also be considered the ideal technique for spinal surgery in this population, as well as in athletes, due to the rapid return to physical and everyday activities and may have a protective factor for optimal recovery because practitioners of physical activity have greater muscle conditioning than sedentary patients. As with athletes, this conditioning facilitates recovery and makes it faster and more effective. Besides that, physical activity plays a protective effect against peripheral insult. This protective state often results from regular physical activity and is not obtained in physically inactive individuals [79].

5. Rehabilitation after ESS and RTP aspects

Due to minimally invasive surgeries that have been developing in recent years, many patients with LDH have already been efficiently treated with ESS [80]. This procedure leads to a faster recovery because it requires minimal soft tissue injury [80, 81]. The main problem is that LDH provokes nerve root compression and lower kinetic chain dysfunction [80, 82]. For this reason, postoperative rehabilitation should give priority to avoid the recurrence of LDH, improve function and return to the patient's routine more quickly by permitting a more accelerated protocol compared to open surgery protocols. When the procedure (ESS) withdraws the herniated intervertebral disc, the correspondent ligamentum flavum and articular process, it naturally leads to modified kinematics of the total kinetic chain and a reduced capability to combat abnormal external forces. For this reason, physical therapy and rehabilitation are necessary to reach important postoperative goals like strengthening the low back muscles to recompense the surgical damage and to avoid degeneration and instability of the adjacent segments. In the case of ESS, this technique does not cause relevant damage that impedes physiotherapy. The hypothesis that spine rehabilitation accentuates the whole movement is suitable for postoperative rehabilitation because it has the aim of improving surgical effectiveness, reducing postoperative complications and pain, in addition to restore patients to maximum physical function [80]. Nonetheless, physical therapy and rehabilitation after lumbar decompression surgery are useful regarding the functional recovery of individuals [80, 83–86]. When talking about rehabilitation, several modalities are included. The main ones are exercise therapy, strength and mobility training, multidisciplinary programs (MP), and physiotherapy [87]. The main modalities of rehabilitation used after spine surgery are standard physiotherapy and MP.

Some studies show a close relationship between disc degeneration and paraspinal muscle weakness [88–90]. For this reason, it is important to increase lumbar stability and because of this, core muscle training is usually performed after lumbar spinal surgery. Optimal human core strength also helps normal dynamic stability to produce forces and counteract unusual stresses [80]. In this context, McKenzie therapy is a broadly recognized nonsurgical therapy for low BP [91, 92], mainly by physical therapists. This therapy has some principles such as returning the spinal joints to a better position through significant posture training and exercise and preventing movements or postures that favor disc herniation or re-herniations [80, 91, 93]. This treatment is effective in aligning the spine, so it avoids the recurrence of LDH in the surgical segment after ESS and prevents the degeneration of the adjacent segment [80].

Therefore, it is important that the individual begins rehabilitation as soon as possible after spine surgery. However, the time at which postoperative rehabilitation is applied is not well known due to the lack of consistency of the results [80] but a review published in 2014 reports that an immediate rehabilitation program for patients who underwent LDH surgery and cognitive intervention with positive reinforcement at the same time is an efficient treatment. Early postoperative physical therapy or rehabilitation results are usually excellent and do not involve complications [94], but it is important to take into account the diagnosis and surgical procedure used to develop rehabilitation programs to relieve pain and help functional recovery [80].

When the patient is a professional athlete or a practitioner of physical activity, the objective is the same: re-establish strength, performance, normal movement patterns, and the highest level of function, in addition to the least amount of pain and return to work or RTP.

Another important observation to be pointed out is that adherence to treatment is barely addressed in the studies. The literature is quite controversial in this respect since the variability is high. One study found that 86% of the patients attended all rehabilitation sessions of the 8-week program and 83% of patients did only home exercises during this period [95]. Erdogmus et al. found worse indexes, that during the rehabilitation period of 3 months, only 50% of patients frequently performed exercises at home [96]. In long-term rehabilitation, it is necessary an intensive supervision to maintain patient's motivation and besides that, it is important to consider patient preferences for treatment [87]. Ivarsson et al. concluded that successful RTP after a sport injury is related to rehabilitation adherence and a low level of negative affective response [97]. Athletes tend to have better adherence to rehabilitation programs than the general population, mainly due to the fact they have important championships to participate in and sponsor [98].

After spine surgery, the athletic population demands different criteria such as RTP rate, career longevity, and performance-based results [99]. RTP is widely discussed in the terms of recovery from injuries suffered while playing a sport [100]. RTP guidelines have significant importance for professional athletes and are also effective for the treatment of non-athlete patients who want to RTP their favorite recreational activities. In spite of many years of study, there is still a lack of universal guidelines for the management of the cervical, thoracic, and lumbar spine and about the return to sport. Randomized controlled clinical trials are absent in the literature, so the guidelines are driven by case reports, case series, reviews, and expert opinions. General recommendations are that an athlete should have a painless active range of motion, painless for specific exercises, and total strength without neurological deficit [100]. Regarding cervical spine surgery, RTP is indicated in cases of a single-level anterior cervical discectomy and fusion, in the lack of neurological deficits and normal cervical range of motion [101–103]. In case of multilevel fusion or other surgical options like laminoplasty, posterior laminectomy and fusion or laminoforaminotomy, there is no consensus about RTP. In the athlete population, available data about RTP after cervical surgery is narrow because other factors other than health issues should be considered, such as personal finances and team performance [101]. As thoracic injuries are not common, there is no case report or case series in the literature regarding ESS of thoracic levels in athletes or practitioners of physical activity, therefore, there is no consensus about RTP in these cases. For traditional open surgery, the estimated time is approximately 3 months [50]. For the lumbar spine, Reiman and colleagues (2016) published a meta-analysis involving 14 studies. The surgical treatment included was any form of discectomy (traditional open or minimally invasive). The authors concluded that the RTP rate was 81% pooled across all studies for surgical intervention and a pooled RTP of 76% in athletes managed conservatively. Nevertheless, the authors acknowledged that due to the low methodological quality and heterogeneity of the studies involved in the analysis, the correct rate of RTP could not be precisely determined [99]. The time to RTP ranged from 5.2 [104] to 8.7 months [105] for professional athletes and from 7.5 [106] to 6 months for non-athletes [107].

In addition, there is an important variability of RTP rates between sports after spinal surgery. According to Cook and Hsu [58], baseball players have a significantly higher RTP rate than other sports, and football players have the lowest RTP rate when they underwent open microdiscectomy. They also concluded that open microdiscectomy was associated with a significantly shorter career in baseball players when compared with nonoperative controls. It is also important to point out that different intrinsic physical demands of some particular sports may influence RTP rates for athletes [58]. **Table 1** shows that there is no clinical study to date evaluating RTP aspects in athletes. All literature is based on case reports and case series, but it is noteworthy that 127 patients underwent ESS and were able to return to normal work a few weeks after the procedure, except one weightlifter that had commitment of cervical and two lumbar segments. This athlete returned to sport 3 months after surgery and competed in the 2016 Rio Olympics 7 months after the procedure, winning the gold medal. Besides that, 3 patients could not RTP and only 1 patient did not return to previous performance. Moreover, these data are limited due to the lack of homogeneity and low sample size but they can sustain the concept that ESS provides advantages over traditional open surgery regarding RTP rates, time, and also in terms of performance. Considering ESS, RTP rates are greater and in better physical conditions and performance, considering case reports and case series in the literature.

6. Considerations and future perspectives

Back pain seems to be more associated with some types of sport than others, due to different spinal overload requirements. In the context of athletes, baseball seems to be associated with spinal injuries.

ESS may be considered a very useful tool because the spine surgeon can access the spinal pathology using various surgical techniques. For practitioners of physical activity, ESS may also be considered the ideal technique for spinal surgery in this population, as well as in athletes, due to the rapid return to physical and everyday activities and this may have a protective factor for optimal recovery because practitioners of physical activity have greater muscle conditioning than sedentary patients. This muscle conditioning facilitates recovery and makes rehabilitation faster and more effective.

Rehabilitation is a key part of the ESS because it is important to increase lumbar stability. Optimal human core strength may help normal dynamic stability to produce forces and counteract unusual stresses, but adherence to rehabilitation programs appears to be an indispensable factor for very rapid RTP. Athletes usually have a better adherence to the rehabilitation programs than the general population. RTP after ESS may be faster than in open techniques and athletes usually return to the same performance, maybe due to some factors such as the early start of the rehabilitation process, previous privileged muscular condition, and psycho-socio-economic factors.

However, there is a necessity of clinical trials in this area to evaluate the role of ESS for athletes and practitioners of physical activity in the context of a larger population of athletes and practitioners of physical activity.

Author details

João Paulo Machado Bergamaschi*, Marcelo Botelho Soares de Brito,
Ariel Falbel Lugão, Thiago Queiroz Soares, Gustavo Vitelli Depieri,
Edgar Takao Utino, Fábio da Silva Forti, Kai-Uwe Lewandrowski and Fernanda Wirth
Atualli Spine Care Clinic, São Paulo, SP, Brazil

*Address all correspondence to: jberga@clinicaatualli.com.br

References

[1] Fiani B, Runnels J, Taylor A, et al. Prevalence of sports-related spinal injury stratified by competition level and return to play guidelines. Reviews in the Neurosciences. 2021;**32**(2):169-179. DOI: 10.1515/revneuro-2020-0080

[2] Abdalkader M, Guermazi A, Engebretsen L, et al. MRI-detected spinal disc degenerative changes in athletes participating in the Rio de Janeiro 2016 Summer Olympics games. BMC Musculoskeletal Disorders. 2020;**21**(1):45. DOI: 10.1186/s12891-020-3057-3

[3] Gause PR, Godinsky RJ, Burns KS, Dohring EJ. Lumbar disk herniations and radiculopathy in athletes. Clinics in Sports Medicine. 2021;**40**(3):501-511. DOI: 10.1016/j.csm.2021.04.001

[4] DePalma MG. Red flags of low back pain. JAAPA. 2020;**33**(8):8-11. DOI: 10.1097/01.JAA.0000684112.91641.4c

[5] Li Y, Hresko MT. Lumbar spine surgery in athletes: Outcomes and return-to-play criteria. Clinics in Sports Medicine. 2012;**31**(3):487-498. DOI: 10.1016/j.csm.2012.03.006

[6] Graw BP, Wiesel SW. Low back pain in the aging athlete. Sports Medicine and Arthroscopy. 2008;**16**(1):39-46. DOI: 10.1097/JSA.0b013e318163be67

[7] Maeda T, Takamatsu N, Hashimoto A, et al. Return to play in professional baseball players following transforaminal endoscopic decompressive spine surgery under local anesthesia. Journal of Spine Surgery. 2020;**6**(Suppl. 1):S300-S306. DOI: 10.21037/jss.2019.11.09

[8] Sivakanthan S, Williams JR, Feroze AH, et al. Endoscopic spine surgery in athletes: Case series and review of literature. World Neurosurgery. 2021;**145**:702-707. DOI: 10.1016/j.wneu.2020.08.211

[9] Hasan S, Härtl R, Hofstetter CP. The benefit zone of full-endoscopic spine surgery. Journal of Spine Surgery. 2019;**5**(Suppl. 1):S41-S56. DOI: 10.21037/jss.2019.04.19

[10] Jang JW, Lee DG, Park CK. Rationale and advantages of endoscopic spine surgery. International Journal of Spine Surgery. 2021;**15**(Suppl. 3):S11-S20. DOI: 10.14444/8160

[11] Cooke PM, Lutz GE. Internal disc disruption and axial back pain in the athlete. Physical Medicine and Rehabilitation Clinics of North America. 2000;**11**(4):837-865

[12] Eck JC, Riley LH 3rd. Return to play after lumbar spine conditions and surgeries. Clinics in Sports Medicine. 2004;**23**(3):367-379, viii. DOI: 10.1016/j.csm.2004.03.002

[13] Khandge AV, Sharma SB, Kim JS. The evolution of Transforaminal endoscopic spine surgery. World Neurosurgery. 2021;**145**:643-656. DOI: 10.1016/j.wneu.2020.08.096

[14] Mayer HM. A history of endoscopic lumbar spine surgery: What have we learnt? BioMed Research International. 2019;**2019**:1-8. DOI: 10.1155/2019/4583943

[15] Syed ON, Foley KT. In: Phillips F, Lieberman I, Polly D, editors. History and Evolution of Minimally Invasive Spine Surgery BT—Minimally Invasive Spine Surgery: Surgical Techniques and Disease Management.

New York: Springer; 2014. pp. 3-13. DOI: 10.1007/978-1-4614-5674-2_1

[16] Giubilei DB, Santos DR d, Gomes MJ, Carvalho MOP d. Endoscopic interlaminar spine surgery guided by portable ultrasound: A new technique. Coluna/Columna. 2022;**21**(2):e260083. DOI: 10.1590/s1808-185120222102260083

[17] Yue JJ, Long W. Full endoscopic spinal surgery techniques: Advancements, indications, and outcomes. International Journal of Spine Surgery. 2015;**9**:17. DOI: 10.14444/2017

[18] Hasan S, Hofstetter CP. Endoscopic spine surgery past, present, and future. Bulletin/Hospital for Joint Diseases. 2019;**77**(1):75-84

[19] Hagan MJ, Remacle T, Leary OP, et al. Navigation techniques in endoscopic spine surgery. BioMed Research International. 2022;**2022**:8419739. DOI: 10.1155/2022/8419739

[20] Sairyo K, Chikawa T, Nagamachi A. State-of-the-art transforaminal percutaneous endoscopic lumbar surgery under local anesthesia: Discectomy, foraminoplasty, and ventral facetectomy. Journal of Orthopaedic Science: Official Journal of the Japanese Orthopaedic Association. 2018;**23**(2):229-236. DOI: 10.1016/j.jos.2017.10.015

[21] Lee DY, Shim CS, Ahn Y, Choi YG, Kim HJ, Lee SH. Comparison of percutaneous endoscopic lumbar discectomy and open lumbar microdiscectomy for recurrent disc herniation. Journal of Korean Neurosurgical Association. 2009;**46**(6):515-521. DOI: 10.3340/jkns.2009.46.6.515

[22] Sivakanthan S, Hasan S, Hofstetter C. Full-endoscopic lumbar discectomy. Neurosurgery Clinics of North America. 2020;**31**(1):1-7. DOI: 10.1016/j.nec.2019.08.016

[23] Yang L, Pan YL, Liu CZ, Guo DX, Zhao X. A retrospective comparative study of local anesthesia only and local anesthesia with sedation for percutaneous endoscopic lumbar discectomy. Scientific Reports. 2022;**12**(1):7427. DOI: 10.1038/s41598-022-11393-4

[24] Wan Q, Zhang D, Li S, et al. Posterior percutaneous full-endoscopic cervical discectomy under local anesthesia for cervical radiculopathy due to soft-disc herniation: A preliminary clinical study. Journal of Neurosurgery. Spine. 2018;**29**(4):351-357. DOI: 10.3171/2018.1.SPINE17795

[25] Sen RD, White-Dzuro G, Ruzevick J, et al. Intra- and perioperative complications associated with endoscopic spine surgery: A multi-institutional study. World Neurosurgery. 2018;**120**:e1054-e1060. DOI: 10.1016/j.wneu.2018.09.009

[26] Fan N, Yuan S, Du P, et al. Complications and risk factors of percutaneous endoscopic transforaminal discectomy in the treatment of lumbar spinal stenosis. BMC Musculoskeletal Disorders. 2021;**22**(1):1041. DOI: 10.1186/s12891-021-04940-z

[27] Gushcha A, Vershinin A, Arestov S, et al. Advantages and weaknesses of percutaneous endoscopic lumbar discectomy: Algorithm selection. Coluna/Columna. 2018;**17**(3):200-205. DOI: 10.1590/s1808-185120181703191839

[28] Zemková E, Zapletalová L. The role of neuromuscular control of postural and core stability in functional movement and athlete performance. Frontiers in Physiology. 2022;**13**:796097. DOI: 10.3389/fphys.2022.796097

[29] Chen X, Chamoli U, Lapkin S, Castillo JV, Diwan AD. Complication rates of different discectomy techniques for the treatment of lumbar disc herniation: A network meta-analysis. European Spine Journal: Official Publication of the European Spine Society, the European Spinal Deformity Society, and the European Section of the Cervical Spine Research Society. 2019;**28**(11):2588-2601. DOI: 10.1007/s00586-019-06142-7

[30] Yoshimoto M, Takebayashi T, Ida K, Tanimoto K, Yamashita T. Microendoscopic discectomy in athletes. Journal of Orthopaedic Science: Official Journal of the Japanese Orthopaedic Association. 2013;**18**(6):902-908. DOI: 10.1007/s00776-013-0442-x

[31] Yamashita K, Higashino K, Sakai T, et al. Revision percutaneous endoscopic lumbar discectomy under the local anesthesia for the recurrent lumbar herniated nucleus pulposus in a high class athlete: A case report. The Journal of Medical Investigation. 2016;**63**(1.2): 135-139. DOI: 10.2152/jmi.63.135

[32] Yamashita K, Tezuka F, Manabe H, et al. Successful endoscopic surgery for L5 radiculopathy caused by far-lateral disc herniation at L5-S1 and L5 isthmic grade 2 spondylolisthesis in a professional baseball player. International Journal of Spine Surgery. 2018;**12**(5):624-628. DOI: 10.14444/5077

[33] Sairyo K, Kitagawa Y, Dezawa A. Percutaneous endoscopic discectomy and thermal annuloplasty for professional athletes. Asian Journal of Endoscopic Surgery. 2013;**6**(4):292-297. DOI: 10.1111/ases.12055

[34] Manabe H, Yamashita K, Tezuka F, et al. Thermal annuloplasty using percutaneous endoscopic discectomy for elite athletes with discogenic low back pain. Neurologia Medico-Chirurgica (Tokyo). 2019;**59**(2):48-53. DOI: 10.2176/nmc.oa.2018-0256

[35] Ball JR, Harris CB, Lee J, Vives MJ. Lumbar spine injuries in sports: Review of the literature and current treatment recommendations. Sports Medicine—Open. 2019;**5**(1):26. DOI: 10.1186/s40798-019-0199-7

[36] Kraemer W, Denegar C, Flanagan S. Recovery from injury in sport: Considerations in the transition from medical care to performance care. Sports Health. 2009;**1**(5):392-395. DOI: 10.1177/1941738109343156

[37] Bergamaschi JPM, de Araújo FF, Soares TQ, et al. Dural injury treatment with a full-endoscopic transforaminal approach: A case report and description of surgical technique. Lyons MK, ed. Case Reports in Orthopedics. 2022;**2022**:1-5. DOI: 10.1155/2022/6570589

[38] Bergamaschi JPM, Costa CAM, Sandon LH. Full-endoscopic resection of osteoid osteoma in the thoracic spine: A case report. International Journal of Spine Surgery. 2021;**14**(s4):S78-S86. DOI: 10.14444/7169

[39] Ahn Y. Endoscopic spine discectomy: Indications and outcomes. International Orthopaedics. 2019;**43**(4):909-916. DOI: 10.1007/s00264-018-04283-w

[40] Parihar VS, Yadav N, Ratre S, Dubey A, Yadav YR. Endoscopic anterior approach for cervical disc disease (disc preserving surgery). World Neurosurgery. 2018;**115**:e599-e609. DOI: 10.1016/j.wneu.2018.04.107

[41] Ruetten S, Hahn P, Oezdemir S, et al. Full-endoscopic uniportal decompression

in disc herniations and stenosis of the thoracic spine using the interlaminar, extraforaminal, or transthoracic retropleural approach. Journal of Neurosurgery. Spine. 2018;**29**(2):157-168. DOI: 10.3171/2017.12.SPINE171096

[42] Goldberg JL, Hussain I, Sommer F, Härtl R, Elowitz E. The future of minimally invasive spinal surgery. World Neurosurgery. 2022;**163**:233-240. DOI: 10.1016/j.wneu.2022.03.121

[43] Hofstetter CP, Ahn Y, Choi G, et al. AOSpine consensus paper on nomenclature for working-channel endoscopic spinal procedures. Global Spine Journal. 2020;**10**(Suppl. 2): 111S-121S. DOI: 10.1177/2192568219887364

[44] Kambin P, Sampson S. Posterolateral percutaneous suction-excision of herniated lumbar intervertebral discs. Report of interim results. Clinical Orthopaedics and Related Research. 1986;(207):37-43

[45] Page PS, Ammanuel SG, Josiah DT. Evaluation of endoscopic versus open lumbar discectomy: A multi-center retrospective review utilizing the American College of Surgeons' National Surgical Quality Improvement Program (ACS-NSQIP) database. Cureus. 2022;**14**(5):e25202. DOI: 10.7759/cureus.25202

[46] Chen Z, Zhang L, Dong J, et al. Percutaneous transforaminal endoscopic discectomy compared with microendoscopic discectomy for lumbar disc herniation: 1-year results of an ongoing randomized controlled trial. Journal of Neurosurgery. Spine. 2018;**28**(3):300-310. DOI: 10.3171/2017.7.SPINE161434

[47] Il JC. Technical considerations of the transforaminal approach for lumbar disk herniation. World Neurosurgery. 2021;**145**:597-611. DOI: 10.1016/j.wneu.2020.08.229

[48] Evins AI, Banu MA, Njoku IJ, et al. Endoscopic lumbar foraminotomy. Journal of Clinical Neuroscience: Official Journal of the Neurosurgical Society of Australasia. 2015;**22**(4):730-734. DOI: 10.1016/j.jocn.2014.10.025

[49] Chen KT, Tseng C, Sun LW, Chang KS, Chen CM. Technical considerations of Interlaminar approach for lumbar disc herniation. World Neurosurgery. 2021;**145**:612-620. DOI: 10.1016/j.wneu.2020.06.211

[50] Fiani B, Jarrah R, Wong A, Alamah A, Runnels J. Repetitive traumatic Discopathy in the modern-era tennis player. Cureus. 2020;**12**(8):e9783. DOI: 10.7759/cureus.9783

[51] Schneider C. Overuse injuries of the spine and trunk BT—injury and health risk management in sports: A guide to decision making. In: Krutsch W, Mayr HO, Musahl V, Della Villa F, Tscholl PM, Jones H, editors. Injury and Health Risk Management in Sports. Berlin Heidelberg: Springer; 2020. pp. 179-182. DOI: 10.1007/978-3-662-60752-7_27

[52] Swärd L, Hellstrom M, Jacobsson B, Pëterson L. Back pain and radiologic changes in the thoraco-lumbar spine of athletes. Spine (Phila Pa 1976). 1990;15(2):124-129. doi:10.1097/00007632-199002000-00015

[53] Ong A, Anderson J, Roche J. A pilot study of the prevalence of lumbar disc degeneration in elite athletes with lower back pain at the Sydney 2000 Olympic Games. British Journal of Sports Medicine. 2003;**37**(3):263-266. DOI: 10.1136/bjsm.37.3.263

[54] Perkins RH, Davis D. Musculoskeletal injuries in tennis. Physical Medicine and

Rehabilitation Clinics of North America. 2006;**17**(3):609-631. DOI: 10.1016/j.pmr.2006.05.005

[55] Bono CM. Low-back pain in athletes. The Journal of Bone and Joint Surgery. American Volume. 2004;**86**(2):382-396. DOI: 10.2106/00004623-200402000-00027

[56] Keene JS, Albert MJ, Springer SL, Drummond DS, Clancy WGJ. Back injuries in college athletes. Journal of Spinal Disorders. 1989;**2**(3):190-195

[57] Purcell L, Micheli L. Low back pain in young athletes. Sports Health. 2009;**1**(3):212-222. DOI: 10.1177/1941738109334212

[58] Cook RW, Hsu WK. Return to play after lumbar spine surgery. Clinics in Sports Medicine. 2016;**35**(4):609-619. DOI: 10.1016/j.csm.2016.05.006

[59] Micheli LJ, Allison G. Lesões da coluna lombar no jovem atleta. Revista Brasileira de Medicina do Esporte. 1999;**5**(2):59-65. DOI: 10.1590/s1517-86921999000200005

[60] Chen BL, Guo JB, Zhang HW, et al. Surgical versus non-operative treatment for lumbar disc herniation: A systematic review and meta-analysis. Clinical Rehabilitation. 2018;**32**(2):146-160. DOI: 10.1177/0269215517719952

[61] Gibson JNA, Subramanian AS, Scott CEH. A randomised controlled trial of transforaminal endoscopic discectomy vs microdiscectomy. European Spine Journal: Official Publication of the European Spine Society, the European Spinal Deformity Society, and the European Section of the Cervical Spine Research Society. 2017;**26**(3):847-856. DOI: 10.1007/s00586-016-4885-6

[62] Ruetten S, Komp M, Merk H, Godolias G. Full-endoscopic cervical posterior foraminotomy for the operation of lateral disc herniations using 5.9-mm endoscopes: A prospective, randomized, controlled study. Spine (Phila Pa 1976). 2008;**33**(9):940-948. DOI: 10.1097/BRS.0b013e31816c8b67

[63] Nakamae T, Fujimoto Y, Yamada K, et al. Transforaminal percutaneous endoscopic discectomy for lumbar disc herniation in athletes under the local anesthesia. Journal of Orthopaedic Science: Official Journal of the Japanese Orthopaedic Association. 2019;**24**(6):1015-1019. DOI: 10.1016/j.jos.2019.07.019

[64] Akira, Dezawa KS. Percutaneous endoscopic lumbar discectomy for athletes. Journal of Spine. 2013:S5-006. DOI: 10.4172/2165-7939.s5-006

[65] Ramirez JF, Gabriel J, Ortiz R, et al. Case report how an elite high-performance weightlifter with spine pain became a silver and gold Olympic winner: A case report. Interventional Pain Management Reports. 2019;**3**(5):145-152

[66] Kapetanakis S, Gkantsinikoudis N, Charitoudis G. Implementation of percutaneous transforaminal endoscopic discectomy in competitive elite athletes with lumbar disc herniation: Original study and review of the literature. The American Journal of Sports Medicine. 2021;**49**(12):3234-3241. DOI: 10.1177/03635465211032612

[67] Hayden JA, Ellis J, Ogilvie R, Malmivaara A, van Tulder MW. Exercise therapy for chronic low back pain. Cochrane Database of Systematic Reviews. 2021;**9**(9):CD009790. DOI: 10.1002/14651858.CD009790.pub2

[68] Balling M, Holmberg T, Petersen CB, Aadahl M, Meyrowitsch DW, Tolstrup JS. Total sitting time, leisure time physical

activity and risk of hospitalization due to low back pain: The Danish Health Examination Survey cohort 2007-2008. Scandinavian Journal of Public Health. 2018;**47**(1):45-52. DOI: 10.1177/1403494818758843

[69] Vuori IM. Dose-response of physical activity and low back pain, osteoarthritis, and osteoporosis. Medicine and Science in Sports and Exercise. 2001;**33** (Suppl. 6):S551-S586; discussion 609-10. DOI: 10.1097/00005768-200106001-00026

[70] Coronado RA, Master H, White DK, et al. Early postoperative physical activity and function: A descriptive case series study of 53 patients after lumbar spine surgery. BMC Musculoskeletal Disorders. 2020;**21**(1):1-10. DOI: 10.1186/s12891-020-03816-y

[71] Rao PJ, Phan K, Maharaj MM, Pelletier MH, Walsh WR, Mobbs RJ. Accelerometers for objective evaluation of physical activity following spine surgery. Journal of Clinical Neuroscience: Official Journal of the Neurosurgical Society of Australasia. 2016;**26**:14-18. DOI: 10.1016/j.jocn.2015.05.064

[72] Schwartz CE, Stark RB, Balasuberamaniam P, Shrikumar M, Wasim A, Finkelstein JA. Moving toward better health: Exercise practice is associated with improved outcomes after spine surgery in people with degenerative lumbar conditions. Canadian Journal of Surgery. 2021;**64**(4):E419-E427. DOI: 10.1503/cjs.010620

[73] Wai EK, Rodriguez S, Dagenais S, Hall H. Evidence-informed management of chronic low back pain with physical activity, smoking cessation, and weight loss. The Spine Journal. 2008;**8**(1):195-202. DOI: 10.1016/j.spinee.2007.10.024

[74] Nie H, Jiang D, Ou Y, Quan Z, Bai C, An H. Efficacy and safety of surgery for lumbar disc herniation in patients aged 80 and older. Turkish Neurosurgery. 2011;**21**(2):172-176. DOI: 10.5137/1019-5149.JTN.3869-10.0

[75] Zhang R, Zhang SJ, Wang XJ. Postoperative functional exercise for patients who underwent percutaneous transforaminal endoscopic discectomy for lumbar disc herniation. European Review for Medical and Pharmacological Sciences. 2018;**22**(Suppl. 1):15-22. DOI: 10.26355/eurrev_201807_15354

[76] Kelly GA, Blake C, Power CK, O'Keeffe D, Fullen BM. The impact of spinal cord stimulation on physical function and sleep quality in individuals with failed back surgery syndrome: A systematic review. European Journal of Pain. 2012;**16**(6):793-802. DOI: 10.1002/j.1532-2149.2011.00092.x

[77] Thaler M, Lechner R, Foedinger B, et al. Driving reaction time before and after surgery for lumbar disc herniation in patients with radiculopathy. European Spine Journal: Official Publication of the European Spine Society, the European Spinal Deformity Society, and the European Section of the Cervical Spine Research Society. 2012;**21**(11):2259-2264. DOI: 10.1007/s00586-012-2378-9

[78] Lechner R, Thaler M, Krismer M, Haid C, Obernauer J, Obwegeser A. Driving reaction time before and after anterior cervical fusion for disc herniation: A preliminary study. European Spine Journal: Official Publication of the European Spine Society, the European Spinal Deformity Society, and the European Section of the Cervical Spine Research Society. 2013;**22**(7):1517-1521. DOI: 10.1007/s00586-013-2688-6

[79] Sluka KA, Frey-Law L, Hoeger BM. Exercise-induced pain and analgesia? Underlying mechanisms and clinical translation. Pain. 2018;**159**(Suppl. 1):

S91-S97. DOI: 10.1097/j.pain.0000000000001235

[80] Lyu Z, Bai J, Chen S, Liu J, Yu W. Efficacy of lumbar kinetic chain training for staged rehabilitation after percutaneous endoscopic lumbar discectomy. BMC Musculoskeletal Disorders. 2021;**22**(1):793. DOI: 10.1186/s12891-021-04674-y

[81] Knight MT, Jago I, Norris C, Midwinter L, Boynes C. Transforaminal endoscopic lumbar decompression & foraminoplasty: A 10 year prospective survivability outcome study of the treatment of foraminal stenosis and failed back surgery. International Journal of Spine Surgery. 1 Dec 2014;**8**:21. DOI: 10.14444/1021

[82] Fei H, Li WS, Sun ZR, Ma QW, Chen ZQ. Analysis of Spino-pelvic sagittal alignment in young Chinese patients with lumbar disc herniation. Orthopaedic Surgery. 2017;**9**(3):271-276. DOI: 10.1111/os.12340

[83] Skolasky RL, Riley LH 3rd, Maggard AM, Bedi S, Wegener ST. Functional recovery in lumbar spine surgery: A controlled trial of health behavior change counseling to improve outcomes. Contemporary Clinical Trials. 2013;**36**(1):207-217. DOI: 10.1016/j.cct.2013.06.018

[84] Demir S, Dulgeroglu D, Cakci A. Effects of dynamic lumbar stabilization exercises following lumbar microdiscectomy on pain, mobility and return to work. Randomized controlled trial. European Journal of Physical and Rehabilitation Medicine. 2014;**50**(6):627-640

[85] Ebenbichler GR, Inschlag S, Pflüger V, et al. Twelve-year follow-up of a randomized controlled trial of comprehensive physiotherapy following disc herniation operation. Clinical Rehabilitation. 2015;**29**(6):548-560. DOI: 10.1177/0269215514552032

[86] Rushton A, Wright C, Goodwin P, Calvert M, Freemantle N. Physiotherapy rehabilitation post first lumbar discectomy: A systematic review and meta-analysis of randomized controlled trials. Spine (Phila Pa 1976). 2011;**36**(14):E961-E972. DOI: 10.1097/BRS.0b013e3181f0e8f8

[87] Oosterhuis T, Costa LOP, Maher CG, de Vet HCW, van Tulder MW, Ostelo RWJG. Rehabilitation after lumbar disc surgery. Cochrane Database of Systematic Reviews. 2014;**2014**(3):CD003007. DOI: 10.1002/14651858.CD003007.pub3

[88] Hyun JK, Lee JY, Lee SJ, Jeon JY. Asymmetric atrophy of multifidus muscle in patients with unilateral lumbosacral radiculopathy. Spine (Phila Pa 1976). 2007;**32**(21):E598-E602. DOI: 10.1097/BRS.0b013e318155837b

[89] Beneck GJ, Kulig K. Multifidus atrophy is localized and bilateral in active persons with chronic unilateral low back pain. Archives of Physical Medicine and Rehabilitation. 2012;**93**(2):300-306. DOI: 10.1016/j.apmr.2011.09.017

[90] Ogon I, Takebayashi T, Takashima H, et al. Quantitative analysis concerning atrophy and fat infiltration of the multifidus muscle with magnetic resonance spectroscopy in chronic low back pain. Spine Surgery and Related Research. 2019;**3**(2):163-170. DOI: 10.22603/ssrr.2018-0023

[91] Namnaqani FI, Mashabi AS, Yaseen KM, Alshehri MA. The effectiveness of McKenzie method compared to manual therapy for treating chronic low back pain: A systematic review. Journal of Musculoskeletal &

Neuronal Interactions. 2019;**19**(4):492-499

[92] Clare HA, Adams R, Maher CG. A systematic review of efficacy of McKenzie therapy for spinal pain. The Australian Journal of Physiotherapy. 2004;**50**(4):209-216. DOI: 10.1016/s0004-9514(14)60110-0

[93] Alhakami AM, Davis S, Qasheesh M, Shaphe A, Chahal A. Effects of McKenzie and stabilization exercises in reducing pain intensity and functional disability in individuals with nonspecific chronic low back pain: A systematic review. Journal of Physical Therapy Science. 2019;**31**(7):590-597. DOI: 10.1589/jpts.31.590

[94] Santana-Ríos JS, Chívez-Arias DD, Coronado-Zarco R, Cruz-Medina E, Nava-Bringas T. Postoperative treatment for lumbar disc herniation during rehabilitation. Systematic review. Acta Ortopédica Mexicana. 2014;**28**(2):113-124

[95] Johansson AC, Linton SJ, Bergkvist L, Nilsson O, Cornefjord M. Clinic-based training in comparison to home-based training after first-time lumbar disc surgery: A randomised controlled trial. European Spine Journal: Official Publication of the European Spine Society, the European Spinal Deformity Society, and the European Section of the Cervical Spine Research Society. 2009;**18**(3):398-409. DOI: 10.1007/s00586-008-0826-3

[96] Erdogmus CB, Resch KL, Sabitzer R, et al. Physiotherapy-based rehabilitation following disc herniation operation: Results of a randomized clinical trial. Spine (Phila Pa 1976). 2007;**32**(19):2041-2049. DOI: 10.1097/BRS.0b013e318145a386

[97] Ivarsson A, Tranaeus U, Johnson U, Stenling A. Negative psychological responses of injury and rehabilitation adherence effects on return to play in competitive athletes: A systematic review and meta-analysis. Open Access Journal of Sports Medicine. 2017;**8**:27-32. DOI: 10.2147/OAJSM.S112688

[98] Marshall A, Donovan-Hall M, Ryall S. An exploration of athletes' views on their adherence to physiotherapy rehabilitation after sport injury. Journal of Sport Rehabilitation. 2012;**21**(1):18-25. DOI: 10.1123/jsr.21.1.18

[99] Reiman MP, Sylvain J, Loudon JK, Goode A. Return to sport after open and microdiscectomy surgery versus conservative treatment for lumbar disc herniation: A systematic review with meta-analysis. British Journal of Sports Medicine. 2016;**50**(4):221-230. DOI: 10.1136/bjsports-2015-094691

[100] Fryhofer GW, Smith HE. Return to play for cervical and lumbar spine conditions. Clinics in Sports Medicine. 2021;**40**(3):555-569. DOI: 10.1016/j.csm.2021.04.002

[101] Robben E, Kempeneers K, De Groef A, Depreitere B, Peers K. Guidelines for rehabilitation and return to play after cervical surgery in a general athletic population: A Delphi analysis. Clinical Journal of Sport Medicine: Official Journal of the Canadian Academy of Sport Medicine. 2021;**31**(2):145-150. DOI: 10.1097/JSM.0000000000000729

[102] Molinari RW, Pagarigan K, Dettori JR, Molinari RJ, Dehaven KE. Return to play in athletes receiving cervical surgery: A systematic review. Global Spine Journal. 2016;**6**(1):89-96. DOI: 10.1055/s-0035-1570460

[103] Kang DG, Anderson JC, Lehman RAJ. Return to play after cervical disc surgery. Clinics in Sports Medicine.

2016;**35**(4):529-543. DOI: 10.1016/j.csm.2016.05.001

[104] Watkins RG 4th, Williams LA, Watkins RG 3rd. Microscopic lumbar discectomy results for 60 cases in professional and Olympic athletes. The Spine Journal. 2003;**3**(2):100-105. DOI: 10.1016/s1529-9430(02)00569-7

[105] Earhart JS, Roberts D, Roc G, Gryzlo S, Hsu W. Effects of lumbar disk herniation on the careers of professional baseball players. Orthopedics. 2012;**35**(1):43-49. DOI: 10.3928/01477447-20111122-40

[106] Matsunaga S, Sakou T, Taketomi E, Ijiri K. Comparison of operative results of lumbar disc herniation in manual laborers and athletes. Spine (Phila Pa 1976). 1993;**18**(15):2222-2226. DOI: 10.1097/00007632-199311000-00013

[107] Sakou T, Masuda A, Yone K, Nakagawa M. Percutaneous discectomy in athletes. Spine (Phila Pa 1976). 1993;**18**(15):2218-2221. DOI: 10.1097/00007632-199311000-00012

Section 2

Surgery for Congenital, Spinal Disorders

Chapter 6

Neurulation and the Possible Etiologies of Neural Tube Defect

Noor Us Saba, Mohd Faheem and Punita Manik

Abstract

Neural tube defects (NTDs) are variety of defects which result from abnormal closure of the neural tube during embryogenesis. Various factors are implicated in the genesis of neural tube defects, with contributions from both genetic and environmental factors. The clear understanding of the causes which leads to NTDs is lacking, but several non-genetic risk factors have been identified which can be prevented by maternal folic acid supplementation. Multiple genetic causes and several critical biochemical reactions have been identified whose regulation is essential for the closure of neural tube. Preventive therapies can be developed by identifying potential risk factors in the genesis of NTDs.

Keywords: neural tube defects, neurulation, genetics, neural plate, folic acid

1. Introduction

Neural tube defects (NTDs) are birth defects which result from the abnormal closure of neural tube during embryogenesis [1]. Its etiology is multifactorial; nutritional, environmental, genetic, and exposure to various teratogenic drugs during pregnancy. The severity of NTDs varies from asymptomatic cutaneous manifestations to life threatening conditions where brain and spinal cord is completely exposed to the exterior.

Here authors describe the process of formation of central nervous system (brain and spinal cord) along with the possible etiologies of NTDs.

2. Neurulation

The initial process involved in the formation of nervous system (brain and spinal cord) is known as neurulation. It is further divided into:

a. Primary neurulation

b. Secondary neurulation

2.1 Primary neurulation

Primary neurulation is responsible for the future formation of brain and most part of the spinal cord. The thickened ectoderm, neural plate, elevates to form neural folds and subsequent fusion of neural folds give rise to neural tube (**Figures 1** and **2**). The fusion begins in cervical region and proceeds in cranial and caudal directions. Ends of the neural tube, neural pore, are closed first on the cranial side (21 days post fertilization) followed by the caudal side (28 days post fertilization) (**Figure 3**). Thus, neurulation is a process involved in the formation of neural tube and closure of neuropores by the end of the fourth week of embryo development [2, 3]. The defects resulting from the abnormalities in primary neurulation leads to open neural tube defects [4, 5].

2.2 Secondary neurulation

The formation of spinal cord distal to mid-sacral region is formed by the process of secondary neurulation. Some of the loosely packed cells of tail bud condense to form an epithelial rod, which later canalise and form a tubular lumen for the last part of sacral and coccygeal regions of spinal cord [6–8]. Studies of various pathways at molecular and cellular level in neurulation-stage embryos provide understanding of development of normal or abnormal neural tube [9]. The malformations resulting due to the abnormalities in secondary neurulation results in closed neural tube defects (**Figure 4**).

3. Mechanisms of neurulation

Shaping of the neural plate with mediolateral narrowing and rostro caudal elongation is needed to initiate closure of neural tube [10]. This elongation depends on Wnt signalling pathway via Frizzled (Fzd) membrane receptors [11]. Convergent extension of neural plate takes place through planar cell polarity (PCP) mediators

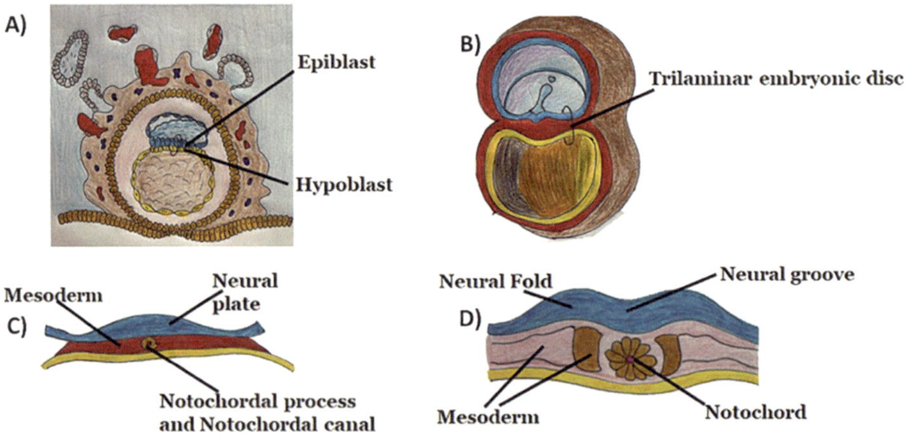

Figure 1.
A—Section of blastocyst of 9 days embryo-epiblast and hypoblast in bilaminar germ disc. B—Transverse section through embryonic disc-trilaminar embryonic disc. C, D—Transverse section of the embryonic disc at approximately 18 days embryo-showing notochord.

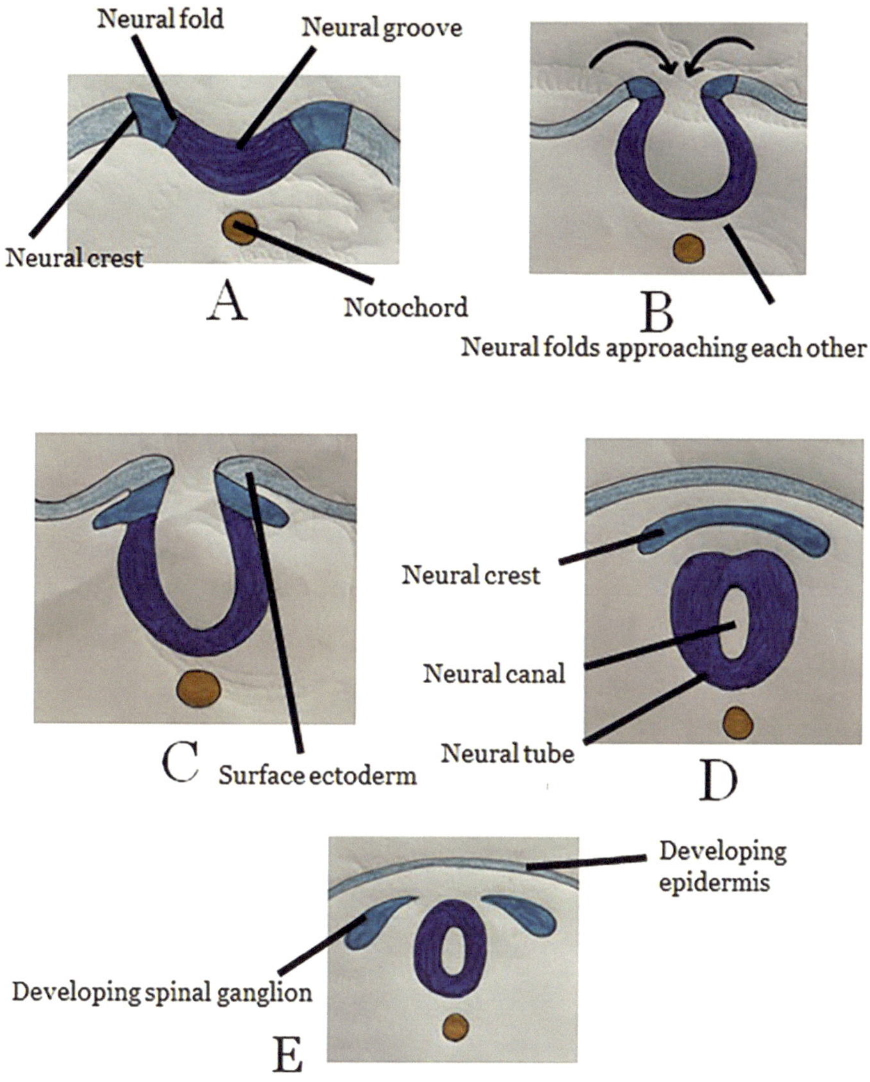

Figure 2.
Illustrations of formation of neural groove, neural folds, neural tube and neural crest in transverse section.

via PCP genes functioning including *Vangl2*, *Celsr1*, *Dvl-1* and *-2*, *Fzd-3* and 6, *Scrb1*, *Ptk7*, and *Sec24b* [12, 13].

Functional failure of PCP mediator genes results in broad neural plate and craniorachischisis due to disruption in the closure of neural plate [14]. Occurrence of closure in the forebrain and part of the midbrain in craniorachischisis implies that PCP-dependent mechanism is not necessary for whole of the brain. Exencephaly developing in mutants of the genes *Fuz* or *Intu* is more likely due to disturbed cilium-dependent hedgehog signaling, than altered regulation of convergent extension for neural tube closure initiation [15]. Thus, there are multiple mechanisms at cellular level on PCP signalling which potentially affects neural tube closure.

Tips of the neural folds approximate each other after bending of neuroepithelium to achieve closure. Median hinge points (MHP) and dorsolateral hinge points (DLHP)

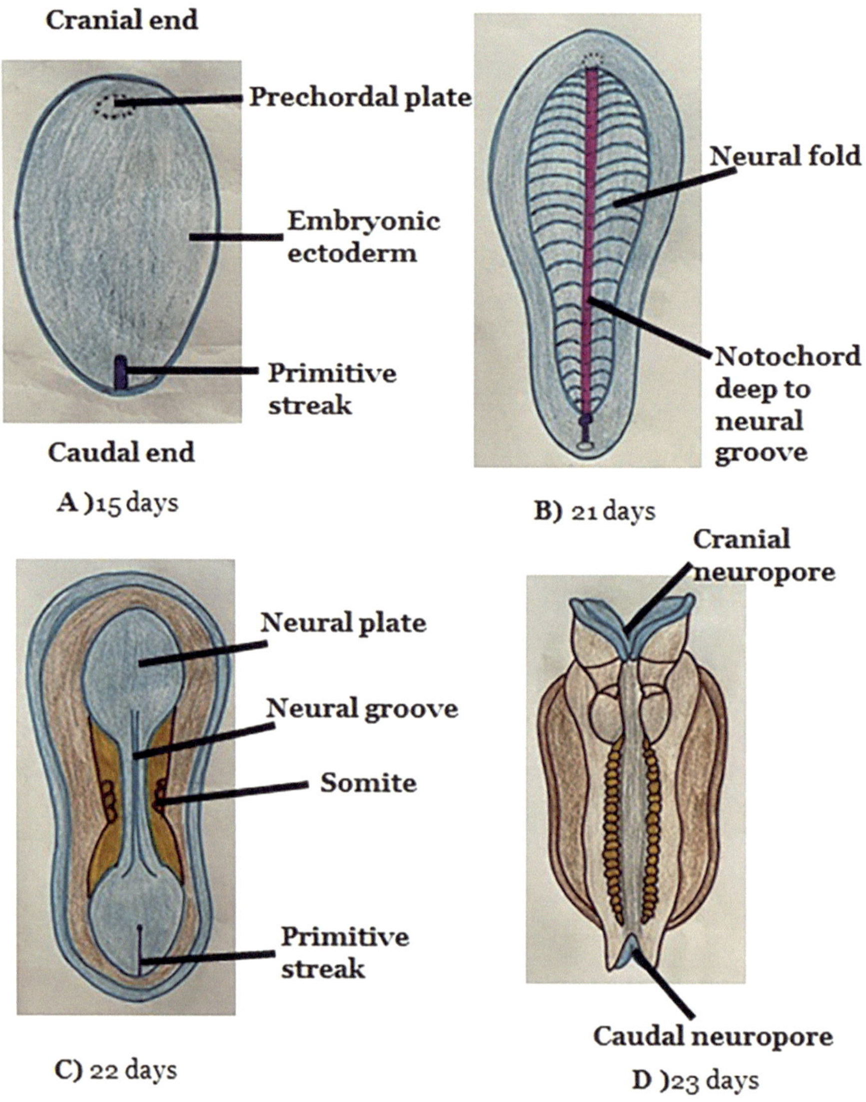

Figure 3.
Dorsal view of embryonic disc.

in a stereotypical manner bring out the bending. Regulating signals for the bending emanate from nonneural tissues around the neural folds. Notochord derived Shh causes induction of floor plate of the neural tube at the MHP. Factors enhancing Shh signals, for example, mutations in cilia-related genes such as *Gli3*, *Rab23*, *Fkbp8*, *Tulp3*, and *Ift40* also results in NTDs [16]. DLHPs take a role for neural tube closure in low spinal region by *Zic2*, expression of BMP antagonist, noggin, sufficiently induces DLHPs in dorsal neural folds [17].

Complexity of cranial neurulation compared to the spinal neurulation appears due to more extensive and sensitive genetic mechanisms. As a result, exencephaly comprises three times of the cases as does spina bifida after induction by teratogens. Disruption of cranial neurulation is contributed by some specific factors;

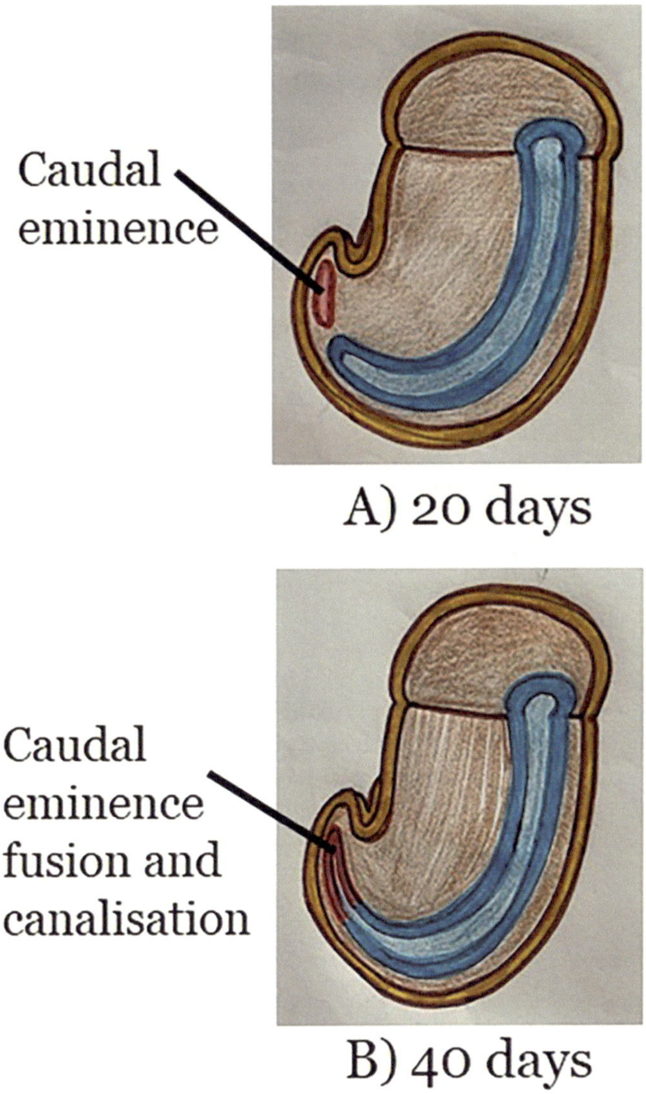

Figure 4.
Secondary neurulation.

mesenchymal expansion under the neural folds, cytoskeleton disruption of actin filaments, and mutant genes (e.g., *n-cofilin*, *vinculin*) of various cytoskeletal components which are not essential for neurulation in spinal region [18].

Meeting of the neural folds in dorsal midline give rise to two different types of epithelial layers, fledgling neural tube and overlying intact surface ectoderm, eventually after process of adhesion, fusion, and remodelling. Ephrin receptors, protease-activated receptors and *Grhl2* expressions, explain this process of adhesion at varying axial levels [19]. Cell proliferation, neuronal differentiation and programmed cell death can be regulated by the genes; *neurofibromin 1*, *nucleoporin*, *Phactr4* for cell cycle progression, Notch pathway genes *Hes1*, *Hes3*, *RBP-Jκ* for neuronal differentiation, and *caspase3* or *Apaf1* genes for characteristic patterns of apoptotic cell death.

NTDs are likely to occur in mutations of these genes, which hampers the regulated cell proliferation, differentiation, and cell death (**Table 1**) [20].

3.1 Type of neural tube defects

NTDs are classically divided into two types:

a. Open neural tube defects

b. Closed neural tube defects

3.1.1 Open neural tube defects

Open NTDs or spina bifida cystica are craniorachischisis, exencephaly-anencephaly and myelomeningoceles (**Figure 5A–F**). Open defects are characterised by the exposure of neural tissue through the skin as well as through the bony defect and is obvious at birth. These defects present with neurological deficit and carries poor prognosis. They can be identified easily during pregnancy due to high levels of α fetoprotein and acetylcholinesterase in amniotic fluid.

Craniorachischisis is the most serious and rare type of open NTD, which involves the defect in both cranial and spinal region. Their reported prenatal terminations range from 0.51 to 10.7 per 10,000 births in different regions of the world. Neural tube gets open from brain stem to spinal cord resulting in anencephaly and spina bifida simultaneously with external exposure of tissue in hindbrain and spinal cord on its posterior aspect. Death of the new-born is certain in craniorachischisis making it a lethal condition [21].

S. No.	Mechanism	Pathways/mediators/genes
1	Shaping and convergent extension of neural plate	Wnt signalling pathway, PCP mediator genes- *Vangl2*, *Celsr1*, *Dvl-1* and *-2*, *Fzd-3* and *-6*, *Scrb1*, *Ptk7*, and *Sec24b*
2	Adhesion, fusion, and remodelling	Ephrin receptors, protease-activated receptors and *Grhl2* expressions
3	Cell proliferation	*neurofibromin 1*, *nucleoporin*, *Phactr4*
	Neuronal differentiation	Notch pathway genes *Hes1*, *Hes3*, *RBP-Jκ*
	Programmed cell death	*caspase3* or *Apaf1* genes for characteristic patterns of apoptotic cell death
4	Induction of floor plate	Notochord derived Shh, cilia-related genes- *Gli3*, *Rab23*, *Fkbp8*, *Tulp3*, and *Ift40*
5	Cranial Neurulation	mesenchymal expansion, genes for cytoskeleton components (e.g., *n-cofilin*, *vinculin*) cilium-dependent hedgehog signalling genes *Fuz* or *Intu*
6	Spinal Neural Tube Closure	by *Zic2*, Expression of BMP antagonist- noggin

Table 1.
Mechanism of neurulation.

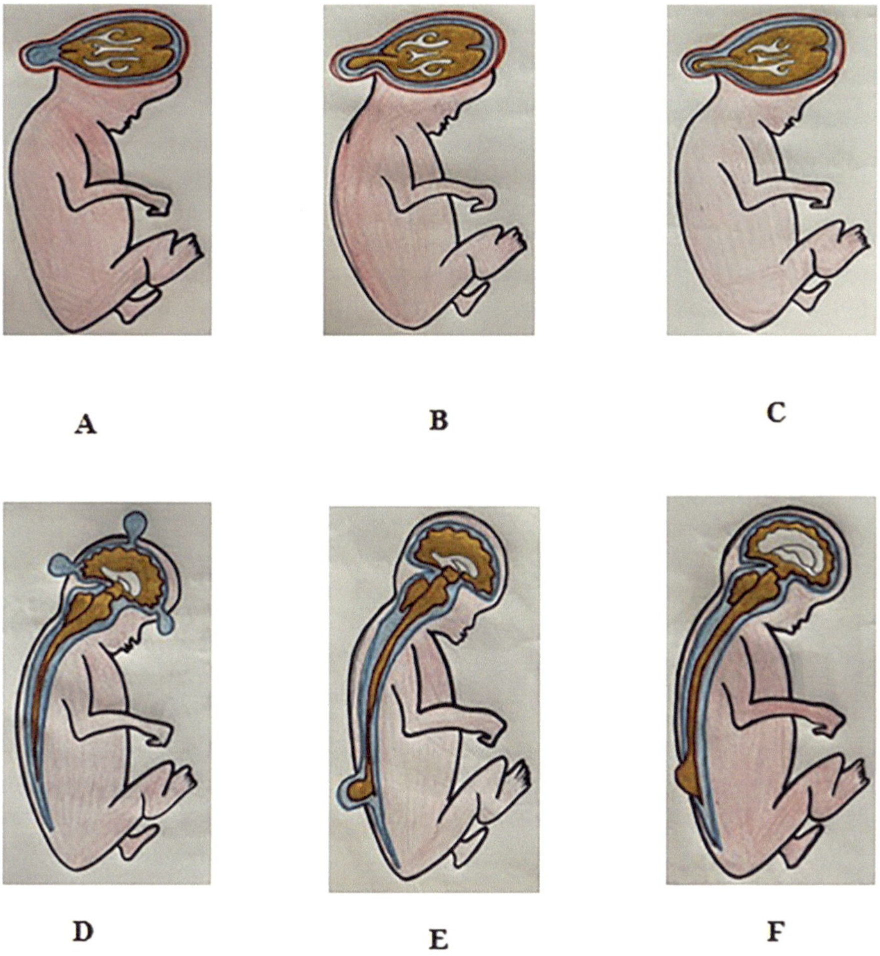

Figure 5.
A–D cephalocele, A—meningocele, B—encephalo-meningocele, C—encephalo-meningo-cystocele, D—anterior, parietal and occipital cephalocele, E—myelomeningocele, F—myelocele.

Anencephaly due to exencephaly involves non closure of only cranial part of the neural tube. Absence of forebrain and the vault of skull with intact skull base can be seen. Forebrain and midbrain are absent, brain stem is less severely involved and pituitary gland is hypoplastic in most of these cases. It is a lethal condition causing death of new-born within few days after birth.

Myelomeningocele results from defect in posterior part of spine usually in the lumbosacral region. Meningeal sac hernia takes place posteriorly, containing cerebrospinal fluid and nervous tissue, through a bony defect in the vertebral arch. Myelocele is a similar open NTD involving the spinal cord without protrusion of meningeal sac. Spinal cord is typically divided into two halves giving an appearance of "open book," which exposes ependymal layer to the surface.

Survival of the babies with open spina bifida depends on the severity and level of the lesion. Some other associated conditions including hydrocephalus, Chiari malformation type II, and vertebral abnormalities make them more complicated [21].

3.1.2 Closed neural tube defects

Closed NTDs or spina bifida occulta are encephalocele, meningocele, lipomeningocoele, diastematomyelia, and tethered filum terminale. Here, the underlying neural defect is masked by the intact overlying skin. The defect lies in the lower lumbar and sacral regions, and represents closed defects with deficient vertebral arches, sacral agenesis, and other skeletal defects. Presence of nevi, depigmentation, haemangiomas, localized hypertrichosis, and lumps including subcutaneous lipomas are some cutaneous stigmata of the lower back, may be the only signs of spina bifida occulta. Symptoms may not develop until late childhood and they possess comparatively better prognosis than open neural tube defects [21].

Encephalocoele is a round, soft, compressible, and nodular sac like protrusion of brain and/or its meningeal covering through an opening in the skull. Majority of encephaloceles pass through the midline calvarial defects and are classified according to the site of herniation; anterior, parietal, and occipital. Among these locations, occipital comprises 75% of the total number of encephaloceles. Hypertrichosis, and bluish translucency could be seen over the lesions during increased intracranial pressure. A comparatively better prognosis is observed if site is more rostral [22].

Meningocoele consists of meningeal herniation through the defect in the vertebral column. The spinal cord in these cases lies within the spinal canal in normal position. Atrophic epidermis of the skin usually covers the pedunculated and compressible lesion of herniated mass. They generally present with normal neurological examination and without any deformity (**Figure 5A–F**).

Lipomyelomeningocele is a form of occult spinal dysraphism where fat herniates through the bony defect. Diastematomyelia refers to a split in the spinal cord by a bony or a fibrous septum. Majority of these patients have cutaneous manifestations (**Table 2**) [23].

4 Aetiology of neural tube defects

NTDs prevalence range from 0.5 to 10 per 1000 pregnancies, thereby poses significant public health problem [1]. Variations in the incidence are due to large variety of risk factors such as:

a. Environmental factors

b. Nutritional deficiencies

c. Genetic causes

4.1 Environment factors

Environmental exposure to air pollution, extremes of temperature, and exposure of toxins to the expectant mothers are some of the known risk factors contributing to the aetiology of NTDs [24]. Study on various animals suggests the effect of teratogens in development of NTDs. Anticonvulsant drug valproic acid and a fungal product fumonism are known teratogens to develop NTDs in humans.

Hyperglycemia in embryos of cultured rodents, maternal obesity and diabetes mellitus are recognised risk factors for NTDs. Increased oxidative stress, change in

Open NTDs- Spina bifida cystica				
S.No	**Type**	**Location of the defect**	**Findings of the defect**	**Prognosis**
1	Craniorachischisis	Cranial and Spinal	Open neural tube from brain stem to spinal cord	Death of the new born, lethal condition
2	Exencephaly-Anencephaly	Cranial	Absent forebrain and skull, thick and flat skull base	Death of the new born, lethal condition
3	Myelomeningoceles	Posterior part of spine, lumbar region	Meningeal sac hernia containing CSF and nervous tissue Associations with hydrocephalus, Chiari malformation type II, and vertebral abnormalities	Survival depends on severity and level of the lesion
Closed NTDs				
1	Encephalocele	Cranial	Hernia through small opening in the skull	Depends on site, lesion more rostral with better prognosis
2	Meningocele	Spinal	Meningeal herniation covered by the skin without its appendages	normal neurological examination and functions of the body
3	Lipomeningocoele	Spinal	Fat along with meninges herniates through the bony defect	Usually have normal neurological function.
4	Diastematomyelia	Spinal	Spinal cord splitting by bony or fibrous septum	Neurological deficit with bowel and bladder involvement
5	Tethered filum terminale	Spinal	Conus medullaris is tethered by filum terminal	Usually become symptomatic in the late childhood

Table 2.
Types of neural tube defects.

Pax3 gene functions, apoptosis of neuroepithelial cell, activation of apoptosis signal-regulating kinase 1(ASK1) enzyme are some effects brought about by the maternal and embryonic hyperglycemia resulting in NTDs (**Table 3**) [25].

4.2 Nutritional deficiencies

Folate is a well recognized vitamin B supplement implicated in the causation of neural tube defects. Poor socioeconomic status with high risk of congenital anomalies focus the scientists to find out the nutritional deficiencies in such cases. In mothers of NTD fetuses, folate was found to be deficient. Mechanism of folic acid in prevention of NTDs was considered when it was seen that blood folic acid levels in some mothers of affected foetuses were normal. It was believed that some suboptimal levels of folate in maternal blood interact with mutated genes, such as *Pax3* to cause NTDs in developing embryos. Neural tube closure requires complex reactions for various nucleotide biosynthesis and methylation. Deficient methylation and abnormal biosynthesis of purine base and thymidylate have been noticed in cases of NTDs [26].

Multifactorial (50%)			
A	S.No.	Non-genetic causes	Examples
	1	Environmental	Air pollution Extremes of temperature Exposure of toxins to the expectant mothers Teratogens; anticonvulsant-valproic acid, fungal product fumonism Hyperglycemia in embryos Maternal obesity and diabetes mellitus
	2	Nutritional	Poor nutritional status and folate deficiency in mothers
B	S.No.	Genetic causes	Examples
	1	Gene-gene interactions	*Dvl1-Dvl2, Cdx1-Cdx2* double knockouts Supplementary sequel of heterozygous mutations *Dvl3* with *Vangl2*^{Lp} Variable phenotypic expressions of *Cecr1* mutation
	2	Effect of modifier genes	Variation in *Lmnb1* in *curly tail* (*Grhl3*) embryos
	3	Implications through experimental models	PCP genes mutations- *CELSR1, VANGL1, VANGL2, FZD6, SCRIB1*, and *DVL2*
	4	Folate one-carbon metabolism in mitochondria	suboptimal levels of folate in maternal blood interact with mutated *Pax3* genes
	5	Histone modifications	Mutations in histone demethylases *Jarid2* and *Fbxl10* Mutations in histone deacetylases *Sirt1* or *Hdac4* Teratogens- Valproic acid and trichostin A
	6	Syndromes	Trisomy 13, Trisomy 18 and Triploidy
Unknown factors (50%)			

Table 3.
Aetiology of neural tube defects.

4.3 Genetics causes

Genetic mutations in the aetiology of NTDs always depend on polygenic and multifactorial inheritance. The causations by gene variants are complicated by the multiple genes, modifier genes, epigenetic factors, and environmental effects. Some recognised mutations of different genes obtained by experiments on animals were found to be the causes in minimal number of NTD cases in humans. Increasing understanding of development of neural tube and NTDs on molecular and cellular level still needs more precision to identify genetic basis of occurrence in individual cases. More than 200 mutations in the genes, and association of the environmental risk affect folate metabolism to causes NTDs. Significance to focus more on individual genes by scientists comes from the fact of having very less percentage of NTD cases in syndromes of chromosomal aberrations as compared to the isolated cases of NTDs. Now a days, data analysis from large-scale genome sequencing of NTD patients is more promising and practicable to mark the contribution of various genes in the patients and mutational burden of associated risks.

4.3.1 Gene interactions and modifier genes

Three wide range mechanisms to explain gene interactions in development of NTDs are; 1—Functional incompetency of two non-comparable genes for example *Dvl1-Dvl2 and Cdx1-Cdx2* double knockouts, 2—supplementary sequel of heterozygous mutations in *Dvl3-Vangl2*, 3—variable phenotypic expressions of inherent mouse strains, *Cecr1* mutation [27]. A remarkable and rare example of modifier gene for growing the tendency of NTDs in curly tail (Grhl3) embryos is variation in *Lmnb1*.

4.3.2 Genetic implications through experimental models

Mutations in PCP genes—*CELSR1*, *VANGL1*, *VANGL2*, *FZD6*, *SCRIB1*, and *DVL2* are well known mutations in mice to cause NTDs. Thus, known to be putative PCP gene mutations can cause multiple types of abnormal births including craniorachischisis, spina bifida, anencephaly, or closed forms of spina bifida in humans. A wide range of NTDs can be seen after combining PCP mutations with other genetic risk factors of NTDs- For example; *VANGL2*, a missense variant, was seen in a spina bifida patient having a putative mutation in *DVL2*.

4.3.3 Genetic factors relation with environmental risk factors

A known environmental risk factor when interacts with genetic alteration in the embryo, could eventually instigate the risk of NTDs. Folate one-carbon metabolism in mitochondria is highly studied category for finding cause of NTDs in such cases and genes related to folate metabolism enlighten the ambience of maternal folate levels.

Enhanced risk of developing spina bifida by the 'risk' genes *GLUT1*, *SOD1*, and *SOD2* conglomerate in foetus of mothers having diabetes and obesity. Some genes related to maternal obesity- *FTO*, *LEP*, and *TCF7L2* were identified as a risk factor for NTDs in embryos.

4.3.4 Gene-regulatory mechanisms and NTDs

Multigenic involvement of NTDs makes it more complicated and difficult to identify due to irregular expressions of genes. Such as, insufficient or excess expression of *Grhl3* and *Grhl2* cause NTDs in mice, positive and negative correlations to explain the relationships among folate status, DNA methylation, and risk of NTDs. Modifications of histone protein or chromatin remodelling are some probable causes of NTDs in mice and in few cases in humans. Histone modifications effectively mis regulate the genes responsible for neurulation. For example, mutations in histone demethylases *Jarid2* and *Fbxl10*, mutations in histone deacetylases *Sirt1* or *Hdac4* and teratogenic inhibition of histone deacetylases by valproic acid and trichostin A.

5. Prevention of neural tube defects

Primary prevention is quite effective in reducing the birth defects related to NTDs. It has been suggested that folic acid supplementation in a dose of 0.4 mg per day prevents large number of NTDs. There is three fold reduction in NTDs recurrence with an intake of 4 mg folic acid per day by the expectant mothers. The exact mechanism of this prevention is yet to be elucidated, but folate plays an important role in numerous chemical reactions, including thymidine and purine production and S- adenosylmethionoine synthesis, which is the methyl donor for DNA, lipids and proteins.

6. Conclusion

The causes of NTDs are multifactorial in humans, including genetic and non-genetic factors. The combination of these factors leads to defective closure of neural tube and subsequent development of malformed fetal appearance. Folic acid supplementation during pregnancy and its awareness through various platforms are necessary to prevent further occurrence of NTDs in children.

Acknowledgements

I am thankful to my family for the support they have provided in writing this chapter.

Conflict of interest

"The authors declare no conflict of interest."

Author details

Noor Us Saba[1*], Mohd Faheem[2] and Punita Manik[1]

1 Department of Anatomy, King George's Medical University, Lucknow, UP, India

2 Department of Neurosurgery, Uttar Pradesh University of Medical Sciences, Saifai, UP, India

*Address all correspondence to: noorussaba83@gmail.com

References

[1] Greene NDE, Copp AJ. Neural tube defects. Annual Review of Neuroscience. 2014;**37**(1):221-242. DOI: 10.1146/annurev-neuro-062012-170354

[2] Sadler TW. Langman's Medical Embryology. 12th ed. Philadelphia: Wolters Kluwer; 2012. p. 63

[3] Moore KL, Persod TVN, Torchia MG. The Developing Human. Clinically Oriented Embryology. 9th ed. Philadelphia, PA: Elsevier Saunders; 2013

[4] O'Rahilly R, Muller F. The two sites of fusion of the neural folds and the two neuropores in the human embryo. Teratology. 2002;**65**:162-170

[5] Sulik KK, Zuker RM, Dehart DB, Cessot F, Delezoide AL, et al. Normal patterns of neural tube closure differ in the human and the mouse. Proceedings of Greenwood Genetics Center. 1998;**18**:129-130

[6] Copp AJ, Brook FA. Does lumbosacral spina bifida arise by failure of neural folding or by defective canalisation? Journal of Medical Genetics. 1989;**26**:160-166

[7] Schoenwolf GC. Histological and ultrastructural studies of secondary neurulation in mouse embryos. The American Journal of Anatomy. 1984;**169**:361-376

[8] Lew SM, Kothbauer KF. Tethered cord syndrome: An updated review. Pediatric Neurosurgery. 2007;**43**(3):236-248

[9] Copp AJ, Greene NDE. Genetics and development of neural tube defects. The Journal of Pathology. 2010;**220**:217-230

[10] Keller R. Shaping the vertebrate body plan by polarized embryonic cell movements. Science. 2002;**298**:1950-1954

[11] Goodrich LV, Strutt D. Principles of planar polarity in animal development. Development. 2011;**138**(10):1877-1892

[12] Juriloff DM, Harris MJ. A consideration of the evidence that genetic defects in planar cell polarity contribute to the etiology of human neural tube defects. Birth Defects Research. Part A, Clinical and Molecular Teratology. 2012a;**94**(10):824-840

[13] Merte J, Jensen D, Wright K, Sarsfield S, Wang Y, et al. Sec24b selectively sorts Vangl2 to regulate planar cell polarity during neural tube closure. Nature Cell Biology. 2010;**12**:41-46

[14] Wallingford JB, Harland RM. Neural tube closure requires Dishevelled-dependent convergent extension of the midline. Development. 2002;**129**(24):5815-5825

[15] Gray RS, Abitua PB, Wlodarczyk BJ, Szabo-Rogers HL, Blanchard O, et al. The planar cell polarity ef- fector Fuz is essential for targeted membrane trafficking, ciliogenesis and mouse embryonic development. Nature Cell Biology. 2009;**11**:1225-1232

[16] Miller KA, Ah-Cann CJ, Welfare MF, Tan TY, Pope K, et al. Cauli: A mouse strain with an ift140 mutation that results in a skeletal ciliopathy modelling Jeune syndrome. PLoS Genetics. 2013;**9**(8):e1003746

[17] Ybot-Gonzalez P, Cogram P, Gerrelli D, Copp AJ. Sonic hedgehog and the molecular regulation of neural tube closure. Development. 2002;**129**:2507-2517

[18] Gurniak CB, Perlas E, Witke W. The actin depolymerizing factor n-cofilin is essential for neural tube morphogenesis and neural crest cell migration. Developmental Biology. 2005;**278**(1):231-241

[19] Pyrgaki C, Liu A, Niswander L. Grainyhead-like 2 regulates neural tube closure and adhesion molecule expression during neural fold fusion. Developmental Biology. 2011;**353**:38-49

[20] Harris MJ, Juriloff DM. An update to the list of mouse mutants with neural tube closure defects and advances toward a complete genetic perspective of neural tube closure. Birth Defects Research: A Clinical Molecular Teratology. 2010;**88**:653-669

[21] Avagliano L, Massa V, George TM, Qureshy S, Bulfamante GP, Finnell RH. Overview on neural tube defects: From development to physical characteristics. Birth Defects Research. 2019;**111**:1455-1467

[22] Pilu G, Buyukkurt S, Youssef A, Tonni G. Cephalocele. Visual Encyclopedia of Ultrasound in Obstetrics and Gynecology - VISUOG. 2014

[23] Ellenberg RG, Abdulrauf SI, Shekhar LN. Spinal Dysraphism and Tethered Cord. 3rd ed. Philadelphia: Elsevier; 2012. pp. 89-90

[24] Carmichael SL, Yang W, Roberts E, Kegley SE, Padula AM, English PB, et al. Residential agricultural pesticide exposures and risk of selected congenital heart defects among offspring in the San Joaquin Valley of California. Environmental Research. 2014;**135**:133-138. DOI: 10.1016/j.envres.2014.08.030

[25] Reece EA. Diabetes-induced birth defects: What do we know? What can we do? Current Diabetes Reports. 2012;**12**(1):24-32

[26] Beaudin AE, Abarinov EV, Noden DM, Perry CA, Chu S, et al. Shmt1 and de novo thymidylate biosynthesis underlie folate-responsive neural tube defects in mice. The American Journal of Clinical Nutrition. 2011;**93**:789-798

[27] Davidson CE, Li Q, Churchill GA, Osborne LR, McDermid HE. Modifier locus for exencephaly in Cecr2 mutant mice is syntenic to the 10q25.3 region associated with neural tube defects in humans. Physiological Genomics. 2007;**31**:244-251

Chapter 7

Osteogenic Cells and Microenvironment of Early Bone Development and Clinical Implication

Kee D. Kim and Charles C. Lee

Abstract

This chapter provides an overview of the complex biological processes involved in bone development and regeneration. The skeletal system serves crucial functions such as structural support, mineral storage, and organ protection. Bone development encompasses diverse cell types, matrices, and signals from embryonic stages to adulthood, with age-related decline in regeneration requiring additional support for large defects. Intramembranous and endochondral ossification processes are explored, involving differentiation of mesenchymal cells into osteoblasts and cartilage formation replaced by bone, respectively. Collagen and proteoglycans, particularly collagen I and II and heparan sulfates, play vital roles in the microenvironment for bone formation and mineralization. Signaling molecules such as BMPs, FGFs, IGFs, and PDGFs important for proliferation and differentiation of bone precursors, embryonic development, growth and maintenance of mature bone include regeneration and angiogenesis. Cell-based approaches, microenvironment-based technologies, and signal-based technologies utilizing growth factors are explored as bone regeneration strategies. Understanding these processes, factors, and technologies is pivotal in improving the treatment of conditions such as osteoporosis, fractures, and bone reconstruction, ultimately developing new technologies.

Keywords: osteogenesis, osteoinductive signals, microenvironment, bone development, bone regeneration

1. Introduction

A remarkable cascade of biological events takes place from mesenchymal condensation during early embryonic development to postnatal maturation, providing the body with the skeletal system for structural support and stability, mineral storage, and protection of vital organs. The process involves various cell types, extracellular matrices ("microenvironment"), and biological signals that orchestrate the formation of the bone in the microenvironment throughout early developmental and maturation stages, even into adulthood. This process may provide a unique insight into developing novel technologies for regenerating and repairing bone defects or bridging bony gaps to achieve a solid fusion as required in fusion surgeries. Bone is able to regenerate and repair itself in healthy individuals as long as the defect is less than a critical size although the regenerative potential declines with aging. While there is no clear definition of a critical-sized bone defect [1], it is generally referred to as the distance of the boney gap that the body is unable to bridge with new bone spontaneously. A critical-sized bone defect would need an additional osteogenic (stem and progenitor cells), osteoinductive (biological signals), and/or osteoconductive (microenvironment) support for full bone regeneration and repair. Obesity, diabetes, osteoporosis, metabolic disorders, extended use of steroids, poor nutrition, advancing age, and drinking and smoking may lead to pseudoarthrosis, which is defined as a chronic condition where a broken bone has failed to heal after a fracture or surgical procedure. Patients with these risk factors and/or those who have been diagnosed with pseudoarthrosis may require a surgical intervention that includes a regenerative approach. Thus, it may be critical to understand how the body utilizes different biological components for developing the skeletal system and apply such understanding in designing an optimal regenerative approach for patients in need.

2. Cells in embryonic bone development

2.1 Intramembranous ossification

Embryonic epithelial and mesenchymal cells undergo a series of sequential and reciprocal communications to initiate mesenchymal condensation through a signaling pathway, which induces the expression of neural cell adhesion molecules (NCAM) and N-cadherin and mediates cell-cell adhesion during intramembranous ossification [2, 3]. The epithelial-mesenchymal crosstalk at the cellular and molecular levels appears to be the first event that leads to the condensation and migration of presumptive skeletogenic cells that are derived from the neural crest or mesoderm. The role of epithelial cells in mesenchymal condensation is clearly identified for intramembranous ossification [4–6]. Interestingly, mandibular bones failed to form in the absence of mandibular epithelium in the chicken (HH 24) and mouse (day 10) embryos, suggesting the crucial role of the epithelium in early bone development. Mesenchymal cells derived from the neural crest proliferate and differentiate directly into the osteogenic lineage without going through the intermediary chondrogenic transition by condensing into compact nodules during intramembranous ossification (**Figure 1**). These condensing mesenchymal cells differentiate into osteoblasts with activation of transcription factors such as CBFA1, which appears to trigger the expression of genes associated with the production of osteopontin, osteocalcin, and extracellular matrices that support bone development [7]. Additional factors such as extracellular signal-regulated kinase (ERK), p38 (MAPK), Akt, p65 (NF-kB), and bone morphogenetic proteins (BMPs) in addition to the activation of transcription factors such as CBFA1 [8].

Mesenchymal cells originating from the neural crest undergo a series of biochemical and cellular events, including proliferation and condensation, leading to the formation of compact nodules (**Figure 2**). Within these nodules, the cells undergo differentiation toward either capillaries or osteoblasts—specialized bone precursor cells responsible for generating collagen and proteoglycan matrix, crucial for calcium

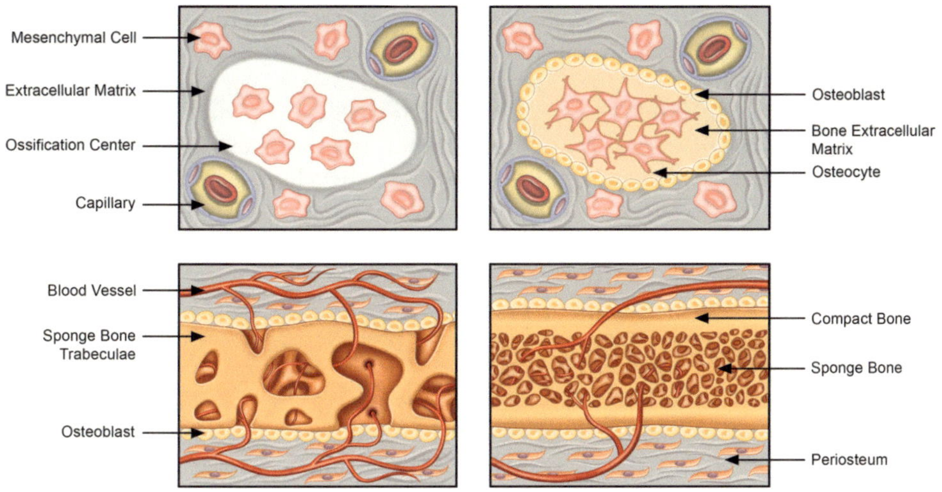

Figure 1.
Intramembranous ossification. The stages of intramembranous ossification include: (i) undifferentiated mesenchymal cells cluster and differentiation into osteoblasts. The ossification centers also emerge wherein the osteoblasts secrete osteoid, containing collagen precursors and other proteins, and entrapping the osteoblasts, which then transform into osteocytes. The clusters of osteoid are invaded by the blood vessels to form the trabecular matrix, whereas osteoblasts on the surface of the newly formed spongy bone form the periosteum. The periosteum then leads to the development of the compact bone superficial to the spongy trabecular bone.

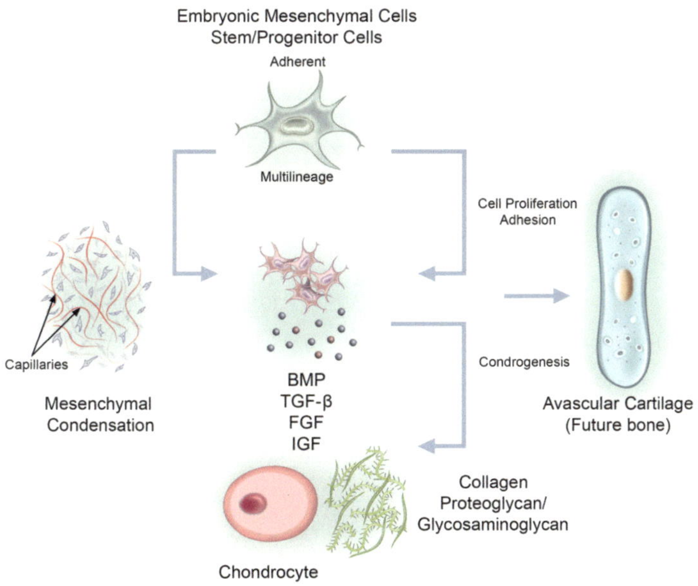

Figure 2.
Embryonic bone development. Multilineage embryonic stem/progenitor cells aggregate into chondrogenic clusters driven by cellular processes including mesenchymal condensation, proliferation, and adhesion. These events are driven by growth factors such as bone morphogenetic proteins (BMP), transforming growth factor-β (TGF-β), fibroblast growth factors (FGF), and insulin-like growth factor (IGF). The developing chondrocytes secrete or modify matrix proteins including collagen, proteoglycans or glycosaminoglycans to initiate avascular cartilage formation, forming a template for future bone development.

binding [9]. Through this process, the osteoid matrix, an initial form of bone, is generated. Over time, this matrix becomes calcified, resulting in the formation of primitive bone. While actively producing the osteoid matrix, osteoblasts maintain proximity to the calcification site. As they become embedded within the calcified matrix, osteoblasts undergo further differentiation and transform into osteocytes. Meanwhile, mesenchymal cells aggregate around the developing calcified bone matrix, forming the periosteum—an outer layer surrounding the bone [10]. The periosteum contributes to bone growth by generating additional osteoblasts and producing osteoid matrix, positioned adjacent to the bone's spicules.

2.2 Endochondral ossification

Endochondral ossification is a highly intricate process involving the differentiation of mesenchymal cells into chondrocytes, leading to the formation of cartilage that is subsequently replaced by bone (**Figure 3**). The initiation of this process is mediated by paracrine signaling from neighboring mesodermal cells, which induces

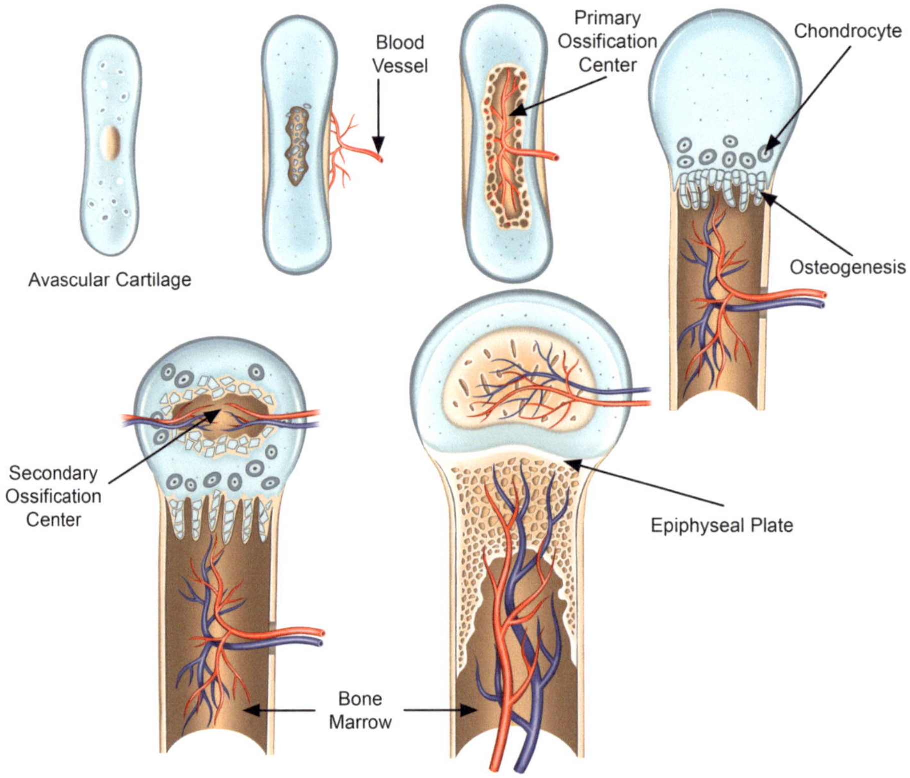

Figure 3.
Endochondral ossification. Endochondral ossification is marked by the formation of cartilage, which in later stages is replaced by bone. Bone formation process is initiated in the primary ossification center by the differentiation of mesenchymal cells into chondrocytes. The primary ossification center leads to the development of the diaphysis of the long bones, and the secondary ossification center leads to the development of the epiphysis. During late differentiation, the chondrocytes undergo apoptosis, forming a mineralized scaffold, which is invaded by the osteoblasts (brought in by the supplying blood vessels). This results in osteogenesis and lengthening of the bone along with the formation of the bone marrow cavity. Endochondral ossification occurs at the growth plate, which is responsible for longitudinal growth; it is also vital for the elongation of the long bones.

the expression of key transcription factors such as Scleraxis (SCX) and Pax 1 in mesenchymal cells [11, 12]. These transcription factors play a crucial role in driving the differentiation of mesenchymal cells into chondrocytes, initiating the formation of cartilage. Notably, SCX is particularly important during the early stages of cartilaginous condensation and any mutations in this gene can result in skeletal deformities [11]. The condensation and maintenance of chondrocytes is facilitated by the involvement of N-cadherin and N-CAM [13], which play significant roles in initiating and sustaining the cellular condensation process. During the proliferative and condensation stage, chondrocytes undergo a remarkable transformation, transitioning from actively dividing cells to hypertrophic chondrocytes. As they undergo hypertrophy, these chondrocytes undergo profound changes in the composition of extracellular matrix (ECM). They modify ECM by incorporating additional fibronectin and collagen X [14], which are crucial for enabling the subsequent mineralization of the cartilage matrix through the deposition of calcium carbonate. The lifecycle of hypertrophic chondrocytes culminates in apoptosis, creating space for the invasion of blood vessels and the establishment of bone marrow [15].

Simultaneously, surrounding cells undergo differentiation into osteoblasts, which are responsible for synthesizing and depositing the bone matrix onto the remnants of degraded cartilage. This gradual replacement of cartilage by bone matrix ultimately leads to the complete substitution of the original cartilaginous template. In the context of long bones, endochondral ossification occurs in a directional manner, spreading outward from the center of the bone. At the ends of long bones, specialized regions known as epiphyseal growth plates play a pivotal role in enabling continued bone growth [16]. These growth plates consist of distinct regions, including a zone of chondrocyte proliferation, a zone of mature chondrocytes, and a zone of hypertrophic chondrocytes. Chondrocytes within the growth plates undergo a carefully orchestrated series of events involving proliferation, maturation, and hypertrophy, contributing to the expansion of the bone structure. As long as the epiphyseal growth plates retain their capacity to produce chondrocytes, the process of bone growth persists, allowing for the longitudinal growth of bones.

3. Microenvironment

3.1 Collagen

The precise arrangement and composition of collagen types play a fundamental role in the intricate process of bone development (**Figure 2**). During embryonic bone formation, two main mechanisms are involved: endochondral ossification and intramembranous ossification, originating from distinct cell sources such as the paraxial and lateral plate mesoderm or neural crest. Collagen I is the predominant type found in mature bone, while Collagen II is predominantly present in developing cartilage [17]. In endochondral ossification, bone tissue replaces a pre-existing cartilaginous scaffold, whereas intramembranous ossification occurs directly from mesenchymal cells [18]. Notably, during the initiation phase and subsequent differentiation into osteoblasts, Collagen II and Collagen IX mRNA expression is observed in osteoblasts of mice and chicks [19, 20]. Furthermore, Collagen X is expressed during the terminal differentiation of chondrocytes, serving as a hallmark of hypertrophy in endochondral ossification.

In the case of intramembranous ossification, Collagen I is a primary collagen type involved [18]. Collagen X production primarily occurs in hypertrophic chondrocytes within the region of the endochondral growth plate dedicated to matrix mineralization. Additionally, Collagen X expression is observed at the edges of epiphyseal cartilage during fracture repair, osteoarthritis, and within the intervertebral disc [21]. As the cartilaginous extracellular matrix (ECM) rich in Collagen X is replaced by the collagenous ECM abundant in Collagen I, a crucial transition from cartilage to bone occurs. Collagen XIII, another collagen type, influences bone formation and potentially plays a role in connecting the regulation of bone mass to mechanical use [22]. Collagen XXIV, in turn, acts as a marker for osteoblast differentiation and bone formation. Collagen XXVII is predominantly found in cartilage even in adulthood [23]. It is associated with cartilage calcification and is believed to contribute to the conversion of cartilage to bone during skeletogenesis. This involvement in skeletogenesis has been established in zebrafish, where Collagen XXVII is essential for vertebral mineralization and postembryonic axial growth [24].

Matrix metalloproteinases (MMPs) are a group of zinc-dependent endopeptidases classified within the metzincin superfamily. These enzymes play a vital role in the degradation of the extracellular matrix (ECM) and collectively possess the ability to degrade various ECM proteins [17]. MMPs are involved in both physiological processes, such as development and tissue repair, and pathological conditions, including tumorigenesis and metastasis. Particularly, they are the primary enzymes responsible for collagen degradation [17]. Understanding the roles and interactions of these collagen types and MMPs provides valuable insights into the intricate processes involved in bone development and maintenance.

3.2 Proteoglycan

Proteoglycans, situated within the extracellular matrix (ECM) among collagen fibrils, play a significant role by providing a high negative charge, which generates osmotic pressure and attractive forces for cations like calcium [25]. Furthermore, glycosaminoglycans, particularly heparan sulfates, facilitate the binding of growth factors (**Figure 2**). The ECM consists of approximately three dozen proteoglycans that contribute to the filling and lubrication of the ECM space. In adult bone, biglycan and decorin promote the formation of bone and collagen fibrils, while keratocan enhances the rate of mineral deposition [9]. During embryonic ossification, proteoglycans also play crucial roles in osteoblast proliferation and differentiation. Poole et al. [26] discovered that proteoglycans become encapsulated within calcified cartilage during mineralization, providing a scaffold for osteoid and bone formation. Fisher et al. [27] identified a small proteoglycan localized to developing bone trabeculae and dentin, as well as osteoblasts and osteoprogenitor cells adjacent to areas undergoing rapid osteogenesis. Proteoglycan desulfation, as identified by Settembre et al. [28], serves as a critical regulator of chondrogenesis preceding endochondral bone formation. Simonet et al. [29] identified osteoprotegerin, a novel secreted glycoprotein acting as an anti-osteoclastogenic decoy receptor, aiding in bone formation by reducing bone resorption.

Perlecan, a ubiquitous and multifunctional molecule, is upregulated in hypertrophic chondrocytes that establish the primary and secondary ossification centers. Functioning as a heparan sulfate proteoglycan (HS) or HS/chondroitin sulfate hybrid, perlecan acts as a pressure sensor in bone development and remodeling [30]. Depletion of chondroitin sulfate results in irregular deposition and aggregation of collagen fibers, impairing connective tissue organization and impeding intramembranous ossification [31]. Matrix metalloproteinases (MMPs) and A disintegrin and metalloproteinase with thrombospondin motifs (ADAMTSs) are involved in the degradation of proteoglycans such as aggrecan, versican, and brevican. Heparan sulfate proteoglycan binds to various growth factors and facilitates ligand-receptor interactions, while betaglycan (TGF-β type III receptor), an integral membrane proteoglycan, binds to TGF-β and presents it to the core type II receptor [32]. Decorin, a small leucine-rich proteoglycan, provides a physical linkage that enhances the adhesion and assembly of aggrecan [33]. In the process of endochondral ossification, chondrocytes synthesize proteoglycans such as aggrecan and decorin, which are then deposited into the ECM along with collagen type II, forming a cartilaginous template for bone formation. These proteoglycans regulate chondrocyte proliferation, differentiation, and ECM mineralization. In summary, proteoglycans and related molecules play essential roles in embryonic ossification, including osteoblast proliferation and differentiation, and are crucial for bone development and remodeling throughout life.

4. Osteoinductive signals

4.1 Bone morphogenetic proteins

Bone morphogenetic proteins (BMPs) are the signaling molecules or growth factors belonging to the transforming growth factor-β (TGF-β) superfamily of proteins. They act as morphogens inducing embryogenesis and development (such as cardiogenesis, somite formation, somatic chondrogenesis, eye formation, digit apoptosis, neurogenesis, and musculoskeletal development). Thus, BMPs play a significant role in bone and cartilage formation (**Figure 4**). They are also multi-functional and are continuously expressed in adulthood to regulate the maintenance of tissue homeostasis (such as joint integrity, vascular remodeling, intramembranous and endochondral ossification) [34, 35]. BMPs occur in different subtypes and play critical roles in bone development. BMP-2 is crucial for chondrocyte proliferation and maturation during endochondral bone development; it is essential for appropriate osteogenesis, chondrogenesis, and adipogenesis. BMP-2 also promotes angiogenesis and is essential for initiating fracture healing [34–36]. It can also stimulate the differentiation of multipotent fibroblastic C3H10T1/2 cells into osteoblasts, chondrocytes, and adipocytes [37]. BMP-2 also enhances the expression of osteogenic markers including alkaline phosphatase, osteocalcin, and osteopontin [36]. BMP-4 coordinates the formation of the apical ectodermal ridge and digit patterning. BMP-5 mutant mice have shorter and weaker bones whereas BMP-6 mutant mice show delayed sternal ossification and shorter bones (specifically the long bones). BMP-7 and BMP-11 have a significant role in skeletal patterning during development. BMP-12, BMP-13, and BMP-14 are also crucial in the formation of bones, joints, tendons, and ligaments. BMP-12 is important in maintaining the structural integrity of the bone, and BMP-14 regulates bone and joint formation during digit development. In contrast to other BMPs, BMP-3 acts as a negative regulator of bone density. Along with bone formation, BMPs also regulate the development of cartilage [34].

During the formation of a new bone, mesenchymal stem cells (MSCs) differentiate into osteoblasts (under the influence of BMP-2) and secrete the organic matrix of the bone. Some osteoblasts get embedded in the bone (as osteocytes), leading to the development of the bone structure. The BMP signal transduction occurs via type I and II BMP receptors and Smad1, 5, and 8 proteins [situated downstream to the BMP receptors (BMPR)]. BMP-2 is secreted by pre-existing osteocytes, osteoblasts, and

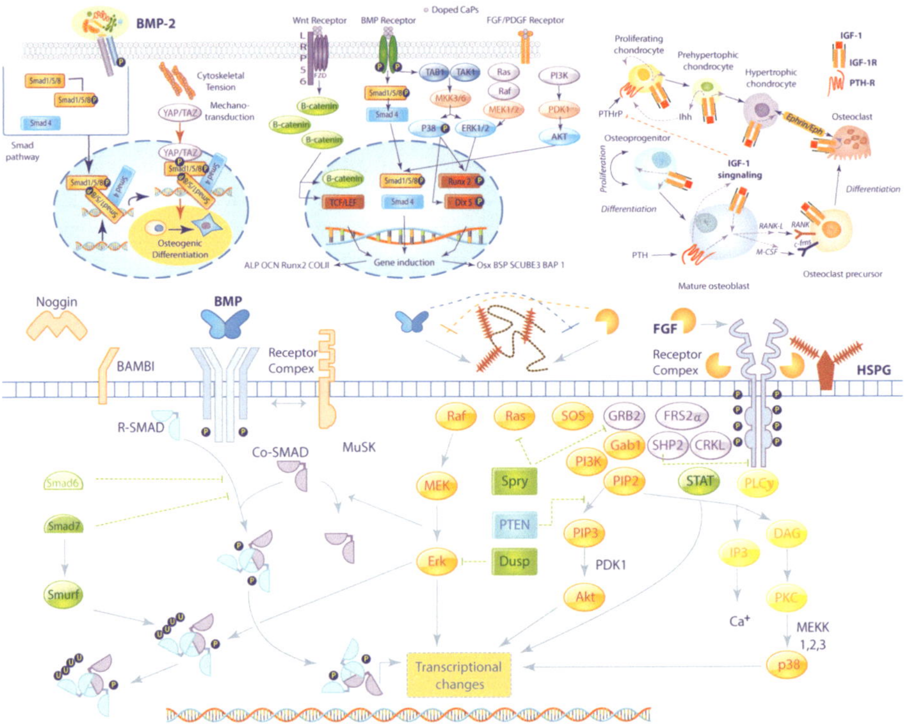

Figure 4.
Growth factors for bone formation. Growth factors and other signaling factors act on osteogenic precursors to drive bone morphogenesis and repair. Bone morphogenetic proteins (BMPs) play critical roles in chondrocyte proliferation and maturation and are essential to the formation of bones, joints, ligaments, and tendons. BMPs bind to cell-surface receptors driving intracellular signaling processes in tandem with SMAD and Wnt signaling pathways to induce transcription of osteogenic genes. Fibroblast growth factors (FGFs) and their receptors (FGFRs) are expressed in specific spatiotemporal patterns during development. The FGF-FGFR complex, in coordination with heparin sulfate proteoglycans at the cell surface, act via intracellular tyrosine kinase signaling to influence osteoblast proliferation, differentiation, and survival. Other anabolic factors, such as growth hormone (GH) and insulin-like growth factor (IGF), act as potent mitogens and differentiation signals which promote bone ossification during early development and bone maintenance and remodeling throughout growth, maturation, and aging processes.

endothelial cells into the bone matrix or bloodstream. Upon secretion, BMP-2 binds with type I or type II serine/threonine kinase receptors present on the MSCs, activating either canonical (Smad) or non-canonical (non-Smad) signaling pathways that lead to bone, cartilage, and fat development. Upon phosphorylation, Smad1, 5, and 8 molecules get complexed with Smad4. This complex is then translocated into the nucleus, activating the osteogenic genes such as Runt-Related Transcription Factor 2 (RUNX2) and Osterix (Osx) in osteoblasts [35, 38, 39]. Alternative non-canonical (non-Smad) signaling via BMP/BMPR interaction may be mediated through the activation of p38, or c-Jun N-terminal kinases via mitogen-activated protein kinase (MAPK), or extracellular signal-related kinase (ERK), phosphatidylinositol 3-kinase (PI3K), and the transforming growth factor-β-activated kinase 1/binding protein 1 (TAB1/TAK1) pathways. All of these pathways result in an increased differentiation of MSCs into osteoblasts [35, 39]. BMPs also show tremendous potential for their use as therapeutic agents to prevent osteoporosis, heal bone fractures, treat periodontal bone defects, and heal patients requiring bone reconstruction [40]. Studies show that subcutaneous injection of BMP-2 can stimulate the formation of ectopic bone nodules, and its expression in fibroblasts may help to repair acute bone defects in the calvaria [41]. Recombinant human BMP-2 has been approved by the Food and Drug Administration (FDA) for clinical use and is available as therapeutic in lumbar spinal fusions (within tapered or cylindrical interbody cages), but the use is limited to due cost and concerns for adverse reactions. Research suggests that developing novel therapeutics targeting BMP-signaling pathways may have clinical implications in the treatment of various disorders (osteoporosis, cardiovascular disease, cancer, etc.) without any adverse side effects [35].

4.2 Fibroblast growth factors

Fibroblast growth factors (FGFs) are a family of 18 signaling molecules known for their role in many developmental processes including skeletal development (**Figure 4**) [42, 43]. As a family, the FGFs have a homologous core region flanked by variations in the amino (N-) and carboxyl (C-) terminal tails which provide the structural basis for varying biological effects which are directed by activation of FGF receptors (FGFRs) in paracrine or endocrine mechanisms [44]. Most of the FGFs are expressed in specific spatiotemporal patterns in the developing embryo where diffusion and FGFR activation is regulated by the presence of heparan sulfate proteoglycans [45]. FGFR1 and FGFR2 are expressed in undifferentiated distal limb bud mesenchyme where they are activated by FGFs produced by the apical ectodermal ridge to induce promixo-distal outgrowth of the limb bud [46].

In endochondral mesenchymal condensation, FGFR3 expression is first activated as the condensed mesenchyme differentiates into chondrocytes, then decreased as central chondrocytes begin hypertrophy [47]. FGFR2 expression is decreased with chondrocyte differentiation while FGFR1 expression increases as chondrocytes mature and hypertrophy [47]. In trabecular bone, mesenchymal progenitors express FGFR1, differentiating osteoblasts express FGFR2, while chondrocyte progenitors express FGFR3 [48]. Early stages of intramembranous bone formation are characterized by expression of FGF2, FGF4, FGF9, FGF18, FGFR1, FGFR2, and FGFR3 [49]. The interaction of FGF18 with FGFR2 regulates early intramembranous ossification [50], while at later stages FGF18 and FGF9 are expressed in differentiating osteoblasts [49, 51]. Osteoblast proliferation, differentiation, and survival are dependent on FGF9 and FGF18 interactions with heparin sulfate proteoglycans, FGFR1, and FGFR2 through downstream tyrosine kinase signaling. Mutations in FGFRs1-3 have been identified in craniosynostosis, while mutations of FGFR3 are implicated in achondroplasia or hypochondroplasia (skeletal dwarfism), and skeletal overgrowth and scoliosis syndromes are associated with inactivation of FGFR3 [52, 53]. Mutations in FGFR2 affect the appendicular skeleton and are implicated in bent bone dysplasia, as well as premature cranial ossification due to accelerated maturation of osteoblasts [54].

4.3 Insulin-like growth factor

Growth Hormone (GH) and Insulin-like growth factors (IGF-1 and IGF-2) are the anabolic hormones that play an important role as potent mitogens and differentiation factors; consequently, promoting bone ossification (during early development), and bone remodeling or maintenance (throughout growth and aging) (**Figure 4**) [55, 56]. The mode of action of GH and IGF-1 occurs either in an endocrine, autocrine, or paracrine manner. GH controls the IGF-1 serum concentrations via its action in the liver, which contributes 75% of serum IGF-1. Elevated serum IGF-1 concentration further regulates GH concentration via the negative feedback control mechanism. IGF-1 and IGF-2 are the most abundant growth factors secreted by osteoblasts, and stored in bone. Serum GH and IGF-1 concentrations rise and peak during postnatal growth and puberty (phases witnessing peak bone mass accrual) [56, 57]. GH and IGF-1 predominantly promote the proliferation of osteoprogenitors and mesenchymal stem cells and stimulates their differentiation into osteoblasts and chondrocytes by inhibiting lipogenic genes, activating the PI3K/PDK-1/Akt pathway, and increasing Wnt (Wingless and INT-1) signaling [55, 57]. In addition to promoting osteoblastogenesis, IGF-1 also decreases osteoblast apoptosis by stabilizing β-catenin; thus, increasing Wnt-dependent activity. The Wnt proteins have a significant impact on embryonic development as well as postembryonic tissue homeostasis [55].

GH and IGF-1 also stimulate the expression of bone morphogenetic proteins that function in skeletal patterning. A signaling cascade is stimulated via IGF-1 binding and activation of the IGF-1 receptor present on mesenchymal stem cells that eventually elevates *RUNX2* gene expression resulting in an increased production of runt-related transcription factor 2 (Runx2). Runx2 is a major transcription factor having its role in osteoblast differentiation, and transformation of mesenchymal stem cells into osteoprogenitors [58, 59]. Furthermore, Runx2 also activates osterix, another important transcription factor that activates osteoblast differentiation and bone mineralization. This osteoblast differentiation is accompanied by a high alkaline-phosphatase activity and an increased collagen synthesis [60]. IGF-1 also stimulates the production of proinflammatory cytokines such as IL-6, and TNF-α in osteoblasts, which further mediate the stimulation of osteoclastogenesis [57]. Furthermore, animal studies involving the inactivation of the IGF-1 receptor revealed the specific role of IGF-1 in bone mineralization. Animal studies have also revealed the role of IGF-1 in osteoclast differentiation and function. IGF-1 deficient mice showed skeletal deformities, decreased chondrocyte proliferation, and increased chondrocyte apoptosis [55]. Bone remodeling involves the coupling of osteoblasts and osteoclasts activity, which is also found to be mediated by IGF via ephrinB2/Eph4 expression (a membrane-bound ligand/ receptor system) [56]. The administration of IGF-1 promotes longitudinal bone growth in animal models [55].

4.4 Platelet-derived growth factor

Platelet-derived growth factors (PDGFs) are potent angiogenesis factors as well as the mitogenic, chemo-attractive, and vascular docking agents that regulate processes such as embryonic development and tissue regeneration (**Figure 4**) [61–63]. They are expressed by platelets, osteoblasts, macrophages, and fibroblasts. PDGFs also function as osteoanabolics and enhance bone regeneration. They are secreted in various isoforms (AA, BB, AB, CC, and DD) that mediate their action via two distinct dimerized receptors [PDGFRs (α and β): members of receptor tyrosine kinases]. PDGF-AA predominantly activates PDGFR-α whereas PDGF-BB predominantly activates PDGFR-β [64]. Among all isoforms, PDGF-BB is considered the most common PDGF due to its varied physiological roles attributed to its ability to bind with all receptor isotypes [62, 63]. PDGF-BB is actively involved in angiogenesis, osteogenesis, and mesengenesis. It functions as a significant connector of these pathways and has the potential to be utilized as a potent therapeutic agent for bone regeneration and repair [63].

The formation of bone involves the formation of microvasculature. The rapidly dividing endothelial cells (present in the microvasculature) stimulate angiogenesis and secrete PDGF-BB that mediates its signal via PDGFR-β interaction, recruiting pericyte precursors into the region of new vessel formation. Pericytes are the perivascular or mural cells of mesenchymal origin. A majority of pericytes are mesenchymal stem cells (MSCs) having osteogenic potential. The PDGF-BB/PDGFR-β signaling pathway also regulates pericyte attachment on the vasculature, their maturation, destabilization, and detachment [62, 63].

PDGF-BB also stimulates vascular endothelial growth factor (an angiogenic factor) expression by pericytes, further promoting angiogenesis. PDGF-BB thus mediates the release of pericytes and MSCs from their abluminal sites in the active angiogenic locations; consequently, giving rise to free MSCs. These local or free MSCs divide rapidly under the influence of PDGF-BB; thus, elevating the pool of osteochondral precursors. In the presence of osteogenic factors such as Wnt signaling and BMPs, these osteochondral progenitors further differentiate into osteoblasts; this signaling process is modulated by PDGF-BB. Furthermore, in the presence of PDGF-BB, the remaining non-differentiated MSCs are repositioned in the perivascular space, stabilizing the newly formed blood vessels and leading to efficient bone formation (during embryonic bone formation and bone injury/fracture repair). In summary, PDGF-BB mediates the production of osteoprogenitor cells at a specific site, induces their multiplication, modifies their responsiveness to osteogenic factors, and assures the structural stability of the newly formed blood vessels [62, 63].

The isoform PDGF-AA is primarily produced and secreted by epithelial cells. It mediates its action on mesoderm-derived cells (via PDGFR-α), and stimulates mesenchyme expansion and angiogenesis. In contrast to PDGF-BB, PDGF-AA can stimulate MSC osteogenic differentiation by the BMP-Smad1/5/8-Runx2/Osx signaling pathway. The activation of BMP-Smad1/5/8 signaling by PDGF-AA occurs by down-regulating PDGFR-α (feedback control), which allows the free BMPR-I to get complexed with BMPR-II. The BMPR-I-BMPR-II complex further activates smad1/5/8 using BMP molecules, thereby promoting MSC differentiation and migration [64].

The isoform PDGF-BB has also been recognized as a significant paracrine factor involved in early bone healing. A study conducted on osteoblast-like cell-cultures also proposed the potential use of a combination of PDGF-BB and synthetic peptides (AC-100, p-15, TP508) for accelerating bone healing [65]. Another study conducted on animal models and periosteal cell cultures showed that PDGF-BB/PDGFR-β signaling inhibits BMP-2-induced osteogenesis (by attenuating Smad1/5/8 phosphorylation) [62]. Both PDGF-BB and BMP-2 are anabolic agents; however, when used in combination, they inhibit osteogenesis, suggesting a sequential use of both growth factors for better bone healing [62]. Contrary to PDGF-BB, there exists a link between PDGF-AA and BMP pathways that stimulates MSC osteogenic differentiation and migration [64]. These findings suggest the potential clinical implications of PDGF-AA along with BMP.

5. Bone growth and maturation

During fetal development, mineralization of the skeleton is a critical process, facilitated by the active involvement of the placenta in transporting essential minerals like calcium, magnesium, and phosphorus from the maternal circulation [66]. By the 8th week of gestation, the human fetus establishes a complete cartilaginous framework, and primary ossification centers begin to form between the 8th and 12th weeks, primarily in vertebrae and long bones. However, it is during the third trimester when the majority of mineralization occurs, with approximately 80% of the ash weight and mineral content being accreted [67]. Additional secondary ossification centers develop in the femur around the 34th week. The differentiation of osteoblasts into osteocytes occurs as they become embedded within the extracellular matrix, while other osteoblasts align along the bone surface, increasing in size. The interconnected trabeculae gradually form woven bone as growth progresses [66]. The primary center of ossification serves as the focal point for bone growth, and osteons, the fundamental units of compact bone, play a significant role in bone structure. Osteoblasts establish interconnections through cytoplasmic processes, which transform into the canaliculi of osteons. The transformation to compact bone involves the reduction of the perivascular space due to bone spicule formation around blood vessels. Consequently, the blood vessel assumes the role of the central canal within the osteon [68]. Adequate mineral delivery is crucial for normal skeletal development and mineralization in the fetus and neonate. The rate of mineral accretion intensifies significantly, with a notable surge from around 60 mg per day at week 25 to over 300 mg per day from the 35th through the 38th weeks. This acceleration slightly diminishes in the final 2 weeks before birth [67]. The turnover of the skeleton helps maintain a robust calcium level in the fetal circulation, as evident in cases of severe maternal hypocalcemia resulting from hypoparathyroidism, where skeletal resorption increases in response [17, 69].

Mineral and bone metabolism operate differently during the fetal development compared to adulthood [67]. The placenta plays a crucial role in providing essential minerals from the maternal circulation to the fetus, resulting in higher concentrations of these minerals in the fetal bloodstream for proper skeletal development. Hormones like parathyroid hormone (PTH) and PTH-related protein are crucial in regulating fetal bone development and serum mineral levels, while factors like vitamin D/calcitriol, fibroblast growth factor-23, calcitonin, and sex steroids have minimal impact [69, 70]. In the neonatal phase, there is a transition in the regulation of mineral homeostasis. Initially, serum calcium levels decrease while phosphorus levels rise, gradually reaching adult values within 24–48 hours [67, 70]. During this phase, the neonate's intestines become the primary source of minerals, kidneys reabsorb minerals, and bone turnover contributes to mineral supply. This transition is triggered by the loss of the placenta and a decline in serum calcium levels after birth. Subsequently, there is an increase in PTH secretion, followed by an elevation in calcitriol levels [67, 70]. Intestinal calcium absorption shifts from a passive process facilitated by lactose to an active and calcitriol-dependent process. However, increasing dietary calcium intake or administering calcium through parenteral routes can bypass the role of calcitriol in regulating mineral and bone metabolism [71].

Endochondral ossification is a fundamental process responsible for the development of the majority of bones in the skeletal system, known as endochondral bones. It involves several key stages that span over several weeks. Initially, the bones take the form of hyaline cartilage models. The process begins with the formation of a bone collar around the middle of the cartilage model, followed by the degeneration of the underlying cartilage. Concurrently, capillaries and osteoprogenitor cells invade the resulting ossification center from the periosteum. Osteoblasts subsequently deposit osteoid, which undergoes calcification, leading to the formation of woven bone. This woven bone is later remodeled into compact bone. Osteoblasts secrete bone matrix, while osteoclasts in the ossification center remove a portion of the newly formed bone, contributing to the creation of the bone marrow cavity [72, 73].

The primary ossification center initially forms in the diaphysis, the middle region of each developing bone. Subsequently, secondary ossification centers develop in the epiphyses through a similar process. Following ossification, the primary and secondary ossification centers are separated by a segment of cartilage called the epiphyseal growth plate, which remains between the epiphysis and diaphysis, enabling continued bone elongation. Ossification of the growth plate persists until around the age of 20 years. The growth plate facilitates bone lengthening by sustaining the growth of cartilage. The two ossification centers eventually merge when the epiphyseal plate disappears, which typically signifies the attainment of full stature [74]. The epiphyseal plates exhibit lower biomechanical properties compared to adjacent mature bone, ligaments, and tendons. A fracture in the growth plate can occur in children from a similar mechanical insult that would result in a join sprain in adults. Growth plate fractures impact the layer of developing tissue near the ends of a child's bones, with higher prevalence observed in the fingers, forearm, and lower leg. The majority of growth plate fractures heal successfully without negatively impacting future bone growth. However, in some cases, the fracture may cause alterations in the growth plate, leading to potential complications later on. These complications can include mild misalignment of the bone, resulting in slight deviation or marginal differences in length compared to the expected outcome. Growth plate fractures are significantly common among children, accounting for approximately 15–30% of all fractures in this age group. Moreover, they occur twice as frequently in boys compared to girls.

6. Aging bone changes

Skeletal mass increases with growth and maturational changes in bone density and dimensions. The most rapid period of bone growth occurs during adolescence with skeletal mass doubling during the pubertal growth spurt. Males showing greater bone strength with increased volume, trabecular number and thickness than females from mid-puberty onward due to the action of testosterone on periosteal apposition [75, 76]. Peak total bone mineral content and total bone mineral density is 22 years for females and 23–26 years for males [77]. The amount of bone present in the skeleton at the end of the maturation process, known as peak bone mass, is a key indicator of bone mass in the elderly [78, 79]. Normal bone homeostasis, a delicate balance of bone formation and resorption is disrupted with aging. Declines in bone mineral density are observed before midlife in trabecular and cortical bone in women but several decades later in men [80, 81]. Noninvasive imaging studies demonstrate greater loss of cortical bone and increases in cortical bone porosity compared with trabecular bone with advancing age [82, 83]. Bone loss in both sexes is driven by declines in estrogen and other steroid hormones. Women experience a period of marked cancellous bone loss with the onset of menopause, followed by a slower phase of loss that continues through the lifespan [84]. Estrogen loss is thought to increase osteoclast recruitment and activation and decrease osteoclast apoptosis, creating a shift toward increased bone resorption [85]. Cellular senescence, a factor in reduced osteoblast proliferation and differentiation, may contribute to a shift in production of osteogenic progenitors in the bone marrow, further exacerbating the shift toward bone resorption in the aged population [86, 87].

7. Factors affecting bone health

Bone health is determined by many factors including genetics, gender, nutrition, hormonal status, bodyweight, age, exercise, metabolic diseases such as diabetes, and lifestyle choices including smoking and alcohol consumption. From birth to adulthood, and perhaps most importantly in the aged, bone health is essential to well-being and quality of life. Bone mineral density is a key factor linked with healthy, normal bones in adulthood. Low bone mineral density is associated with reduced strength of bones and conditions such as fractures and osteoporosis. In contrast, abnormal and excessive growth of new bone tissue on the other end of the spectrum may be just as debilitating. Heterotopic ossification, the formation of extra-skeletal bone in muscle and soft tissues, or Paget's disease characterized by large bones with irregular structure prone to fractures, bowing and deformities are examples of bone overgrowth conditions.

7.1 Smoking

While genetics account for 50–90% of bone mineral density variation in humans [88, 89], many lifestyle factors are controllable and exert a strong influence on bone health. Cigarette smoking is one of the most prevalent and preventable risk factors for osteoporosis and bone fractures and has significant adverse effects on bone healing [90, 91]. Smoking is associated with lower bone mineral density in both men and women over age 50, increased risk of fractures [92, 93], and slower rates of bone repair [94]. The mechanisms by which smoking affects bone health are poorly understood but may be related to changes in hormone status (estrogen, adrenal cortical hormones), impaired calcium absorption, reduced vitamin D availability, impaired vascularization, and/or increased free radical production [95].

7.2 Alcohol consumption

Another widespread and avoidable risk factor with negative consequences for bone health is alcohol consumption [96–98], although many epidemiological studies find minimal effects on fracture risk or bone mineral density with moderate alcohol use [99–101]. Chronic alcohol abuse or heavy binge-drinking is associated with an increased incidence of fractures from falls and delays in fracture healing [97, 102]. In rodent models, chronic alcohol administration reduced serum concentrations of the active form of vitamin D3 [103]. This finding was mitigated with vitamin D supplementation [104]. Loss of bone mineral density, trabecular volume and compressive strength were observed in a study of binge-alcohol treatment in rats [105] as well as chronic alcohol consumption [106]. Further, excessive drinking is associated with an increase in bone resorption that disrupts normal bone homeostatic turnover and leads to increases in cortical bone porosity [107, 108]. Studies to date appear to implicate alterations in bone remodeling, via increase in osteoclast activity and inhibition of osteoblast differentiation as possible mechanisms through which alcohol influences bone health [109, 110].

7.3 Diabetes

The long-term exposure to metabolic changes related to diabetes has profound effects on bone metabolism and molecular alterations in bone structure. Type 1 diabetes mellitus (T1DM) patients experience reduced cortical bone size and inadequate peak bone mass most likely attributable to suppression of osteoblast differentiation and activity. Younger patients at the time of onset were observed with greater deficits in bone accrual, bone mineral density, and compressive bone strength in the radius and tibia [111, 112]. Hip fracture risk increases 5–8% in T1DM patients compared with non-diabetic controls, despite similar measures of bone mineral density in the lumbar spine [113]. The proposed mechanisms underlying these changes include insulin deficiency, accumulation of advanced glycation end products, reduced bone deposition and turnover, inflammation, and osteocyte dysfunction [114]. Patients with type 2 diabetes mellitus (T2DM) are frequently observed with normal or even increased bone mineral density but are predisposed to fragility fractures due to increased cortical porosity, smaller cortical area, and decreased bone material strength. Serum markers of bone turnover were reduced compared with non-diabetic controls, suggesting impairment of normal bone remodeling mechanisms [115]. Another hypothesis proposes that prolonged high circulating glucose concentrations lead to advanced glycation end-products in circulation and resulting in collagen crosslinks in bone. Like bisphosphonate therapy, prolonged low bone turnover and changes in the biomechanical properties in T2DM create a more brittle bone that contributes to increased fracture risk [115, 116].

7.4 Genetics

Senescent cells show genetic alterations like telomere shortening, impaired DNA repair and damage response [117]. The up-regulation of GATA4 by DNA damage response (DDR) stimulates NF-κB and senescence-associated secretory phenotype (SASP) production [118]. The bone microenvironment in aged cells like osteoblast precursors and osteocytes develops a SASP, tissue degeneration, and enhanced expression of senescence-associated markers like p16Ink4a, p21 and p53 [119]. The expression of cytokines like IL1 also activates SASP in osteocytes of older bones. Accumulation of Poly [ADP-ribose] polymerase 1 (PARP1) in senescent cells causes bone mineralization, vasodilation triggered by DDR, and excessive extracellular matrix calcification [120]. Ataxia-telangiectasia-mutated (ATM) gene encoding for a Ser/Thr kinase is involved in DNA repair of double-strand break and its inactivation causes short telomeres, decreased bone formation, and defective osteoblasts with enhanced bone resorption [121]. Xeroderma pigmentosum-type D (XPD) gene is found to be crucial for DNA repair and its alteration causes osteoporosis and kyphosis [122]. Mutation in autophagy-related 7 (ATG7) gene, a key component of autophagy can lead to bone loss. Mutations in the mtDNA polymerase gamma (Polg), the DNA polymerase in mitochondria causes osteoporosis with reduced osteogenesis and increased osteoclastogenesis [123].

7.5 Obesity

Obesity is defined at a body mass index ≥ 30 kg/m^2 with excessive body fat and has increasingly been affecting global health. Specifically, obesity has been shown to result in higher blood loss during lumbar fusion procedures, longer hospital stay, greater complication rates, and worse functional outcomes compared to nonobese patients [124]. While various factors such as environment, metabolism, genetics, and behavior interplay in the onset and development of obesity, the imbalance between high food intake and low energy expenditure ultimately lead to the accumulation of excessive body fat. Proinflammatory factors such as TNF-a, IL1b, IL6, resistin, and leptin has been shown to upregulate in the adipose tissue, resulting in their release to the bloodstream and a systemic low-grade inflammatory state in other organs including the skeletal system [125]. In addition, hyperlipidemia decreases the osteogenic capability of bone precursors, potentially due to the disturbance in the balance between adipogenesis and osteogenesis toward adipogenesis [126]. Obese patients show a significantly lower lumbar fusion rate as well as a series of post-operative complications compared to nonobese patients [127]. As with patients with other risk factors as described above, a more advanced approach may be needed for successful bone repair and regeneration, which includes appropriate cells, microenvironment, and biological signals.

8. Bone regeneration technologies

Bone regeneration technologies and approaches aims at repairing or replacing damaged or lost bone tissue. These technologies can help restore the structure, function, and integrity of bones affected by trauma, disease, or congenital abnormalities. A comprehensive approach to an efficient bone repair and regeneration may include stem and progenitor cells (exogenous, endogenous), proper microenvironment (collagen, proteoglycan), and signals (growth factors) (**Figure 5**).

8.1 Cell-based approaches

Cell-based bone regeneration technologies involve the use of living cells to repair and regenerate damaged or lost bone tissue. These approaches aim to overcome the

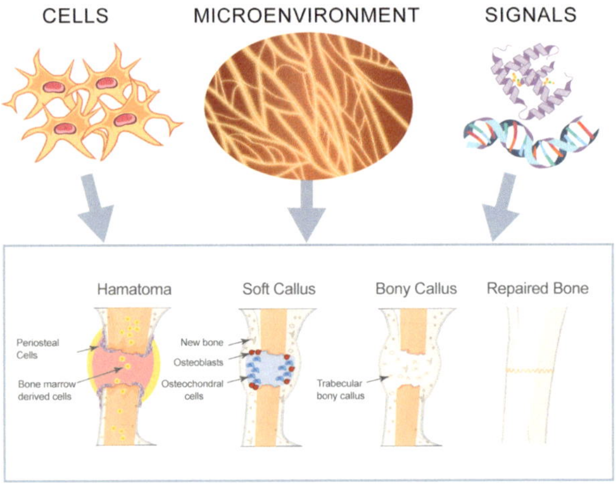

Figure 5.
Stages of bone repair and regeneration. 1. Hematoma formation: The broken blood vessels and hemorrhage at the break site result in the formation of a hematoma or clotted blood. 2. The soft callus formation: Phagocytic cells invade the hematoma, and clear the dead cells. Fibroblasts and osteoblasts also invade the region and initiate the bone reformation process. Fibroblasts synthesize collagen fibers whereas osteoblasts form the spongy bone. The resultant repaired tissue (between the broken bone ends) is known as the soft or fibrocartilaginous callus. 3. Bony callus formation: The soft callus is converted into a bony callus of spongy bone. This process is similar to the endochondral ossification of bone. 4. Repaired bone: The osteoblasts and osteoclasts then carry out bone remodeling to convert the bony callus to create bone tissue similar to the original bone. The entire bone repair process is influenced by the infiltration of the bone cells (osteoblast and osteoclast), the microenvironment of the bone, and the availability of external signals (mediated by growth factors and cytokines).

limitations of traditional bone grafting techniques by harnessing the regenerative potential of cells. Cell-based bone regeneration technologies utilize a variety of cells, including mesenchymal stem cells (MSCs) [128, 129], osteoprogenitors [130], induced pluripotent stem cells (iPSCs) [131, 132], endothelial progenitor cells (EPCs), and periosteal cells [133], to facilitate the regeneration and repair of bone tissue. MSCs, derived from sources like bone marrow or adipose tissue, can differentiate into bone-forming cells and secrete regenerative molecules. Stem cells are classically defined as cells that can self-renew and differentiate into multiple cellular lineages. Osteoprogenitors, found in the bone marrow, contribute to bone formation and repair. iPSCs, generated by reprogramming adult cells, can differentiate into osteoblasts. EPCs promote vascularization, while periosteal cells, obtained from the outer bone layer, possess regenerative potential and can differentiate into various bone-related cell types. Collectively, these cells offer promising approaches for advancing cell-based bone regeneration if challenges in delivery and retention of cells can be overcome.

However, it is important to note that a typical cell population cultured in a laboratory may contain different cell types, which can significantly confound the identification of "true" stem cells. For example, only about 7% of cells in a typical MSC culture possess the stem cell-like characteristics at a clonal level, suggesting 93% of cells in a typical MSC culture are not stem/progenitor cells [134]. Interestingly, there has been no stem cell-based treatment modality approved by the U.S. FDA for the repair and regeneration of damaged bone. While MSCs may need further identification and characterization to obtain a cell population that can provide a better clinical outcome, it is feasible to postulate that stem and progenitor cells may need a niche resembling the environment of early bone development. MSCs, for example, may not differentiate into functional bone without going through the developmental stages (intramembranous or endochondral ossification) through mesenchymal condensation in a properly formulated microenvironment as discussed above. This may be particularly true as MSCs have been known to be very responsive to their microenvironment [135].

8.2 Microenvironment-based technologies

Microenvironment-based bone regeneration technologies utilize a range of materials, including hydroxyapatite/calcium phosphate, polymers, ceramics, bioglasses, metals, and composites, to create an ideal environment for bone regeneration. Hydroxyapatite and calcium phosphate mimic the structure of natural bone mineral and support osteogenesis. Polymers like poly(lactic-co-glycolic acid) (PLGA) and polycaprolactone (PCL) provide biocompatible scaffolds that mimic the extracellular matrix and promote cell growth. Ceramics such as calcium phosphate ceramics offer excellent biocompatibility and act as bone substitutes. Bioglasses stimulate bone regeneration by releasing bioactive ions. Metals like titanium and its alloys provide mechanical support and can be modified to enhance bioactivity. Composites combine different materials to optimize properties. These microenvironment-based approaches, in the form of scaffolds, coatings, or fillers, aim to enhance bone regeneration and restore function in patients with bone defects or injuries.

In a therapeutic context, the condition of the implant site can have a significant impact on the fate of transplanted stem and progenitor cells [136]. Factors such as cytokines, growth factors, endogenous cells, enzymes, and mechanical stimuli play a role in maintaining the balance between anabolic and catabolic processes in a healthy intervertebral disc. However, a degenerating disc characterized by decreased proteoglycans and collagen II, increased proteinases and cytokines, and decreased pH can create an unfavorable microenvironment for stem cells used in therapy [136]. The success of interbody fusion surgeries, such as anterior cervical discectomy and fusion (ACDF) or lumbar spine fusion procedures, depends on a favorable microenvironment at the disc [135]. If fusion fails, patients may experience persistent or new pain, and the implanted devices may fail, necessitating additional surgeries. The microenvironment in posterolateral fusion in the lumbar spine can pose even more challenges to successful fusion [135]. Autologous bone grafting, where bone is harvested from a non-load bearing site like the iliac crest, is considered the gold standard for bone repair due to the presence of both stem cells and their native microenvironment [135]. However, this approach has limitations and risks, including donor site morbidity, fracture, infection, increased blood loss, prolonged operative time, and nerve damage. As a result, bone graft substitutes have gained popularity as alternatives to autografts. These substitutes, which include allografts, ceramics, polymers, and biologics, have shown potential in bone regeneration [135].

Corticocancellous allograft and demineralized bone matrix (DBM) are examples of allograft-based bone graft substitutes that have osteoconductive and osteoinductive properties [137]. DBM, in particular, provides a scaffold for bone stem and progenitor cells and has been shown to upregulate osteogenic genes and mineralization [137]. Mechanical stress, vascularity, and surface characteristics of graft materials can influence the microenvironment and stimuli experienced by mesenchymal stem cells (MSCs) and affect their osteogenic differentiation [138]. Ceramic-based substitutes like hydroxyapatite (HA) and β-tricalcium phosphate (β-TCP) have demonstrated varying degrees of ectopic bone formation and cell attachment [139]. Surface modifications and coating can improve the compatibility and performance of calcium phosphate ceramics [140]. Synthetic substitutes such as poly-l-lactic acid (PLLA), polyglycolic acid (PGA), and PLGA have shown compatibility with MSCs but may degrade too quickly to bridge critical-sized bone defects [141, 142]. Polysaccharide-based materials, including cellulose, alginate, chitosan, and glycosaminoglycans, have been investigated for bone regeneration and have shown promise as scaffolds for tissue engineering [143–146]. Recent studies have highlighted the potential of carbohydrate-based polymers including the hyper-crosslinked carbohydrate polymer in enhancing bone formation (**Figure 6**) [147, 148]. While bone graft substitutes aim to create an conducive environment for bone regeneration, they may not be sufficient for high-risk patient populations, such as those with diabetes, who have shown lower rates of bone regeneration [149, 150]. Additional therapeutic approaches and considerations such as inclusion of growth factors and cell-based approaches are necessary to address the microenvironmental challenges in these cases.

8.3 Signal-based technologies

Signals, such as growth factors, can also be used to stimulate bone regeneration. Growth factors are proteins that promote the growth, division, and differentiation of cells. Growth factors can be delivered to the site of injury using a variety of methods, including injections, gels, and membranes. Infuse™ Bone Graft (Medtronic, Minneapolis, MN) is a bone regeneration technology that utilizes the bone morphogenetic protein-2 (BMP-2) signal to stimulate bone healing. This technique involves implanting a collagen sponge soaked with recombinant human BMP-2 into the site of bone defect or fracture. The advantage of this approach includes enhanced bone healing, minimally invasive delivery, elimination of autograft harvesting, reduced pain and morbidity. However, there are also cons to consider, such as potential side effects

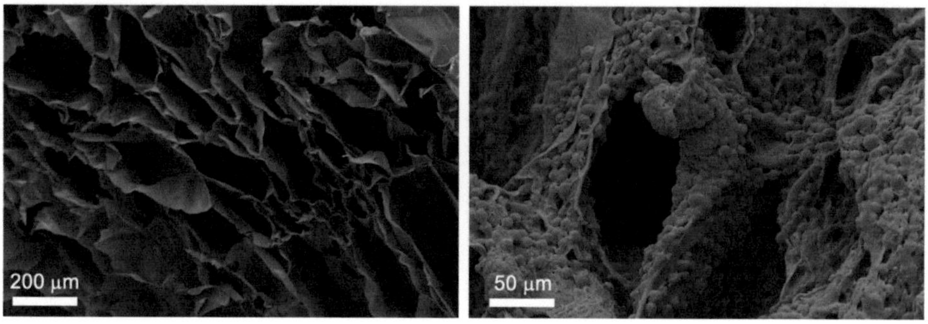

Figure 6.
Carbohydrate-based microenvironment. The hyper-crosslinked carbohydrate polymer (HCCP) scaffold is characterized by high-density, interconnected pores with extraordinary surface area for cell adhesion and space for nutrient transfer (left panel, SEM image, scale bar = 200 µm). Mesenchymal stem cells (MSC) and CD34+ hematopoietic cells show exceptional adherence to HCCP. Biocompatibility is demonstrated via normal cellular growth, migration, and expansion patterns (left panel, SEM image, scale bar = 50 µm).

like excessive bone growth and inflammation, concerns with off-label use, higher cost compared to traditional grafting, and the need for more long-term safety data. Careful evaluation by medical professionals is necessary to weigh the benefits and risks to ensure its appropriate use in clinical practice. Augment Bone Graft (Wright Medical Technology, Inc) employs recombinant human PDGF-BB with a β-tricalcium phosphate carrier to improve healing in ankle and foot fusion surgeries [151, 152]. Approved by the FDA since 2015, this product is also in use in dental and neuropathic ulceration applications. In a sheep model, Augment Bone Graft was comparable with autograft bone for promoting spinal fusion suggesting this combination may be a viable alternative in the clinical setting [153].

9. Conclusion

Bone development, growth, and maturation are complex processes dependent on progenitor cells, hormones, and growth factors. Under normal physiological conditions, peak bone mass is achieved in early adulthood. Thereafter, bone homeostasis is maintained through a balance of resorption and deposition that is influenced by many environmental factors including nutrition, age, disease status, drinking, and smoking, to name a few. Loss of bone mineral density begins about menopause in women, several decades earlier than men, but continues throughout the aging process in both sexes. Bone fragility in the elderly is most likely due to a physiological shift in favor of bone resorption activity creating less bone density, as well as reduced activity of the progenitor cell populations. Bone regeneration technologies are still in their early stages of development but have the potential to revolutionize the way we treat bone diseases and injuries. New technologies patterned using cues from embryonic bone development may provide patients with new and improved options for bone repair and regeneration.

Conflict of interest

Charles Lee is an inventor of the hyper-crosslinked carbohydrate polymer discussed in this chapter and founder of Molecular Matrix, Inc.

Author details

Kee D. Kim[1] and Charles C. Lee[2]*

1 Department of Neurological Surgery, School of Medicine, University of California, Davis, CA, USA

2 Department of Cell Biology and Human Anatomy, School of Medicine, University of California, Davis, CA, USA

*Address all correspondence to: cglee@ucdavis.edu

References

[1] Nauth A, Schemitsch E, Norris B, Nollin Z, Watson JT. Critical-size bone defects: Is there a consensus for diagnosis and treatment? Journal of Ortopaedic Trauma. 2018;**32**(Suppl. 1):S7-S11

[2] Long F, Ornitz DM. Development of the endochondral skeleton. Cold Springer Harbour Perspectives Biology. 2013;**5**(1):a008334

[3] Giffin JL, Gaitor D, Franz-Odendaal TA. The forgotten Skeletogenic condensations: A comparison of early skeletal development amongst vertebrates. Journal of Developmental Biology. 2019;**7**(1):4

[4] Hall BK, Tremaine R. Ability of neural crest cells from the embryonic chick to differentiate into cartilage before their migration away from the neural tube. The Anatomical Record. 1979;**194**(3):469-475

[5] Dunlop LL, Hall BK. Relationships between cellular condensation, preosteoblast formation and epithelial-mesenchymal interactions in initiation of osteogenesis. The International Journal of Developmental Biology. 1995;**39**(2):357-371

[6] Hall BK. Tissue interactions and the initiation of osteogenesis and chondrogenesis in the neural crest-derived mandibular skeleton of the embryonic mouse as seen in isolated murine tissues and in recombinations of murine and avian tissues. Journal of Embryology and Experimental Morphology. 1980;**58**:251-264

[7] Huang W, Yang S, Shao J, Li YP. Signaling and transcriptional regulation in osteoblast commitment and differentiation. Frontiers in Bioscience. 2007;**12**:3068-3092

[8] Ducy P, Zhang R, Geoffroy V, Ridall AL, Karsenty G. Osf2/Cbfa1: A transcriptional activator of osteoblast differentiation. Cell. 1997;**89**(5):747-754

[9] Lin X, Patil S, Gao YG, Qian A. The bone extracellular matrix in bone formation and regeneration. Frontiers in Pharmacology. 2020;**11**:757

[10] Breeland G, Sinkler MA, Menezes RG. Embryology, Bone Ossification. Treasure Island, FL: StatPearls Publishing; 2023. Available from: http://www.ncbi.nlm.nih.gov/books/NBK539718/

[11] Alberton P, Popov C, Prägert M, Kohler J, Shukunami C, Schieker M, et al. Conversion of human bone marrow-derived mesenchymal stem cells into tendon progenitor cells by ectopic expression of scleraxis. Stem Cells and Development. 2012;**21**(6):846-858

[12] Wallin J, Wilting J, Koseki H, Fritsch R, Christ B, Balling R. The role of Pax-1 in axial skeleton development. Development. 1994;**120**(5):1109-1121

[13] Tavella S, Raffo P, Tacchetti C, Cancedda R, Castagnola P. N-CAM and N-cadherin expression during in vitro chondrogenesis. Experimental Cell Research. 1994;**215**(2):354-362

[14] Wilson R, Norris EL, Brachvogel B, Angelucci C, Zivkovic S, Gordon L, et al. Changes in the chondrocyte and extracellular matrix proteome during post-natal mouse cartilage development. Molecular & Cellular Proteomics. 2012;**11**(1):M111

[15] Yang L, Tsang KY, Tang HC, Chan D, Cheah KSE. Hypertrophic chondrocytes can become osteoblasts and osteocytes in endochondral bone formation. Proceedings of the National Academy of Sciences of the United States of America. 2014;**111**(33):12097-12102

[16] Karimian E, Chagin AS, Sävendahl L. Genetic regulation of the growth plate. Frontiers in Endocrinology (Lausanne). 2011;**2**:113

[17] Ricard-Blum S. The collagen family. Cold Spring Harbor Perspectives in Biology. 2011;**3**(1):a004978

[18] Galea GL, Zein MR, Allen S, Francis-West P. Making and shaping endochondral and intramembranous bones. Developmental Dynamics. 2021;**250**(3):414-449

[19] Nah HD, Pacifici M, Gerstenfeld LC, Adams SL, Kirsch T. Transient chondrogenic phase in the intramembranous pathway during normal skeletal development. Journal of Bone and Mineral Research. 2000;**15**(3):522-533

[20] Kulyk WM, Coelho CN, Kosher RA. Type IX collagen gene expression during limb cartilage differentiation. Matrix. 1991;**11**(4):282-288

[21] Kielty CM, Grant ME. The collagen family: Structure, assembly, and Organization in the Extracellular Matrix. In: Royce PM, Steinmann B, editors. Connective Tissue and its Heritable Disorders [Internet]. Hoboken, NJ, USA: John Wiley & Sons, Inc.; 2002. pp. 159-221. DOI: 10.1002/0471221929.ch2

[22] Ylönen R, Kyrönlahti T, Sund M, Ilves M, Lehenkari P, Tuukkanen J, et al. Type XIII collagen strongly affects bone formation in transgenic mice. Journal of Bone and Mineral Research. 2005;**20**(8):1381-1393

[23] Plumb DA, Dhir V, Mironov A, Ferrara L, Poulsom R, Kadler KE, et al. Collagen XXVII is developmentally regulated and forms thin fibrillar structures distinct from those of classical vertebrate fibrillar collagens. The Journal of Biological Chemistry. 2007;**282**(17):12791-12795

[24] Gaudreault P, Beland M, Girodias JB, Thivierge RL. Single daily doses of trimethoprim/sulphadiazine for three or 10 days in urinary tract infections. Acta Paediatrica. 1992;**81**(9):695-697

[25] Hynes RO, Naba A. Overview of the matrisome: An inventory of extracellular matrix constituents and functions. Cold Spring Harbor Perspectives in Biology. 2012;**1**(1):a004903

[26] Poole AR, Pidoux I, Rosenberg L. Role of proteoglycans in endochondral ossification: Immunofluorescent localization of link protein and proteoglycan monomer in bovine fetal epiphyseal growth plate. The Journal of Cell Biology. 1982;**92**(2):249-260

[27] Fisher LW, Termine JD, Dejter SW, Whitson SW, Yanagishita M, Kimura JH, et al. Proteoglycans of developing bone. The Journal of Biological Chemistry. 1983;**258**(10):6588-6594

[28] Settembre C, Arteaga-Solis E, McKee MD, de Pablo R, Al Awqati Q, Ballabio A, et al. Proteoglycan desulfation determines the efficiency of chondrocyte autophagy and the extent of FGF signaling during endochondral ossification. Genes & Development. 2008;**22**(19):2645-2650

[29] Simonet WS, Lacey DL, Dunstan CR, Kelley M, Chang MS, Lüthy R, et al. Osteoprotegerin:

A novel secreted protein involved in the regulation of bone density. Cell. 1997;**89**(2):309-319

[30] Hayes AJ, Farrugia BL, Biose IJ, Bix GJ, Melrose J. Perlecan, a multi-functional, cell-instructive, matrix-stabilizing proteoglycan with roles in tissue development has relevance to connective tissue repair and regeneration. Frontiers in Cell and Development Biology. 2022;**10**:856261

[31] Ida-Yonemochi H, Morita W, Sugiura N, Kawakami R, Morioka Y, Takeuchi Y, et al. Craniofacial abnormality with skeletal dysplasia in mice lacking chondroitin sulfate N-acetylgalactosaminyltransferase-1. Scientific Reports. 2018;**8**(1):17134

[32] Sarrazin S, Lamanna WC, Esko JD. Heparan sulfate proteoglycans. Cold Springer Harbor Perspective Biology. 2011;**3**(7):a004952

[33] Han B, Li Q, Wang C, Patel P, Adams SM, Doyran B, et al. Decorin regulates the Aggrecan network integrity and biomechanical functions of cartilage extracellular matrix. ACS Nano. 2019;**13**(10):11320-11333

[34] Wang RN, Green J, Wang Z, Deng Y, Qiao M, Peabody M, et al. Bone morphogenetic protein (BMP) signaling in development and human diseases. Genes Diseases. 2014;**1**(1):87-105

[35] Halloran D, Durbano HW, Nohe A. Bone morphogenetic Protein-2 in development and bone homeostasis. Journal of Developmental Biology. 2020;**8**(3):19

[36] Chen D, Harris MA, Rossini G, Dunstan CR, Dallas SL, Feng JQ, et al. Bone morphogenetic protein 2 (BMP-2) enhances BMP-3, BMP-4, and bone cell differentiation marker gene expression during the induction of mineralized bone matrix formation in cultures of fetal rat calvarial osteoblasts. Calcified Tissue International. 1997;**60**(3):283-290

[37] Date T, Doiguchi Y, Nobuta M, Shindo H. Bone morphogenetic protein-2 induces differentiation of multipotent C3H10T1/2 cells into osteoblasts, chondrocytes, and adipocytes in vivo and in vitro. Journal of Orthopaedic Science. 2004;**9**(5):503-508

[38] Chen D, Zhao M, Mundy GR. Bone morphogenetic proteins. Growth Factors. 2004;**22**(4):233-241

[39] Ingwersen LC, Frank M, Naujokat H, Loger K, Bader R, Jonitz-Heincke A. BMP-2 long-term stimulation of human pre-osteoblasts induces osteogenic differentiation and promotes Transdifferentiation and bone Remodeling processes. International Journal of Molecular Sciences. 2022;**23**(6):3077

[40] Sykaras N, Opperman LA. Bone morphogenetic proteins (BMPs): How do they function and what can they offer the clinician? Journal of Oral Science. 2003;**45**(2):57-73

[41] Chen G, Xu H, Yao Y, Xu T, Yuan M, Zhang X, et al. BMP Signaling in the development and regeneration of cranium bones and maintenance of Calvarial stem cells. Frontiers in Cell and Development Biology. 2020;**8**:135

[42] Ornitz DM, Marie PJ. Fibroblast growth factor signaling in skeletal development and disease. Genes & Development. 2015;**29**(14):1463-1486

[43] Beenken A, Mohammadi M. The FGF family: Biology, pathophysiology and therapy. Nature Reviews. Drug Discovery. 2009;**8**(3):235-253

[44] Mohammadi M, Olsen SK, Ibrahimi OA. Structural basis for fibroblast growth factor receptor activation. Cytokine & Growth Factor Reviews. 2005;**16**(2):107-137

[45] Wu ZL, Zhang L, Yabe T, Kuberan B, Beeler DL, Love A, et al. The involvement of heparan sulfate (HS) in FGF1/HS/FGFR1 signaling complex. The Journal of Biological Chemistry. 2003;**278**(19):17121-17129

[46] Kimura I, Pancho LR, Isoi Y, Kimura M. Diabetes-induced enhancement of prostanoid-stimulated contraction in mesenteric veins of mice. Japanese Journal of Pharmacology. 1989;**51**(3):403-410

[47] Peters KG, Werner S, Chen G, Williams LT. Two FGF receptor genes are differentially expressed in epithelial and mesenchymal tissues during limb formation and organogenesis in the mouse. Development. 1992;**114**(1):233-243

[48] Jacob AL, Smith C, Partanen J, Ornitz DM. Fibroblast growth factor receptor 1 signaling in the osteo-chondrogenic cell lineage regulates sequential steps of osteoblast maturation. Developmental Biology. 2006;**296**(2):315-328

[49] Ornitz DM, Marie PJ. FGF signaling pathways in endochondral and intramembranous bone development and human genetic disease. Genes & Development. 2002;**16**(12):1446-1465

[50] Eswarakumar VP, Monsonego-Ornan E, Pines M, Antonopoulou I, Morriss-Kay GM, Lonai P. The IIIc alternative of Fgfr2 is a positive regulator of bone formation. Development. 2002;**129**(16):3783-3793

[51] Reinhold MI, Naski MC. Direct interactions of Runx2 and canonical Wnt signaling induce FGF18. The Journal of Biological Chemistry. 2007;**282**(6):3653-3663

[52] Ornitz DM, Itoh N. The fibroblast growth factor signaling pathway. Wiley Interdisciplinary Reviews: Developmental Biology. 2015;**4**(3):215-266

[53] Vajo Z, Francomano CA, Wilkin DJ. The molecular and genetic basis of fibroblast growth factor receptor 3 disorders: The achondroplasia family of skeletal dysplasias, Muenke craniosynostosis, and Crouzon syndrome with acanthosis nigricans. Endocrine Reviews. 2000;**21**(1):23-39

[54] Holmes G, Rothschild G, Roy UB, Deng CX, Mansukhani A, Basilico C. Early onset of craniosynostosis in an Apert mouse model reveals critical features of this pathology. Developmental Biology. 2009;**328**(2):273-284

[55] Kawai M, Rosen CJ. The insulin-like growth factor system in bone: basic and clinical implications. Endocrinology Metabolic Clinical North America. 2012;**41**(2):323-333

[56] Dixit M, Poudel SB, Yakar S. Effects of GH/IGF axis on bone and cartilage. Molecular and Cellular Endocrinology. 2021;**519**:111052

[57] Locatelli V, Bianchi VE. Effect of GH/IGF-1 on bone metabolism and Osteoporsosis. International Journal of Endocrinology. 2014;**2014**:235060

[58] Kawane T, Qin X, Jiang Q, Miyazaki T, Komori H, Yoshida CA, et al. Runx2 is required for the proliferation of osteoblast progenitors and induces proliferation by regulating Fgfr2 and Fgfr3. Scientific Reports. 2018;**8**(1):13551

[59] Kim WJ, Shin HL, Kim BS, Kim HJ, Ryoo HM. RUNX2-modifying enzymes: Therapeutic targets for bone diseases. Experimental & Molecular Medicine. 2020;**52**(8):1178-1184

[60] Liu Q, Li M, Wang S, Xiao Z, Xiong Y, Wang G. Recent advances of Osterix transcription factor in osteoblast differentiation and bone formation. Frontiers in Cell and Development Biology. 2020;**8**:601224

[61] Balamurugan K, Koehler L, Dürig JN, Hempel U, Rademann J, Hintze V, et al. Structural insights into the modulation of PDGF/PDGFR-β complexation by hyaluronan derivatives. Biological Chemistry. 2021;**402**(11):1441-1452

[62] Novak S, Madunic J, Shum L, Vucetic M, Wang X, Tanigawa H, et al. PDGF inhibits BMP2-induced bone healing. NPJ. Regenerative Medicine. 2023;**8**(1):3

[63] Caplan AI, Correa D. PDGF in bone formation and regeneration: New insights into a novel mechanism involving MSCs. Journal of Orthopaedic Research. 2011;**29**(12):1795-1803

[64] Li A, Xia X, Yeh J, Kua H, Liu H, Mishina Y, et al. PDGF-AA promotes osteogenic differentiation and migration of mesenchymal stem cell by down-regulating PDGFRα and derepressing BMP-Smad1/5/8 signaling. PLoS One. 2014;**9**(12):e113785

[65] Vordemvenne T, Paletta JRJ, Hartensuer R, Pap T, Raschke MJ, Ochman S. Cooperative effects in differentiation and proliferation between PDGF-BB and matrix derived synthetic peptides in human osteoblasts. BMC Musculoskeletal Disorders. 2011;**12**:263

[66] Kovacs CS. Bone development in the fetus and neonate: Role of the calciotropic hormones. Current Osteoporosis Reports. 2011;**9**(4):274-283

[67] Kovacs CS. Bone development and mineral homeostasis in the fetus and neonate: Roles of the calciotropic and phosphotropic hormones. Physiological Reviews. 2014;**94**(4):1143-1218

[68] Florencio-Silva R, da Sasso GR, Sasso-Cerri E, Simões MJ, Cerri PS. Biology of bone tissue: Structure, function, and factors that influence bone cells. BioMed Research International. 2015;**2015**:421746

[69] Viljakainen HT, Korhonen T, Hytinantti T, Laitinen EKA, Andersson S, Mäkitie O, et al. Maternal vitamin D status affects bone growth in early childhood—A prospective cohort study. Osteoporosis International. 2011;**22**(3):883-891

[70] Zhang R, Lu Y, Ye L, Yuan B, Yu S, Qin C, et al. Unique roles of phosphorus in endochondral bone formation and osteocyte maturation. Journal of Bone and Mineral Research. 2011;**26**(5):1047-1056

[71] Katagiri T, Takahashi N. Regulatory mechanisms of osteoblast and osteoclast differentiation. Oral Diseases. 2002;**8**(3):147-159

[72] Seeman E. Bone modeling and remodeling. Critical Reviews in Eukaryotic Gene Expression. 2009;**19**(3):219-233

[73] Szulc P, Seeman E, Duboeuf F, Sornay-Rendu E, Delmas PD. Bone fragility: Failure of periosteal apposition to compensate for increased endocortical resorption in postmenopausal women. Journal of Bone and Mineral Research. 2006;**21**(12):1856-1863

[74] Burr DB, Allen MR, editors. Basic and Applied Bone Biology. Amsterdam: Elsevier/Academic Press; 2013. p. 373

[75] Kirmani S, Christen D, van Lenthe GH, Fischer PR, Bouxsein ML, McCready LK, et al. Bone structure at the distal radius during adolescent growth. Journal of Bone and Mineral Research. 2009;**24**(6):1033-1042

[76] Farr JN, Khosla S. Skeletal changes through the lifespan—From growth to senescence. Nature Reviews. Endocrinology. 2015;**11**(9):513-521

[77] Lu J, Shin Y, Yen MS, Sun SS. Peak bone mass and patterns of change in Total bone mineral density and bone mineral contents from childhood into young adulthood. Journal of Clinical Densitometry. 2016;**19**(2):180-191

[78] Hernandez CJ, Beaupré GS, Carter DR. A theoretical analysis of the relative influences of peak BMD, age-related bone loss and menopause on the development of osteoporosis. Osteoporosis International. 2003;**14**(10):843-847

[79] Rizzoli R, Bianchi ML, Garabédian M, McKay HA, Moreno LA. Maximizing bone mineral mass gain during growth for the prevention of fractures in the adolescents and the elderly. Bone. 2010;**46**(2):294-305

[80] Riggs BL, Melton LJ, Robb RA, Camp JJ, Atkinson EJ, McDaniel L, et al. A population-based assessment of rates of bone loss at multiple skeletal sites: Evidence for substantial trabecular bone loss in young adult women and men. Journal of Bone and Mineral Research. 2008;**23**(2):205-214

[81] Riggs BL, Melton Iii LJ, Robb RA, Camp JJ, Atkinson EJ, Peterson JM, et al. Population-based study of age and sex differences in bone volumetric density, size, geometry, and structure at different skeletal sites. Journal of Bone and Mineral Research. 2004;**19**(12):1945-1954

[82] Zebaze RMD, Ghasem-Zadeh A, Bohte A, Iuliano-Burns S, Mirams M, Price RI, et al. Intracortical remodelling and porosity in the distal radius and post-mortem femurs of women: A cross-sectional study. Lancet. 2010;**375**(9727):1729-1736

[83] Nicks KM, Amin S, Atkinson EJ, Riggs BL, Melton LJ, Khosla S. Relationship of age to bone microstructure independent of areal bone mineral density. Journal of Bone and Mineral Research. 2012;**27**(3):637-644

[84] Riggs BL, Khosla S, Melton LJ. Sex steroids and the construction and conservation of the adult skeleton. Endocrine Reviews. 2002;**23**(3):279-302

[85] Clarke BL, Khosla S. Physiology of bone loss. Radiologic Clinics of North America. 2010;**48**(3):483-495

[86] Farr JN, Xu M, Weivoda MM, Monroe DG, Fraser DG, Onken JL, et al. Targeting cellular senescence prevents age-related bone loss in mice. Nature Medicine. 2017;**23**(9):1072-1079

[87] Khosla S, Farr JN, Kirkland JL. Inhibiting cellular senescence: A new therapeutic paradigm for age-related osteoporosis. The Journal of Clinical Endocrinology and Metabolism. 2018;**103**(4):1282-1290

[88] Eisman JA. Genetics of osteoporosis. Endocrine Reviews. 1999;**20**(6):788-804

[89] Ralston SH, de Crombrugghe B. Genetic regulation of bone mass and

susceptibility to osteoporosis. Genes & Development. 2006;**20**(18):2492-2506

[90] Hernigou J, Schuind F. Tobacco and bone fractures: A review of the facts and issues that every orthopaedic surgeon should know. Bone and Joint Research. 2019;**8**(6):255-265

[91] Niu S, Lim F. CE: The effects of smoking on bone health and healing. The American Journal of Nursing. 2020;**120**(7):40-45

[92] Kanis JA, Johnell O, Oden A, Johansson H, De Laet C, Eisman JA, et al. Smoking and fracture risk: A meta-analysis. Osteoporosis International. 2005;**16**(2):155-162

[93] Scolaro JA, Schenker ML, Yannascoli S, Baldwin K, Mehta S, Ahn J. Cigarette smoking increases complications following fracture: A systematic review. The Journal of Bone and Joint Surgery. American Volume. 2014;**96**(8):674-681

[94] Wong PKK, Christie JJ, Wark JD. The effects of smoking on bone health. Clinical Science (London, England). 2007;**113**(5):233-241

[95] Al-Bashaireh AM, Haddad LG, Weaver M, Chengguo X, Kelly DL, Yoon S. The effect of tobacco smoking on bone mass: An overview of pathophysiologic mechanisms. Journal of Osteoporosis. 2018;**2018**:1206235

[96] Hannan MT, Felson DT, Dawson-Hughes B, Tucker KL, Cupples LA, Wilson PW, et al. Risk factors for longitudinal bone loss in elderly men and women: The Framingham Osteoporosis Study. Journal of Bone and Mineral Research. 2000;**15**(4):710-720

[97] Chakkalakal DA. Alcohol-induced bone loss and deficient bone repair. Alcoholism, Clinical and Experimental Research. 2005;**29**(12):2077-2090

[98] Kelsey JL. Risk factors for osteoporosis and associated fractures. Public Health Reports. 1989;**104**:14-20

[99] Williams FMK, Cherkas LF, Spector TD, MacGregor AJ. The effect of moderate alcohol consumption on bone mineral density: A study of female twins. Annals of the Rheumatic Diseases. 2005;**64**(2):309-310

[100] Hansen MA, Overgaard K, Riis BJ, Christiansen C. Potential risk factors for development of postmenopausal osteoporosis—Examined over a 12-year period. Osteoporosis International. 1991;**1**(2):95-102

[101] Yuan S, Michaëlsson K, Wan Z, Larsson SC. Associations of smoking and alcohol and coffee intake with fracture and bone mineral density: A Mendelian Randomization Study. Calcified Tissue International. 2019;**105**(6):582-588

[102] Santori C, Ceccanti M, Diacinti D, Attilia ML, Toppo L, D'Erasmo E, et al. Skeletal turnover, bone mineral density, and fractures in male chronic abusers of alcohol. Journal of Endocrinological Investigation. 2008;**31**(4):321-326

[103] Turner RT, Aloia RC, Segel LD, Hannon KS, Bell NH. Chronic alcohol treatment results in disturbed vitamin D metabolism and skeletal abnormalities in rats. Alcoholism, Clinical and Experimental Research. 1988;**12**(1):159-162

[104] Mercer KE, Wynne RA, Lazarenko OP, Lumpkin CK, Hogue WR, Suva LJ, et al. Vitamin D supplementation protects against bone loss associated with chronic alcohol administration in female mice. The Journal of Pharmacology

and Experimental Therapeutics. 2012;**343**(2):401-412

[105] Callaci JJ, Juknelis D, Patwardhan A, Wezeman FH. Binge alcohol treatment increases vertebral bone loss following ovariectomy: Compensation by intermittent parathyroid hormone. Alcoholism, Clinical and Experimental Research. 2006;**30**(4):665-672

[106] Hogan HA, Argueta F, Moe L, Nguyen LP, Sampson HW. Adult-onset alcohol consumption induces osteopenia in female rats. Alcoholism, Clinical and Experimental Research. 2001;**25**(5):746-754

[107] Turner RT, Kidder LS, Kennedy A, Evans GL, Sibonga JD. Moderatealcoholconsumptionsuppresses bone turnover in adult female rats. Journal of Bone and Mineral Research. 2001;**16**(3):589-594

[108] Díez-Ruiz A, García-Saura PL, García-Ruiz P, González-Calvin JL, Gallego-Rojo F, Fuchs D. Bone mineral density, bone turnover markers and cytokines in alcohol-induced cirrhosis. Alcohol and Alcoholism. 2010;**45**(5):427-430

[109] Luo Z, Liu Y, Liu Y, Chen H, Shi S, Liu Y. Cellular and molecular mechanisms of alcohol-induced osteopenia. Cellular and Molecular Life Sciences. 2017;**74**(24):4443-4453

[110] Eby JM, Sharieh F, Callaci JJ. Impact of alcohol on bone health, homeostasis and fracture repair. Current Pathobiological Reports. 2020;**8**(3):75-86

[111] Shah VN, Joshee P, Sippl R, Pyle L, Vigers T, Carpenter RD, et al. Type 1 diabetes onset at young age is associated with compromised bone quality. Bone. 2019;**123**:260-264

[112] Xu L, Yu J, Wang O, Hou Y, Li W, Zhang H, et al. Comparison of differences in bone microarchitecture in adult- versus juvenile-onset type 1 diabetes Asian males versus non-diabetes males: An observational cross-sectional pilot study. Endocrine. 2021;**71**(1):87-95

[113] Halper-Stromberg E, Gallo T, Champakanath A, Taki I, Rewers M, Snell-Bergeon J, et al. Bone mineral density across the lifespan in patients with type 1 diabetes. The Journal of Clinical Endocrinology and Metabolism. 2020;**105**(3):746-753

[114] Cortet B, Lucas S, Legroux-Gerot I, Penel G, Chauveau C, Paccou J. Bone disorders associated with diabetes mellitus and its treatments. Joint, Bone, Spine. 2019;**86**(3):315-320

[115] Farr JN, Drake MT, Amin S, Melton LJ, McCready LK, Khosla S. In vivo assessment of bone quality in postmenopausal women with type 2 diabetes. Journal of Bone and Mineral Research. 2014;**29**(4):787-795

[116] de Araújo IM, Moreira MLM, de Paula FJA. Diabetes and bone. Archives in Endocrinological Metabolism. 2022;**66**(5):633-641

[117] Corrado A, Cici D, Rotondo C, Maruotti N, Cantatore FP. Molecular basis of bone aging. International Journal of Molecular Sciences. 2020;**21**(10):3679

[118] Kim HN, Chang J, Shao L, Han L, Iyer S, Manolagas SC, et al. DNA damage and senescence in osteoprogenitors expressing Osx1 may cause their decrease with age. Aging Cell. 2017;**16**(4):693-703

[119] Farr JN, Fraser DG, Wang H, Jaehn K, Ogrodnik MB, Weivoda MM, et al. Identification of senescent cells in the bone microenvironment. Journal

of Bone and Mineral Research. 2016;**31**(11):1920-1929

[120] Müller KH, Hayward R, Rajan R, Whitehead M, Cobb AM, Ahmad S, et al. Poly(ADP-ribose) links the DNA damage response and biomineralization. Cell Reports. 2019;**27**(11):3124-3138

[121] Rasheed N, Wang X, Niu QT, Yeh J, Li B. Atm-deficient mice: An osteoporosis model with defective osteoblast differentiation and increased osteoclastogenesis. Human Molecular Genetics. 2006;**15**(12):1938-1948

[122] de Boer J, Andressoo JO, de Wit J, Huijmans J, Beems RB, van Steeg H, et al. Premature aging in mice deficient in DNA repair and transcription. Science. 2002;**296**(5571):1276-1279

[123] Dobson PF, Dennis EP, Hipps D, Reeve A, Laude A, Bradshaw C, et al. Mitochondrial dysfunction impairs osteogenesis, increases osteoclast activity, and accelerates age related bone loss. Scientific Reports. 2020;**10**(1):11643

[124] De la Garza-Ramos R, Bydon M, Abt NB, Sciubba DM, Wolinsky JP, Bydon A, et al. The impact of obesity on short- and long-term outcomes after lumbar fusion. Spine (Phila Pa 1976). 2015;**40**(1):56-61

[125] Forte YS, Renovato-Martins M, Barja-Fidalgo C. Cellular and molecular mechanisms associating obesity to bone loss. Cell. 2023;**12**(4):521

[126] Shapses SA, Pop LC, Wang Y. Obesity is a concern for bone health with aging. Nutrition Research. 2017;**39**:1-13

[127] Katsevman GA, Daffner SD, Brandmeir NJ, Emery SE, France JC, Sedney CL. Complexities of spine surgery in obese patient populations: A narrative review. The Spine Journal. 2020;**20**(4):501-511

[128] Nakamura A, Akahane M, Shigematsu H, Tadokoro M, Morita Y, Ohgushi H, et al. Cell sheet transplantation of cultured mesenchymal stem cells enhances bone formation in a rat nonunion model. Bone. 2010;**46**(2):418-424

[129] Hao C, Wang Y, Shao L, Liu J, Chen L, Zhao Z. Local injection of bone mesenchymal stem cells and fibrin glue promotes the repair of bone atrophic nonunion In vivo. Advances in Therapy. 2016;**33**(5):824-833

[130] Kim SJ, Shin YW, Yang KH, Kim SB, Yoo MJ, Han SK, et al. A multi-center, randomized, clinical study to compare the effect and safety of autologous cultured osteoblast(Ossron) injection to treat fractures. BMC Musculoskeletal Disorders. 2009;**10**:20

[131] Xu X, Shi D, Liu Y, Yao Y, Dai J, Xu Z, et al. In vivo repair of full-thickness cartilage defect with human iPSC-derived mesenchymal progenitor cells in a rabbit model. Experimental and Therapeutic Medicine. 2017;**14**(1):239-245

[132] Rana D, Kumar S, Webster TJ, Ramalingam M. Impact of induced pluripotent stem cells in bone repair and regeneration. Current Osteoporosis Reports. 2019;**17**(4):226-234

[133] Jeffery EC, Mann TLA, Pool JA, Zhao Z, Morrison SJ. Bone marrow and periosteal skeletal stem/progenitor cells make distinct contributions to bone maintenance and repair. Cell Stem Cell. 2022;**29**(11):1547-1561.e6

[134] Lee CCI, Christensen JE, Yoder MC, Tarantal AF. Clonal analysis and hierarchy of human bone marrow

mesenchymal stem and progenitor cells. Experimental Hematology. 2010;**38**(1):46-54

[135] Lee CC, Hirasawa N, Garcia KG, Ramanathan D, Kim KD. Stem and progenitor cell microenvironment for bone regeneration and repair. Regenerative Medicine. 2019;**14**(7):693-702

[136] Huang YC, Leung VYL, Lu WW, Luk KDK. The effects of microenvironment in mesenchymal stem cell-based regeneration of intervertebral disc. The Spine Journal. 2013;**13**(3):352-362

[137] Dozza B, Lesci IG, Duchi S, Della Bella E, Martini L, Salamanna F, et al. When size matters: Differences in demineralized bone matrix particles affect collagen structure, mesenchymal stem cell behavior, and osteogenic potential. Journal of Biomedical Materials Research. Part A. 2017;**105**(4):1019-1033

[138] Vlaikou AM, Kouroupis D, Sgourou A, Markopoulos GS, Bagli E, Markou M, et al. Mechanical stress affects methylation pattern of GNAS isoforms and osteogenic differentiation of hAT-MSCs. Biochimica Biophysica Acta Molecular Cell Research. 2017;**1864**(8):1371-1381

[139] Denry I, Kuhn LT. Design and characterization of calcium phosphate ceramic scaffolds for bone tissue engineering. Dental Materials. 2016;**32**(1):43-53

[140] Chen W, Zhou H, Weir MD, Bao C, Xu HHK. Umbilical cord stem cells released from alginate-fibrin microbeads inside macroporous and biofunctionalized calcium phosphate cement for bone regeneration. Acta Biomaterialia. 2012;**8**(6):2297-2306

[141] Holderegger C, Schmidlin PR, Weber FE, Mohn D. Preclinical in vivo performance of novel biodegradable, electrospun poly(lactic acid) and poly(lactic-co-glycolic acid) nanocomposites: A review. Materials (Basel). 2015;**8**(8):4912-4931

[142] Wu DT, Munguia-Lopez JG, Cho YW, Ma X, Song V, Zhu Z, et al. Polymeric scaffolds for dental, Oral, and craniofacial regenerative medicine. Molecules. 2021;**26**(22):7043

[143] Park S, Park J, Jo I, Cho SP, Sung D, Ryu S, et al. In situ hybridization of carbon nanotubes with bacterial cellulose for three-dimensional hybrid bioscaffolds. Biomaterials. 2015;**58**:93-102

[144] Hung BP, Naved BA, Nyberg EL, Dias M, Holmes CA, Elisseeff JH, et al. Three-dimensional printing of bone extracellular matrix for craniofacial regeneration. ACS Biomaterials Science & Engineering. 2016;**2**(10):1806-1816

[145] Levengood SL, Zhang M. Chitosan-based scaffolds for bone tissue engineering. Journal of Materials Chemistry B. 2014;**2**(21):3161-3184

[146] Mathews S, Mathew SA, Gupta PK, Bhonde R, Totey S. Glycosaminoglycans enhance osteoblast differentiation of bone marrow derived human mesenchymal stem cells. Journal of Tissue Engineering and Regenerative Medicine. 2014;**8**(2):143-152

[147] Lee SS, Fyrner T, Chen F, Álvarez Z, Sleep E, Chun DS, et al. Sulfated glycopeptide nanostructures for multipotent protein activation. Nature Nanotechnology. 2017;**12**(8):821-829

[148] Koleva PM, Keefer JH, Ayala AM, Lorenzo I, Han CE, Pham K, et al. Hyper-Crosslinked carbohydrate polymer

for repair of critical-sized bone defects. Bioresearch Open Access. 2019;**8**(1):111-120

[149] Scott RT, Hyer CF. Role of cellular allograft containing mesenchymal stem cells in high-risk foot and ankle reconstructions. The Journal of Foot and Ankle Surgery. 2013;**52**(1):32-35

[150] Camargo WA, de Vries R, van Luijk J, Hoekstra JW, Bronkhorst EM, Jansen JA, et al. Diabetes mellitus and bone regeneration: A systematic review and Meta-analysis of animal studies. Tissue Engineering. Part B, Reviews. 2017;**23**(5):471-479

[151] Daniels TR, Younger ASE, Penner MJ, Wing KJ, Le ILD, Russell IS, et al. Prospective randomized controlled trial of Hindfoot and ankle fusions treated with rhPDGF-BB in combination with a β-TCP-collagen matrix. Foot & Ankle International. 2015;**36**(7):739-748

[152] Krell ES, DiGiovanni CW. The efficacy of platelet-derived growth factor as a bone-stimulating agent. Foot and Ankle Clinics. 2016;**21**(4):763-770

[153] Gadomski BC, Labus KM, Puttlitz CM, McGilvray KC, Regan DP, Nelson B, et al. Evaluation of lumbar spinal fusion utilizing recombinant human platelet derived growth factor-B chain homodimer (rhPDGF-BB) combined with a bovine collagen/β-tricalcium phosphate (β-TCP) matrix in an ovine model. JOR Spine. 2021;**4**(3):e1166

Section 3

Spinal/Peripheral Nerve Trauma Surgery

Chapter 8

Manual Reduction, Subpedicle Approach, and Body Cages to Treat Burst Fracture

Kung-Chia Li, Yu-Chieh Hsieh, Ching-Hsiang Hsieh and Ting-Hua Liao

Abstract

Thoracolumbar (TL) burst fractures occasionally result in severe instability, acute or delayed neurological dysfunction and require surgical intervention. Burst fractures can be reduced by manual reduction first and the following surgical approaches including anterior, posterior, or both have individual advantages and limitations. Even transpedicular decompression and augmentation with the body cages and short-segment fixation (TpBA) are regarded successful, yet they are limited in their ability to decompress the contralateral spinal cord and bilateral procedures are necessary. Thus, a posterior far-lateral subpedicle approach to open the lateral vertebral cortex window, creating a tunnel to remove retropulsed bony fragments and pass body cages for full-body augmentation (SpBA) to treat burst fracture was herein reported. The characteristics of SpBA include unilateral approach, direct decompression, short operation time, and no posterior instrumentation. While adjacent disc injury and degeneration may occur in burst fractures, Li's short-term results indicate that SpBA is effective in preventing its adverse effects. This chapter describes the detailed advanced techniques and classification of the results obtained by a professional team manual reduction for post-traumatic kyphosis. The unilateral subpedicle approach with body cages and cementation without screw instrumentation rendering a minimally invasive solution for spinal burst fractures was demonstrated.

Keywords: subpedicle approach, Magerl incomplete burst fracture, thoracolumbar burst fractures, spinal trauma, manual reduction, posterior instrumentation, body cage, kyphosis, kyphosis classification

1. Introduction

Thoracolumbar (TL) burst fractures occasionally lead to severe spinal instability and even cause acute or delayed neurological dysfunction, and surgical treatments are required [1–3]. The purpose of surgical intervention is to bring about nerve decompression, reconstruction of the vertebral body, and correction of angular deformity and stability [4]. Traditionally, decompression of the spinal cord and fixation of spinal construct can be performed either by anterior, posterior, or both approaches with individual advantages and limitations [5–8]. A perfect minimally invasive approach with safe and fast procedure and leading to long-term good results and function recovery is still expected.

Transpedicular decompression and body augmentation (TpBA) with body cages combining short-segment fixation after indirect decompression by team manual reduction [9] has been reported to be a successful method to treat high-energy burst fractures or osteoporotic Kümmell's disease [10, 11]. However, transpedicle decompression is limited in its decompression of the contralateral spinal cord, and bilateral procedures are needed. In 2014, Li et al. [12] reported a new approach, that is, unilateral subpedicle window operation: through a posterior far-lateral approach, so that the lateral vertebral cortex window can be opened by pushing the cortex shell laterally and ventrally. The subpedicle cortical window then works as a tunnel to remove all retropulsed bony fragments and passing body cage for full-body augmentation (SpBA). In addition, the screw instrumentation was not needed.

The problem is that adjacent disc injury usually occurs concurrently with burst fracture [13–16], which was reported as the key mechanism for the progress in the kyphosis angle and the post-operative loss of the correction angle [17–19]. However, if the fracture of the endplate can be healed, resettlement of disc does not cause kyphosis progression [20]. The literature [21, 22] also confirmed that adjacent disc degeneration may occur in burst fractures; however, only 13% is severe and related to endplate fractures. According to the short-term results, SpBA was good in prevention of the adverse effects of adjacent disc injury [12]. However, up-to-date, the long-term results have not been reported yet.

This chapter will describe the detailed technique of team manual reduction and provide the classification of the outcome results. This chapter will also retrospectively evaluate the TpBA and SpBA outcomes based on the radiographic and clinical results of SpBA with a minimum 10-year follow-up. We hypothesized that unilateral mini-open SpBA to treat TL burst fractures is able to achieve cord decompression, vertebral reconstruction, and satisfactory long-term results as compatible or even better than TpBA, in particular with a smaller wound and a shorter operation duration.

2. Background of manual reduction

Manual reduction has been successfully applied in the correction of thoracolumbar fractures. From the biomechanical studies of cadaver burst fractures, traction force on the fractured cadaver vertebra can reduce retropulsed bony fragments in the spinal canal, restore anterior and posterior vertebral height, and the extension force is able to correct the kyphotic angles [23, 24]. Clinically, posture reduction in the thoracolumbar fractures has been considered to be safe and effective [25]. In 2003, Li et al. [26] reported a 5-member manual reduction (team-MR) for high-energy burst fracture while the patient was in prone position under general anesthesia with full muscle relaxation. The reduction rate was close to 100% in acute fracture without complications. The prone position was good for manual force control and next surgical approach. In 2004, Li et al. [27] reported team-MR for acute osteoporotic compression fracture and achieved similar results. Li's clinical series have confirmed team-MR to be safe and effective in restoring thoracolumbar vertebral fractures [9–12]. Tropiano [28] reported a reduction frame that was used to reduce the spine fracture without anesthesia. The patient was in supine position receiving cephalic axial traction and lordotic reduction with a strap under the fracture site. Then a thoracolumbar plaster cast was fabricated. The frame use is limited in non-operative acute fracture and cephalic traction force through cervical spine is poor in force quantity and direction adjustment. In 2018, Carlo et al. [29] reported a 3-member manual reduction for acute burst fracture as a technical note; in 2021, Li et al. [30] confirmed the effect of a 3-member manual reduction in acute spine fractures. However, a 3-member manual reduction is weak to correct chronic deformity following spine fracture because it cannot change the patient posture according to the deformity. In addition to acute spine fracture, even the chronic post-traumatic kyphosis was possibly reduced by team-MR by elevating the patient's shoulders if at the thoracic spine or raising the patient's lower limbs if at the low lumbar spine which may increase the extension forces to correct post-traumatic kyphosis (**Figure 1**). The success of manual reduction may prevent further operative decompression procedures or instrumentation reduction, which will decrease the necessity of open surgery in osteoporotic fractures or lessen the implant strain and bone-screw interface stress and prevent potential implant failure if open surgery is needed. In this chapter, we report our experiences of manual reduction for all spine fractures including fresh and old, high-energy and osteoporotic fractures, and ankylosing spondylosis in the past 25 years.

2.1 Techniques of team manual reduction

All the patients received manual reduction, using C-arm fluoroscopy to monitor the reduction if pre-operative MRI showed spinal cord compression and spinal angulation. Most of the patients with spinal fracture were anesthetized and put in a prone position with caution. (*For simple compression fracture, manual reduction can be done without anesthesia if patient's compliance is good.*) Prior to manual reduction, C-arm fluoroscopy was used to locate the index level. Manual reduction was done by a team (**Figure 1-A**): one anesthetist to hold the patient's head and monitor vital signs; two assistants to hold the patient's shoulders (one on each side) and to provide traction and elevation of the trunk; two assistants to hold the patient's legs (one on each side) to prevent upward motion of the body during traction; the surgeon to place his dominant hand on the apex region of the kyphotic deformity. If index level is at thoracic spine, manual reduction is begun with gentle traction and elevation of the trunk by the assistants holding the patient's shoulders, and with the surgeon's both hands gradually and simultaneously increasing the pushing force to counter the elevation force (**Figure 1-B**). If index level is

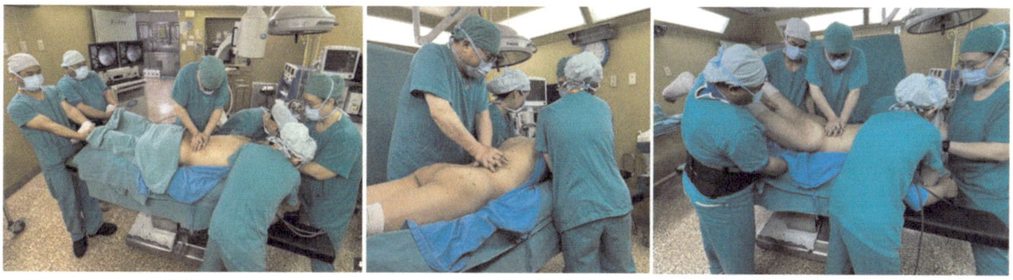

1A 1B 1C

Figure 1.
Photographically shown operation steps; A: Team manual reduction to provide traction force and lordotic force to correct the kyphosis; B: If the thoracic kyphosis is not perfectly corrected, then the advanced step will elevate the shoulder and upper trunk and compression force over the kyphosis apex region, and C: If the lumbar lordosis is not well restored, then the next step will elevate the hip and lower trunk and compression force over the deformity apex point.

at lumbar spine, manual reduction is begun with gentle traction and elevation of pelvic and lower limb by two assistants to hold the patient's hips and legs (one on each side) (**Figure 1-C**). The surgeon places both hands over the apex of kyphosis to counter the elevation force. After completion of manual reduction, C-arm fluoroscopy is repeated to check the kyphosis reduction site and exclude any possibility of cord compression. If the reduction result is unsatisfactory, manual reduction can be repeated as many times as needed. In the acute fractures, usually traction force is enough and the unfixed deformity is easily and completely reduced. In contrast, for the chronic case, the extension force is often needed and sometimes greater compression force by the surgeon is practically ensured to reduce the kyphosis, but the compression force must be well controlled so as not to exceed patient's body weight.

Manual reduction includes traction and extension forces and should be operated step by step. Especially in kyphosis >60 degrees, slow traction without extension component should be applied first, which usually initiates a bony or disc opening. This procedure may last for more than 10 s and can be repeated 2–4 times. After checking in C-arm fluoroscopy, if the reduction is not good enough, then extension force can be followed with caution. The limitation of correction at one site is not more than 50 degrees. If the results of manual reduction were not satisfactory, then osteotomy should be considered as a substitute. There is no need to insist on manual reduction alone to achieve a perfect reduction.

2.2 Results of manual reduction

Twenty hundred and thirty cases of thoracolumbar kyphotic deformities were included in this study from January 1997 to December 2022. The male-to-female ratio was approximately 680:1350, and the mean age of the patients was 65 years (range 21 to 102 years). The inclusion criteria for this study dictated patients to have symptomatic thoracolumbar kyphosis (either primary or secondary, due to diseases, 197 cases) or spinal fracture due to trauma or osteoporosis (1833 cases) who were necessitated to undergo vertebroplasty or surgical intervention.

In the reducible cases, the spinal column height could be restored, and kyphosis corrected by manual reduction. According to the results from manual reduction in thoracolumbar kyphosis, the reduction patterns have been classified as follows and are shown in **Table 1**.

Type I. Opening of the unfused deformed vertebral body and disc was achieved, where the vertebral body fracture has not healed and interbody fusion was not established and could be restored by manual reduction (**Figures 2–4**). The most acute spinal fracture is easily reduced in this mechanism.

Type II. Restoration of the disc space and successful realignment of the deformed vertebral body were achieved, corresponding to Type II kyphosis, where the vertebral body has healed with deformity, resulting in further tilting after the disc degeneration (**Figure 5**). The forces can open the narrowed disc space and correct the deformed vertebral column.

Type III. Iatrogenic open-wedge fracture was induced by the team manual reduction (**Figures 6–9**). Because the healed deformed vertebrae and solid interbody fusion had been established, the force can open neither the original body breakage nor the disc space. When the vertebra was osteoporotic enough, the manual force will create a new open-wedge fracture, either in the originally healed vertebra or in the adjacent intact vertebral body, which can result in restoration of the anterior column height and thus correct the kyphosis.

Kyphosis pattern	Kyphosis diagram	Reduction diagram	Reduction pattern	cases
Type 1: Unhealed deformed body or disc	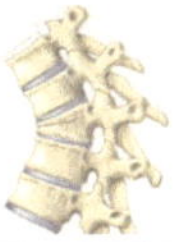	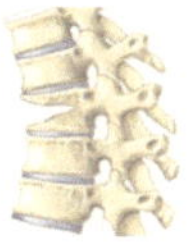	Opening and restoration of the vertebral body and disc spaces	1748 (86%)
Type II: Healed deformed body and unfused disc	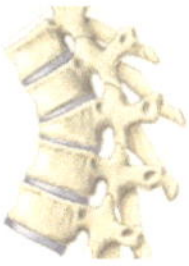	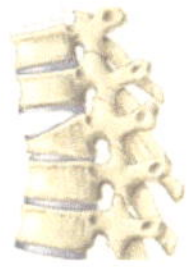	Open wedge of disc space and realignment of the tilt deformed vertebral body	21 (1%)
Type III: Fused deformed body and disc with osteoporosis	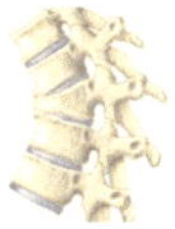	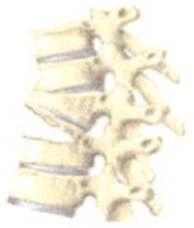	Iatrogenic open-wedge fracture of adjacent body	221 (11%)
Type IV: Fused deformed body and disc without osteoporosis	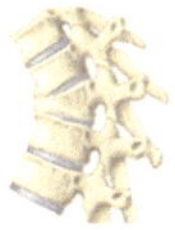		Failure of correction by manual reduction	40 (2%)

Table 1.
Classification of kyphosis based on the results of manual reduction.

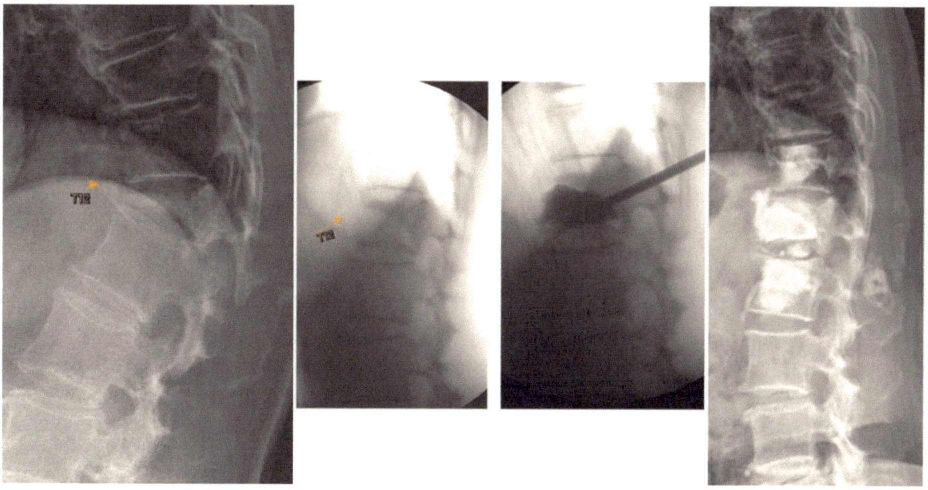

Figure 2.
Demonstrated radiographs of a 77-year-old female with T11-L1 kyphosis, T11-L1 lateral Cobb's angle pre-op: 50′; post-manual reduction: 10′; post-vertebroplasty 10′. Cement vertebroplasties (T11,12,L1) and discoplasty (T12/L1) were done due to simultaneous reduction of vertebral body and disc.

Type IV. Failure of reduction, where solid interbody fusion was found in a non-osteoporotic spine. This type is usually predictable before operation by experienced surgeons.

The new classification of thoracolumbar kyphosis is based on the results of manual reduction and functionally guides the subsequent surgeries. In Type I kyphosis, except in infection case, the vertebroplasty, cement discoplasty, or posterior body

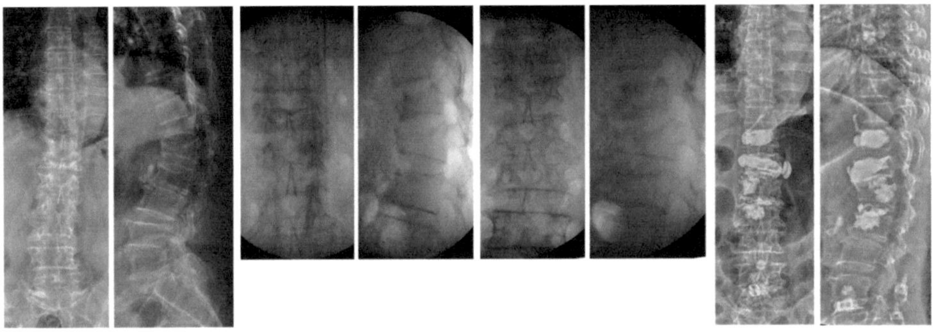

Figure 3.
Demonstrated radiographs of a 71-year-old female with T11-L2 kyphosis, T11-L2 lateral Cobb's angle pre-op: 50'; postural reduction: 34'; post-manual reduction: 19'; post-vertebroplasty 12'. Cement vertebroplasties (T11,12,L1) and discoplasty (T12/L1) were done due to simultaneous reduction of vertebral body and disc.

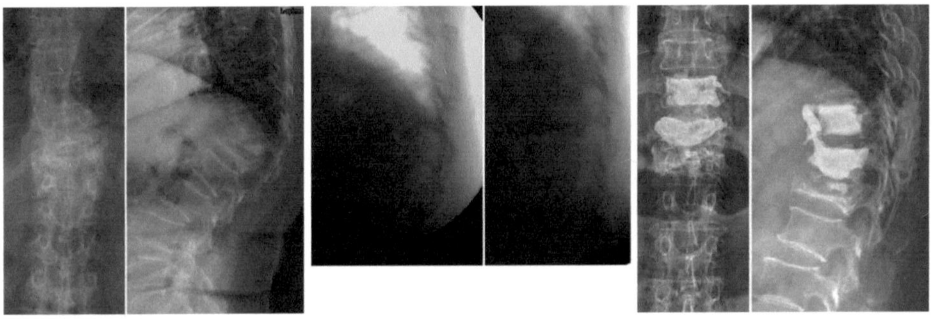

Figure 4.
Demonstrated radiographs of a 67-year-old female with T11–1 kyphosis, T11-L2 lateral Cobb's angle pre-op: 64'; posture reduction: 53'; post-manual reduction: 28'; post-vertebroplasty 27'. Cement vertebroplasties (T11 & T12) and discoplasty (T12/L1) were done due to simultaneous reduction of vertebral body and disc.

reconstruction is the major operation after manual reduction and additional posterior instrumentation is needed if spinal instability is found. In Type II kyphosis, discectomy and interbody fixation are indicated if post manual reduction takes place. In Type III kyphosis, vertebroplasty or body augmentation with body cage with/without posterior instrumentation is indicated if manual reduction succeeds (**Figure 4**). In Type IV kyphosis, open or close osteotomy and posterior fixation are suggested.

Two major complications (0.1%) of manual reduction were found in the early learning curve in 1997. Hypotension and hemothorax were noted after manual reduction in a 78-year-old female with 90^0 kyphosis (**Figure 10**) who received blood transfusion, chest tube insertion, and intensive care unit (ICU) care and finally recovered. Another complication was reflected with iatrogenic L1 pars fracture without neurological injury; this was fixed with posterior instrumentation. After 2000, there were no major complications noted in the past 20 years. The common asymptomatic complication is cement leakage due to the opening of anterior vertebral cortex (**Figure 11**). Right now, if there is open wedge of anterior cortex, the cement vertebroplasty will be divided into two stages; that is, 1 cc liquid cement was first injected to form a thin cement membrane lining on anterior longitudinal ligament and then, 5 min later when the first cement was hard enough to prevent cement leakage,

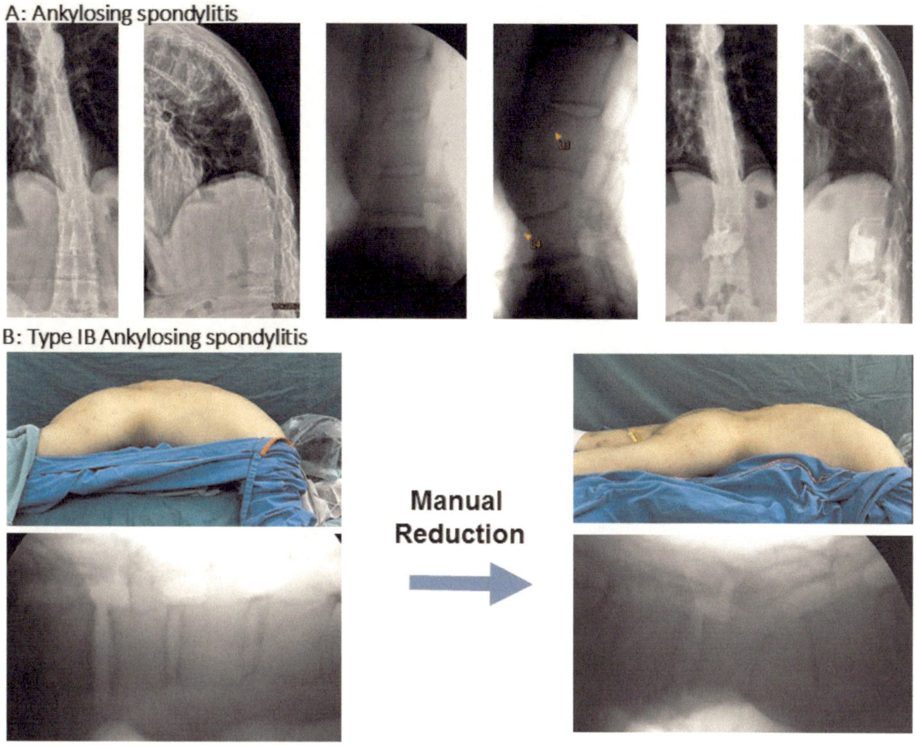

Figure 5.
Ankylosing spondylitis (A) and type 1B ankylosing spondylitis (B); 27YM, ankylosing spondylitis and kyphosis, manual reduction at the force concentrated at L3/4, inducing disc open wedge. L2/L5: Pre-op: 15′ kyphosis, posture reduction: 15′ kyphosis, post-manual reduction: 19′ lordosis; 33′ lordosis was corrected (measured at C-arm films). The interbody cementation was done.

sufficient high viscous cement was injected to fulfill the open spaces, either in vertebral body defect or in disc space.

2.3 Discussion

Based on our 25-year experiences, the manual reduction of thoracolumbar kyphosis is effective and safe. Manual reduction is commonly used in orthopedic practice to manage long bone fractures and reduce limb joint dislocation [31]. Cervical spine injury is usually treated with traction [32]. In this chapter, manual reduction was designed based on basic biomechanical studies [23, 24, 33, 34] and hyperextension postural reduction [35]. Clinical application achieved a high success rate. The learning curve for manual reduction is short and no major complications were observed if the correction was not more than 50 degrees. Classification of thoracolumbar kyphosis was made according to retrospective study of the immediate results after manual reduction. This classification may be influenced by observer bias, since the post-reduction films were evaluated by the surgeons after performing the manual reduction. Since this is a qualitative analysis, the flaw had far less impact than if quantitative comparisons had to be made.

In Type I kyphosis with breakage of the vertebral body, manual reduction has led to a very good restoration of the vertebral body. Reduction of acute burst or

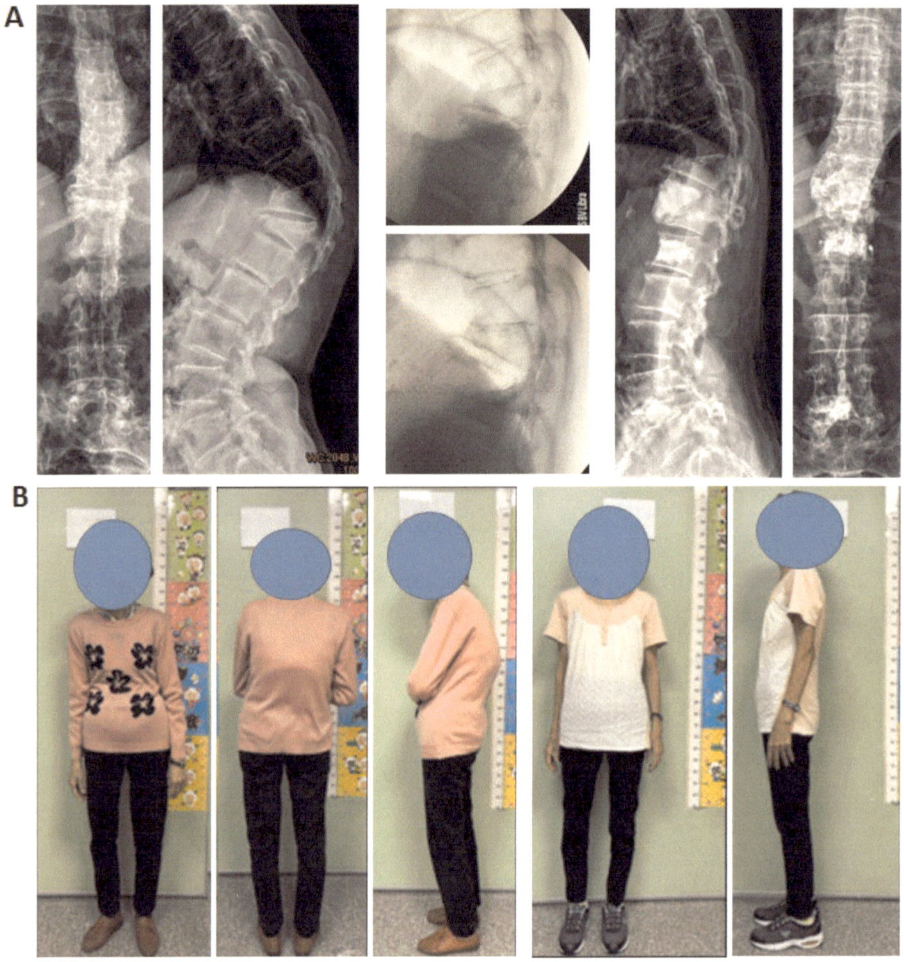

Figure 6.
Demonstrated radiographs of (A) and corresponding pictures (B) of a 78-year-old female with T10-L1 kyphosis, T10-L1 lateral Cobb's angle pre-op: 78′; postural reduction: 77′; post-manual reduction: 34′; post-vertebroplasty 33′. T12 open-wedge reduction was noted. T12 and T11 vertebroplasties were done.

compression fractures [36] was as easy by manual reduction as instrumentation reduction [37], followed by posterior fixation with transpedicle body augmenter [26, 38, 39]. Non-union osteoporotic compression fractures, also known as Kümmell's disease [40–42], were also easily reduced by manual reduction accompanied by posterior body reconstruction with transpedicle body augmenter [27]. Vertebroplasty or kyphoplasty was shown to increase vertebral body height without instrumentation, but the restoration result was limited [36, 43–45]. The difference between manual reduction and postural hyperextension reduction lies in the amount of force used. Manual reduction can be repeated if the reduction is not complete and the forces can be increased to induce restoration close to the anticipated result. Therefore, manual reduction is a safe, effective, and economic method to reduce Type I kyphotic deformity.

Acute secondary body collapse in active spinal tuberculosis, multiple myeloma with compression fracture, or osteolytic metastasis can be easily reduced by the

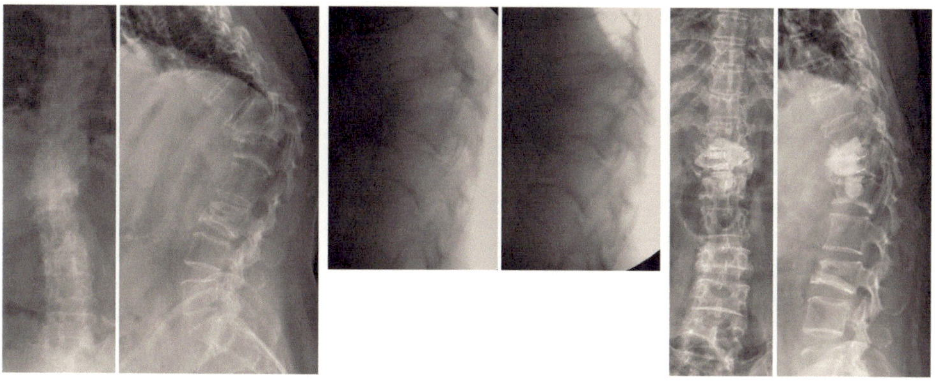

Figure 7.
Demonstrated radiographs of a 54-year-old female with T11-L1 kyphosis, T11-L1 lateral Cobb's angle pre-op: 86′; posture reduction: 58′; post-manual reduction: 34′; post-vertebroplasty 34′. T12 open wedge was induced by manual reduction and restored by subpedicle decompression and body augmentation (SpBA) with cemented two polyetheretherketones (PEEKs).

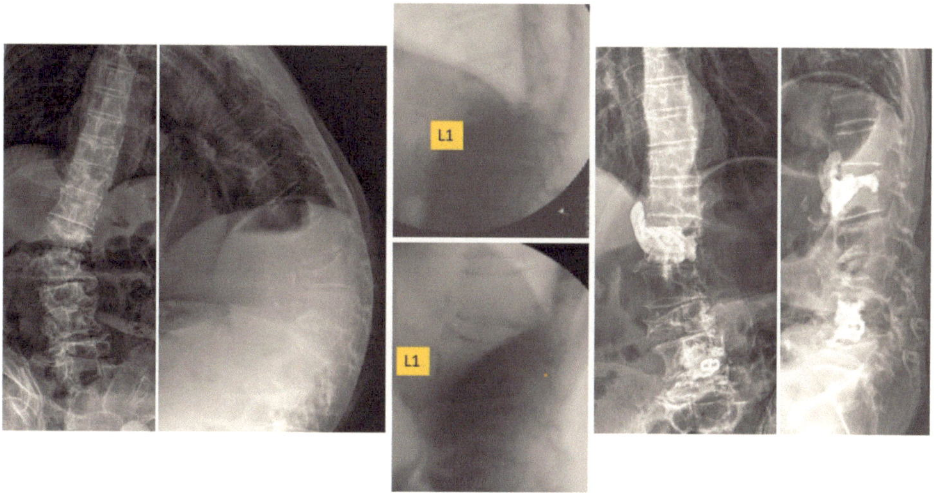

Figure 8.
Demonstrated radiographs of a 79-year-old male with T12-L2 Kypho-scoliosis, L1-L3 lateral Cobb's angle pre-op: 50′; postural reduction: 38′; post-manual reduction: 3′; post-vertebroplasty 3′. L1 open-wedge correction was induced by manual reduction and cementation was done.

manual reduction. This finding may result in a new treatment policy in the future. Traditionally, body collapse with cord compression secondary to active tuberculosis [46] or metastasis [47, 48] has been explored through an anterior approach in order to remove the compression source. But with manual reduction, the kyphosis could be reduced and spinal cord can be decompressed, and confirmed intraoperatively by C-arm myelogram. For tuberculosis (TB) spine with body collapse, subpedicle debridement with bone graft and posterior instrumentation should be sufficient, but this should be followed by medical treatment for tuberculosis. For secondary body collapse due to spinal metastasis, the subpedicle corpectomy and discectomy in combination with posterior fixation should be able to prevent cord compression, and this should be followed with chemotherapy or radiotherapy. Manual reduction and

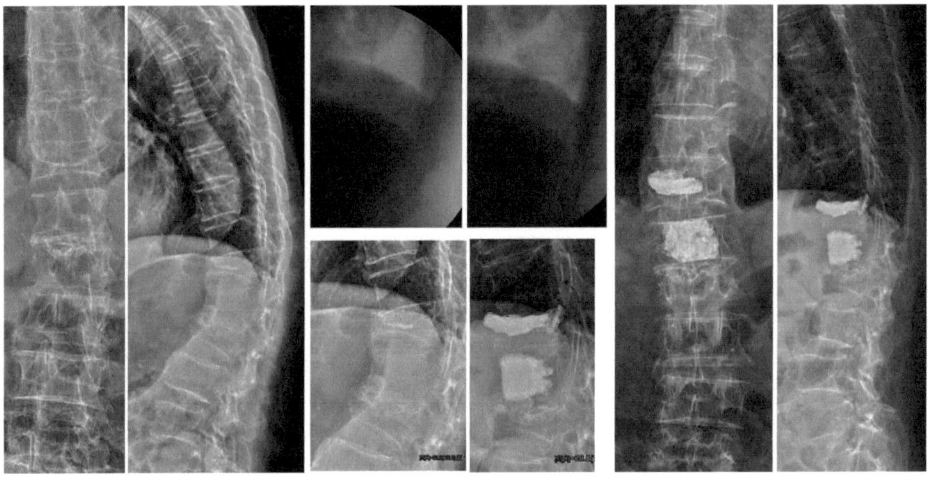

Figure 9.
Demonstrated radiographs of a 92-year-old male with T11-L2 kyphosis, T11-L2 lateral Cobb's angle pre-op: 52'; posture reduction: 50'; post-manual reduction: 30'; post-vertebroplasty: 29' T12 fracture site partial reduction and L1 iatrogenic open-wedge fracture.

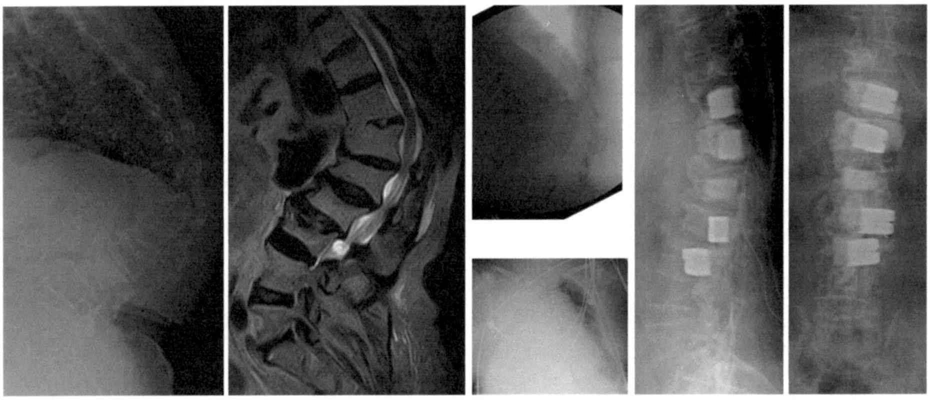

Figure 10.
Demonstrated radiographs of a 71-year-old female with T10-L3 95' post-manual reduction: 24' Hemothorax: T12 open-wedge fracture. Multiple SpBAs were done. SpBA indicates subpedicle decompression and body augmentation.

posterior approach will be much easier than the combination of anterior decompression and posterior fixation.

In Type II kyphosis with healed or deformed body without anterior interbody fusion, manual reduction can open the disc and correct malalignment of the deformed vertebral body. Traditionally, such deformities may necessitate an anterior approach to decompress the cord, followed by anterior or posterior fusion [49]. Because tilting of the vertebra can be corrected by manual reduction, the posterior approach including transpedicle discectomy [50] and interbody fusion with transpedicle body augmenter would be sufficient. Manual reduction can change treatment modalities in Type II kyphosis.

In Type III kyphosis with anterior interbody fusion in osteoporotic spine, the iatrogenic open-wedge fracture can be induced by manual reduction and kyphosis should be corrected. That situation followed by percutaneous vertebroplasty with

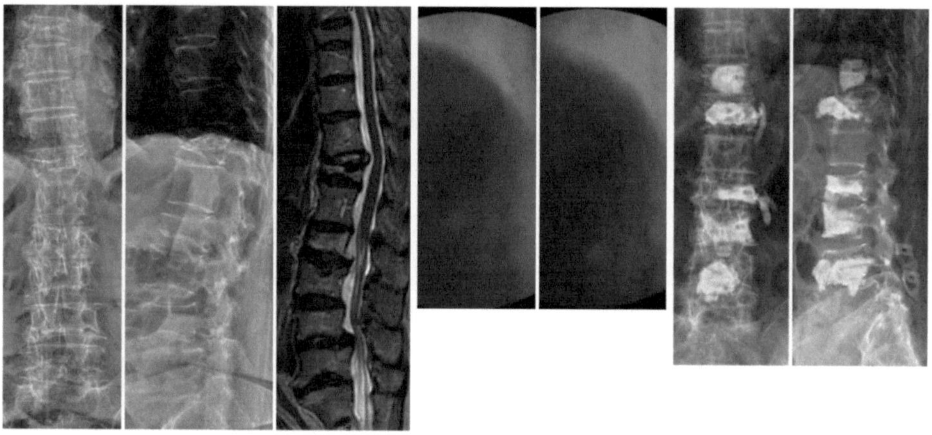

Figure 11.
Demonstrated radiographs of a 70-year-old female with T11-L1 kyphosis, T11-L1 lateral Cobb's angle pre-op: 24′; posture reduction: 23′; post-manual reduction: 3′; post-vertebroplasty 2′. The cement leakage was noted at T12 and L2 vertebroplasties.

sufficient cement vertebral filling will lead to a good result. Usually, the degree of osteoporosis should be evaluated first. The success can be predicted when dual X-ray absorptiometry (DEXA) < −2.5. Theoretically, the force needed to create an iatrogenic open-wedge fracture must increase according to the strength of the vertebrae.

In Type IV kyphosis, if the fusion segment is strong, manual force may not create a new fracture, and thus fail to reduce the kyphosis. In such cases, transpedicular wedge osteotomy [51, 52] or the anterior approach must be needed. But in contrast, success using Type III will lead to simple posterior instrumentation with posterior body reconstruction, which prevents the technically demanding and highly risky transpedicle shortening osteotomy or the anterior approach. Manual reduction can change the selection of traditional operative procedures in Type III kyphosis.

2.4 Summary of team manual reduction

Manual reduction can reduce the thoracolumbar kyphosis through different mechanisms and change the followed treatments. New classifications of kyphosis and new concepts in treating thoracolumbar kyphosis have been developed after the development of team manual reduction.

3. TpBA and SpBA to fix burst fractures following manual reduction

This retrospectively observational, single-institute case series study was approved by the St. Martin De Porres Hospital, Chia-Yi, Taiwan ethics review board [IRB 20C-006].

This retrospective study evaluated patients with TL burst fractures from January 2004 to December 2012. The inclusion criteria were as follows: single-level high-energy non-osteoporotic burst fractures (Type A3.3 according to the classification of Magerl et al. [53] with more than five points graded by the load-sharing mechanism described by Gaines et al. [54], and involving T10–L2 with neurologic function limited to Frankel Grade C, D, or E [25]. Fifty-three non-operatively treated cases or

DEXA < −2.5 and 16 patients with other major organ system or musculoskeletal injuries were excluded. Five patients who sustained multilevel involvement were also excluded. A total of 128 qualified patients completed the procedures. Because the cases with other organ trauma were excluded, the general conditions were stable in enrolled cases. The operation was done within 48 h after the patients were sent to the hospital within 10 days after the fracture happened. All cases were done by the same surgeons.

The clinical results were based on the latest follow-up before December 2022. Four patients died of unrelated medical illnesses and six patients were lost to follow-up. These 10 patients were excluded from this retrospective study. Finally, 118 cases with 41C, 58D, and 19E by the Frankel grading system [25] and average 7.1 ± 0.9 points graded by the load-sharing mechanism were included in this study. The follow-up rate was 92.2%. The male-to-female ratio was 71:47. The mean follow-up was 163.7 ± 27.1 (range, 124–227) months and age at the time of operation, 56.3 ± 6.7 (range, 32–67) years. The mechanisms of injury included fall (47%) and traffic accidents (53%). The demographic data are listed in **Table 2**.

The pre-operative evaluation protocol included anteroposterior (AP) and neutral lateral TL radiographs, and either computed tomography (CT) scans or MRI scans to evaluate fracture sites and cord compression status. The mean follow-up was 173 ± 29 (TpBA) and 156 ± 23 (SpBA) months ($p = 0.001$), and the age at the time of operation was 55.8 ± 6.6 and 56.7 ± 6.9 years ($p = 0.47$). All patients tolerated the TpBA or SpBA surgery smoothly.

In the radiographic analysis, the lateral Cobb's angle was measured as described by Kuklo et al. [55] from the superior endplate of the vertebral body above the fracture to the inferior endplate of the vertebral body below the fracture level. The segment wedge angle was measured from the superior endplate to the inferior endplate of the fractured vertebral body wedge angle of the fractured vertebral body as described previously by Verlaan et al. [22]. The predicted anterior and posterior vertebral body heights were estimated by the mean of the heights of the upper and lower adjacent segments. The angles and body heights were measured on neutral thoracolumbar radiographs before the operation, immediately after surgery, and at the final follow-up. All digitization and measurements were done using EBM-viewer software (EBM Technologies Inc., Taipei, Taiwan) with an accuracy of ±0.1 mm by a graduate student.

Items	TpBA[a]	SpBA[a]
Cases	53	65
Male:female	33:20	38:27
Age (yr)	55.8 ± 6.6	56.7 ± 6.9
T11:T12:L1:L2	7:20:18:8	11:22:23:9
Load-sharing score	7.2 ± 0.9	7.0 ± 1.2
Fall: traffic accident	25:28	31:34
Follow-up (mo)	173 ± 29	156 ± 23
Frankel E:D:C	21:23:9	20:35:10
Final Frankel E:D:C	49:4:0	60:5:0

[a]*TpBA indicates transpedicle body augmentation; SpBA, subpedicle decompression and body augmentation.*

Table 2.
Demographic data of the patients.

Clinical results were assessed by the performance scale (Grades A–E) described by Frankel et al. [25] and also evaluated pains using the Visual Analog Score (VAS).

Student's paired t-tests were done between two groups to evaluate all radiographic and clinical parameters. All the data are presented as mean ± standard deviation. The level of statistical significance was set as $p < 0.05$.

3.1 Operative techniques using transpedicle decompression and transpedicle body augmentation with short-segment fixation (TpBA)

After manual reduction, short-segment fixation was followed. Pedicle screws were placed at the level above and below the fractured vertebrae (two levels, four screws) using the rod screw system (Reduction-Fixation Spinal Pedicle Screw System, Advanced Spine Technology Inc., Oakland, CA, USA; Diapason, Stryker Corporation, Allendale, NJ, USA; and UP spine system, TiTec Medical Co., Ltd., Taipei, Taiwan). Bilateral pedicle tunnels to the vertebral body were made by an awl, followed by serial custom-made trials (8 to 14 mm) to prepare transpedicle tunnel for decompression and body augmentation. The bony defect in the fractured vertebral body was filled through bilateral transpedicle tunnels [9], with autologous bone graft mixed with calcium sulfate (Osteoset, Wright Medical Technology, Arlington, TN, USA) if the autograft from the posterior iliac bone was insufficient. Then the augmenter was inserted into the vertebral body through the pedicle tunnel, and finally, bone graft was used to fill the pedicle tunnel space. Patients wore a thoracolumbar brace for 3 months. After discharge, patients were followed up regularly.

3.2 Operative techniques of subpedicle decompression (TpBA) and body augmentation without screw fixation (SpBA)

In the SpBA group, a paramedian incision of about 1 inch in length was made on the more painful side as reported by the patient. The transverse process was identified with muscle splitting and blunt dissection. The superior part of the transverse process was then punched out to expose the subpedicle region, that is, the pedicle-body junction area, where no nerve or vessel resides (**Figure 12**). A guiding pin was first inserted and confirmed by C-arm fluoroscopy, followed by serial custom-made dilators to prepare for the passage of body augmenters, the residual bone may be pushed into anterior and peripheral region, which served as autogenous bone graft and may help in vertebral fracture healing and anterior ankylosis. The outer vertebral cortex was pushed by the dilators to the lateral side, which then worked as a shield to protect the surrounding structures. After the preparation, a subpedicle working tunnel of about 13 × 22 × 40 mm was created for the removal of retropulsed bony fragments and passing two spacers simultaneously. The upper segmental nerve root was protected by a nerve retractor. Two pile-up body cages of 10 × 13 × 27 mm were inserted into the vertebral body through the subpedicle window. Body cages can be made of polyetheretherketone (PEEK) or titanium, solid or hollow, cylindrical or rectangular. Polymethyl methacrylate (radiopaque bone cement; Howmedica International S. De R.L., Limerick, Ireland) was used to stabilize the body cages and provide the initial partial internal support if stability was not perfectly established after the body cages were inserted or bone quality was not good enough. Usually, patients were able to walk on the same day of the operation. Both groups of patients were asked to wear a thoracolumbar brace for 3 months. After discharge, patients were followed up regularly.

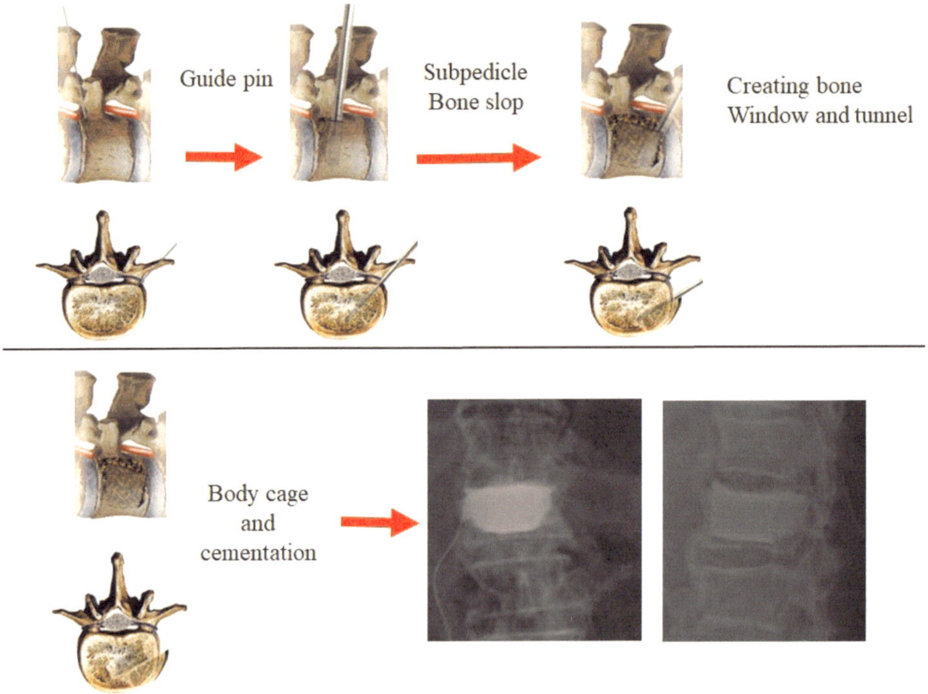

Figure 12.
Subpedicle decompression and body augmentation (SpBA) flowcharts of subpedicle decompression and body augmentation with body cage and cementation as shown in the lateral and transverse views. The first step is the insertion of the guiding pin as confirmed by C-arm fluoroscopy; second, the creation of a bone slop in the cephalocaudal direction; third, creation of the subpedicle bone window and tunnel; fourth, after the removal of retropulsed bone fragments and placement, the body cages with cementation were inserted. SpBA indicates subpedicle decompression and body augmentation.

3.3 Results of TpBA and SpBA

A summary of the results of the operative parameters is shown in **Table 3**. The average blood loss and hospitalization were not different between the two groups. The operation duration was significantly shorter in the SpBA group (40 ± 12 min), only 59% of that for the TpBA group (68 ± 17 min) ($p < 0.001$). All patients in the SpBA group could walk without or with assistance within 24 h after the operation; but ambulation for the TpBA group was achieved 1 to 3 days after the operation. Signs of fracture healing, that is, appearance of anterior vertebral cortical line could be documented radiographically within 3 to 5 months. Initial reduction and maintenance of reduction were mostly achieved in both groups. The final post-operative anterior vertebral restoration rates in the two groups were similar. There was no implant dislodgement in either group. The partial or complete spontaneous anterior or lateral ankylosing bridge was noted in every case of both groups (**Figures 13–16**).

The initial anterior vertebral height correction was 52.2 ± 4.8% (TpBA) versus 57.1 ± 4.2% (SpBA) ($p < 0.001$) and final loss reduction was 2.4 ± 0.8% versus 2.3 ± 0.9% ($p = 0.28$). Initial corrections of the lateral Cobb angle were 23.7° ± 3.9° versus 24.4° ± 4.3°) ($p = 0.41$) and of the final reduction loss were 2.9° ± 2.2° versus 2.8° ± 2.4° ($p = 0.79$).

Adjacent disc degeneration secondary to endplate fracture was noted in every case in the SpBA group; however, no late radiculopathy in the SpBA group was noted. In

	Operative parameters[a]				
	Hospital stay (d)		Blood loss (mL)		Op. time (min)
TpBA	4.7 ± 1.2		228 ± 77		68 ± 17
SpBA	4.4 ± 1.1		211 ± 70		40 ± 12
P	0.34		0.21		<0.001
	Anterior body height (%)				
	Pre-op	Post-op FU	Correction	Final FU	Correction loss
TpBA	43.0 ± 4.4%	95.2 ± 1.9%	52.2 ± 4.8%	92.7 ± 2.0%	2.4 ± 0.8%
SpBA	42.6 ± 4.2%	99.8 ± 1.5%	57.1 ± 4.2%	97.5 ± 1.2%	2.3 ± 0.9%
P	0.69	<0.001	<0.001	<0.001	0.28
	Lateral Cobb's Angle (°)				
	Pre-op	Post-op FU	Correction	Final FU	Correction loss
TpBA	26.4° ± 13.9°	2.5° ± 2.4°	23.7° ± 3.9°	5.5° ± 2.9°	2.9° ± 2.2°
SpBA	26.9° ± 4.2°	2.6° ± 11.9°	24.4° ± 4.3°	5.4° ± 2.3°	2.8° ± 2.4°
P	0.41	0.94	0.41	0.77	0.79

[a]*TpBA indicates transpedicle body augmentation; SpBA, subpedicle decompression and body augmentation.*

Table 3.
Results of operative parameters, anterior body height, and kephotic angle (°).

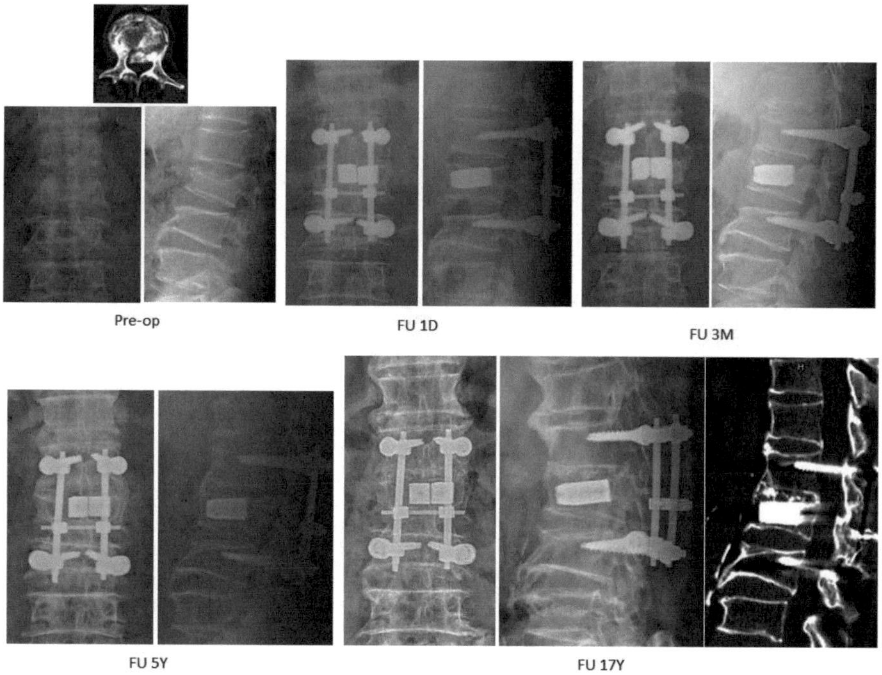

Figure 13.
Demonstrated radiographs of a 58-year-old male who fell from height with L2 burst fracture with Frankel grade D. He was treated with manual reduction and transpedicle body augmentation (TpBA). The fracture was healed with anterior ankylosing bridging 3 months post-operatively. He is still pain free and works at his farm.

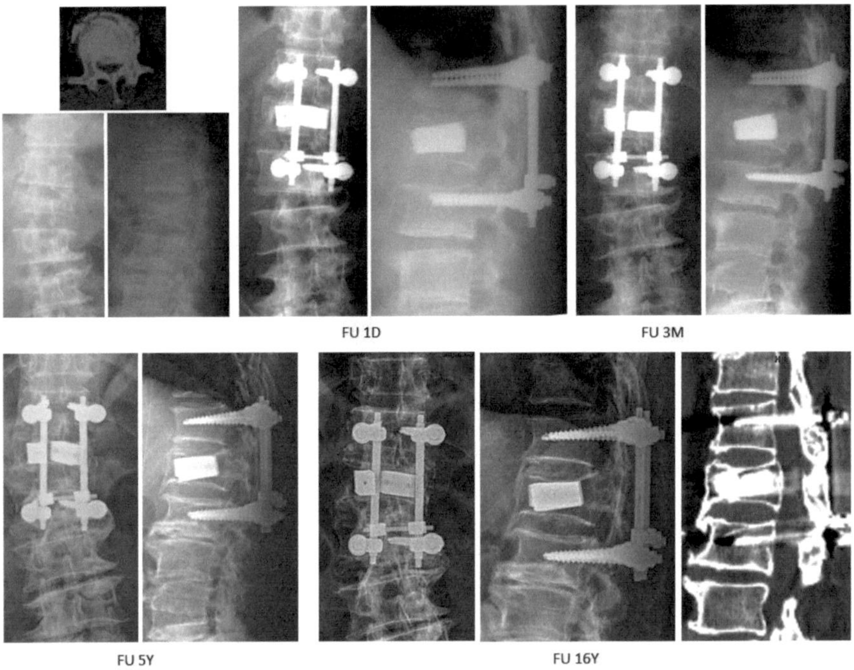

Figure 14.
Demonstrated radiographs of a 62-year-old male who fell from height with L1 burst fracture with Frankel grade D. He was treated with manual reduction and transpedicle body augmentation (TpBA). The fracture was healed smoothly and his previous lumbar degenerative scoliosis seems not to be affected too much by TpBA operation.

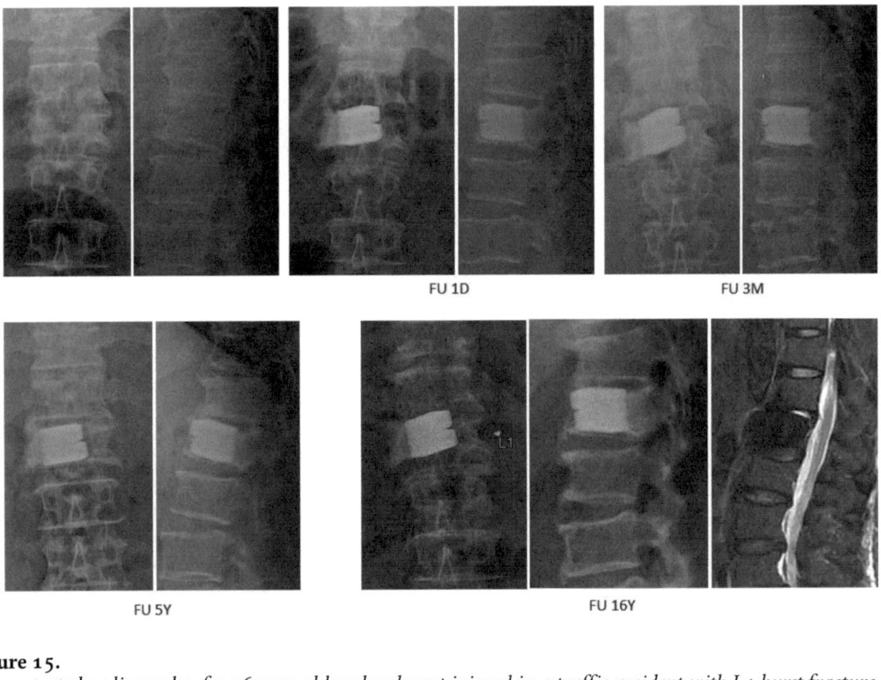

Figure 15.
Demonstrated radiographs of a 56-year-old male who got injured in a traffic accident with L1 burst fracture with Frankel grade E. He was treated with manual reduction, subpedicle decompression, and cement-augmented body cages. The spontaneous anterior ankylosis was noted from 1 month and continued to 16 years post-operatively and he is symptom free.

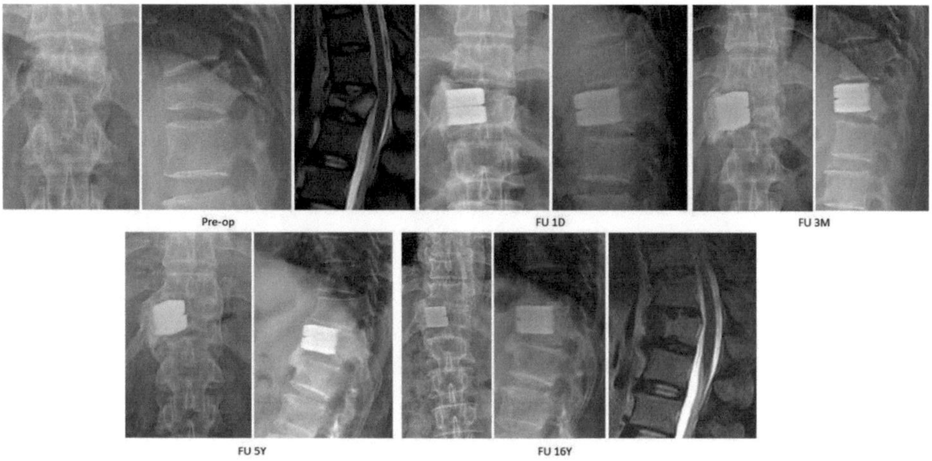

Figure 16.
Demonstrated radiographs of a 46-year-old male MD who had motorcycle accident and resulted in a L2 burst fracture with Frankel grade C with urinary incontinence. He was treated with manual reduction and transpedicle body augmentation (TpBA). He experienced the removal of implant and underwent decompression surgery due to residual spinal stenosis 6 years later. He is still an active physician.

clinical evaluations, there were no significant intergroup statistical differences in VAS at pre-operative status (TpBA vs. SpBA = 7.5 ± 1.4 vs. 7.8 ± 1.3) as well as at the final visit (1.4 ± 0.4 vs. 1.2 ± 0.5). Totally, 109 patients were maintained or recovered to Frankel grade E. Four cases in the TpBA group and five in the SpBA group improved from grade C to grade D.

Complications included three superficial infections in the TpBA group, which were cured by antibiotics management, three post-operative seromas in the TpBA group and one in the SpBA group, which healed after debridement, and two deep vein thromboses in the TpBA group. Two patients in the SpBA group had an intraoperative first lumbar (L1) root overstretch injury, which caused numbness and neuralgia at the left inguinal region and leg weakness, but the symptoms gradually subsided in 4 and 6 weeks later. Three patients in the TpBA group had residual symptoms of incomplete decompression of the spinal stenosis, and laminectomy to decompress the spinal cord was done later (**Figure 17**). Four dura tears, which were caused by the penetration of bony spike, were observed during subpedicle decompression after the removal of retropulsed bony fragments; the tears were sutured or packed with gelatin sponge and healed without neurological impairment.

3.4 Discussion

Traditionally, there are three main surgical methods used for thoracolumbar Magerl incomplete burst fractures: anterior approach, posterior approach, and a combination of both [5–8]. The anterior approach directly decompresses the spinal cord, but it comes with a risk of damaging the lungs, internal organs, and vascular structures. On the other hand, the posterior approach, including laminectomy, can only achieve indirect decompression. In this reported study, manual reduction [9] was used to provide indirect decompression, while the subpedicle approach [12] was used to directly remove the retropulsed bony fragments. This approach combines the advantages of both anterior and posterior decompression, but without the potential

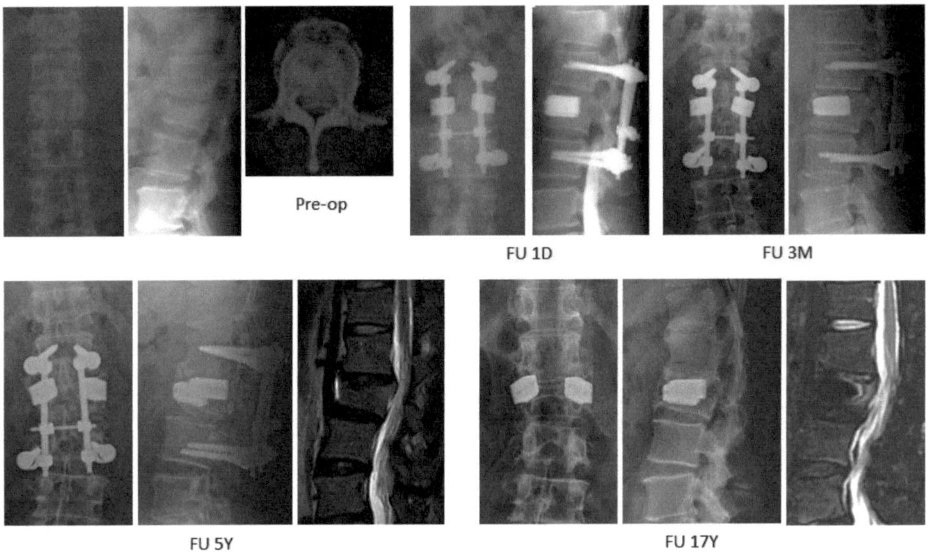

Figure 17.
Demonstrated radiographs of a 46-year-old male MD who had motorcycle accident and resulted in a L2 burst fracture with Frankel grade C with voiding dysfunction. He was treated with manual reduction and transpedicle body augmentation (TpBA). He experienced the removal of implant and underwent decompression surgery due to residual spinal stenosis 6 years later. He is still an active physician.

surgical complications. The study used a posterior far-lateral approach to create a unilateral subpedicle cortical window that served as a tunnel to remove all retropulsed bony fragments and passing body cage for full-body augmentation. The study demonstrated that the unilateral mini-open SpBA method for treating thoracolumbar burst fractures was effective in achieving cord decompression, vertebral reconstruction, and satisfactory long-term results, as good as those seen with TpBA, but with a smaller wound and shorter operation time, as evidenced by the results of a minimum 10-year follow-up.

In interpreting our data, it is important to consider some limitations. First, there may be nonhomogeneous inclusion protocols due to differences in pre-operative fracture classification methods. These protocols were studied and implemented by the trauma team in the emergency department, with some cases using computed tomography and others using MRI. This might result in different severities of neurological symptoms in each group at different times, leading to bias. Second, the study did not have a proper randomized control group. As this was a retrospective study, we performed fewer posterior short-segment fixations after learning that the results of SpBA were satisfactory. Consequently, the follow-up period of SpBA was significantly shorter than that of TpBA. Third, the clinical outcomes were determined by the treating surgeons, which may introduce bias in interpreting the findings. Fourth, all radiographs were obtained in the supine position, which could result in bias when compared to studies using standing radiographs. Finally, blinded evaluation of radiographic results was not possible, as the body cages or posterior screws were visible on the radiographs. However, independent reviewers were used to evaluate other criteria.

The long-term results of SpBA showed that adjacent disc degeneration did occur; however, there was no significant radiculopathy. Burst fractures are often accompanied by various degrees of intervertebral disc injury above the affected vertebrae

[13–15], with reported rates as high as 63.4% [16]. The severity of intervertebral disc injury increased with the degree of fracture [13, 56]. The progression of kyphosis angle and loss of correction angle after surgery were mainly due to more severe intervertebral disc injuries and changes in the intervertebral disc shape [17–19]. However, if the fracture of the endplate can be healed, resettlement of disc does not cause kyphosis progression [20]. The literature [21, 22] also confirmed that adjacent disc degeneration does occur in burst fractures; however, only 13% are severe and related to endplate fractures. In the SpBA group, the vertebral body was fully restored by the body cage and fixed with cement. The endplate was restored and healed as completely as possible. Intervertebral disc injury is not only difficult to recover [57–59], but also increases apoptosis of intervertebral disc tissue [60], leading to intervertebral disc degeneration and spontaneous fusion [61]. Our findings support this, as every case in SpBA had disc degeneration and tended toward anterior ankylosis across the upper disc. Changes in the intervertebral disc angle and height reflect changes in the Cobb angle [19, 62]. Changes in the intervertebral disc morphology, based on the fractured and deformed endplate, may be the primary reason for this angle change [63]. However, body cages with cementation can restore the body and endplate well, and degenerative disc material can still link with the healed flat endplate without causing angle changes, even if the height is decreased. This may explain why Cobb's angle has been maintained well after over a 10-year follow-up.

For high-energy burst fracture, PEEK cages and solid titanium cages lead to the same good clinical results. Originally, we used titanium cylindrical body cage to ensure the endplate reconstruction and prevent disc degeneration as slightly as possible. Later, we found that if cement could fulfill the body and support the endplate well, the PEEK cages, just as a spacer not a fusion device, would have led to the same results of titanium cages (**Figure 18**). The vertebral bone growth around the cage-cement complex was observed and finally stable fracture healing was achieved. Either titanium or PEEK cage would have the same mechanism. Due to interspinal process device being reported to decrease the disc stress [64, 65], the interspinal process device (IPD) (Rocker, Paonan Biotech Co., Ltd., Taiwan) was applied hopefully to decrease the disc stress and prevent the disc degeneration and kyphosis.

This study reveals that cemented body cages lead to similar clinical results as the body cage with short-segment fixation. The body cages are the internal supporter to the vertebral body to reconstruct the body height. The cement can fix the cage to the residual bony structure of the vertebra and prevent the cage dislodgement. The fractured vertebra will heal around the cage-cement complex and restore the spine stability. The long-term clinical results showed that the cemented body cages can work alone and the short-segment fixation is not needed. The cement lumbar interbody fixation without screw instrumentation was reported, leading to novel good clinical results with spontaneous ankylosis shown by a 10-year follow-up in lumbar degenerative spondylolisthesis and 6-year follow-up in degenerative lumbar scoliosis [66, 67]. All these findings suggest that cementation in the spine surgery can provide long-lasting stabilization, potentially inducing spontaneous ankylosis to further stabilize the spine construct over time.

4. Conclusion

This chapter describes the detailed techniques and results of treating post-traumatic kyphosis through team manual reduction, which has been developed and

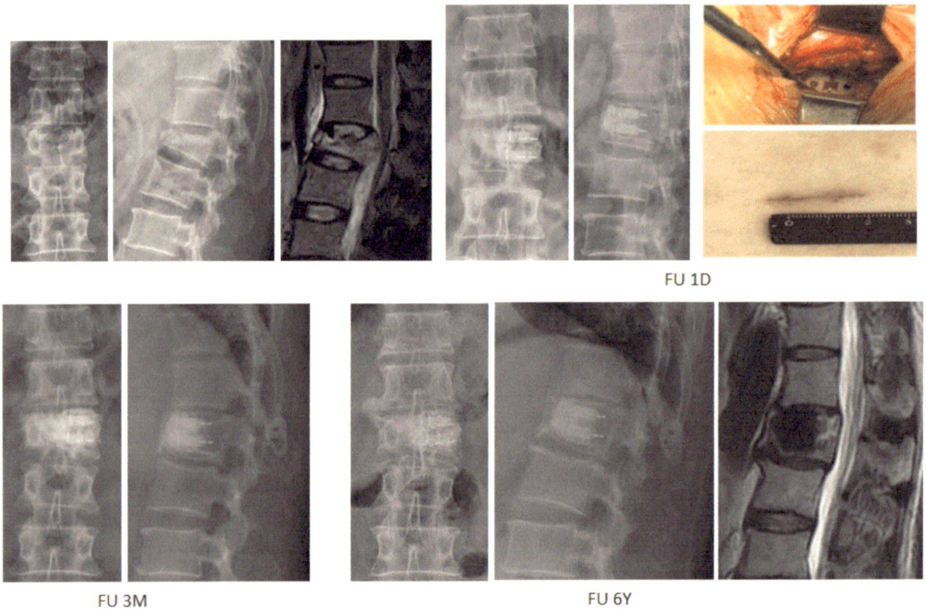

Figure 18.
Demonstrated radiographs of a 47-year-old male who fell from height with L1 burst fracture with Frankel grade D. He was treated with manual reduction, subpedicle decompression, and body cages with interspinal process device (IPD) (rocker, Paonan biotech Co., ltd., Taiwan). The photographs show the final results of cage insertion at the bone window and incision wound. The fracture was healed 3 months post-operatively and the patient returned back to be an active construction worker.

practiced 25 years in over 2000 patients. A practical classification system for thoracolumbar kyphosis was presented based on the results of team manual reduction.

The chapter further reports on surgical procedures used to treat thoracolumbar burst fractures, including TpBA with short-segment fixation and SpBA without instrumentation. The advanced SpBA procedure has advantages of being able to remove retropulsed bony fragments and reconstruct the fractured vertebra with body cages and cementation via a unilateral mini-open subpedicle window approach. The surgical outcomes of SpBA have been reported to be positive, with complete spinal cord decompression, maintenance of reduction, and further ensured fracture healing through anterior or lateral spontaneous interbody ankylosis.

Overall, the chapter concludes that combining team manual reduction and SpBA is a safe and efficient approach for treating thoracolumbar burst fractures, with good clinical outcomes observed in patients with a minimum 10-year follow-up.

Acknowledgements

The authors are grateful to the colleagues in the hospital for their professional contribution and assistance in data collection and analyses.

Conflict of interest

The authors declare no conflict of interest.

Author details

Kung-Chia Li*, Yu-Chieh Hsieh, Ching-Hsiang Hsieh and Ting-Hua Liao
Yang Ming Hospital, Chiayi, Taiwan

*Address all correspondence to: kungchiali@gmail.com

References

[1] Mulcahy MJ, Dower A, Tait M. Orthosis versus no orthosis for the treatment of thoracolumbar burst fractures: A systematic review. Journal of Clinical Neuroscience. 2021;**85**:49-56. DOI: 10.1016/j.jocn.2020.11.044

[2] Yan H, Ni M, Zhai W, Guo J, Huang Z, Zhang J, et al. Balloon kyphoplasty combined with posterior pedicle screw fixation for the treatment of osteoporotic thoracolumbar burst fractures. Annals of Palliative Medicine. 2021;**10**(7):7514-7524. DOI: 10.21037/apm-21-665

[3] Barakat AS, Elattar A, Fawaz K, Sultan AM, Koptan W, ElMiligui Y, et al. A comparative study between the universal spinal system®(USS) and the CD horizon® legacy™(CDH) in the management of thoracolumbar fractures. SICOT-J. 2019;**5**:42. DOI: 10.1051/sicotj/2019039

[4] Liao J-C, Chen W-P, Wang H. Treatment of thoracolumbar burst fractures by short-segment pedicle screw fixation using a combination of two additional pedicle screws and vertebroplasty at the level of the fracture: A finite element analysis. BMC Musculoskeletal Disorders. 2017;**18**:1-8. DOI: 10.1186/s12891-017-1623-0

[5] Piccone L, Cipolloni V, Nasto L, Pripp C, Tamburrelli F, Maccauro G, et al. Thoracolumbar burst fractures associated with incomplete neurological deficit in patients under the age of 40: Is the posterior approach enough? Surgical treatment and results in a case series of 10 patients with a minimum follow-up of 2 years. Injury. 2020;**51**(2):312-316. DOI: 10.1016/j.injury.2019.12.031

[6] De Iure F, Lofrese G, De Bonis P, Cultrera F, Cappuccio M, Battisti S. Vertebral body spread in thoracolumbar burst fractures can predict posterior construct failure. The Spine Journal. 2018;**18**(6):1005-1013. DOI: 10.1016/j.spinee.2017.10.064

[7] Tan T, Rutges J, Marion T, Gonzalvo A, Mathew J, Fitzgerald M, et al. Anterior versus posterior approach in traumatic thoracolumbar burst fractures deemed for surgical management: Systematic review and meta-analysis. Journal of Clinical Neuroscience. 2019;**70**:189-197. DOI: 10.1016/j.jocn.2019.07.083

[8] Wang T, Wang Z, Ji P, Zhang J, Zhang C, Zhang L. The efficacy and safety of anterior versus posterior approach for the treatment of thoracolumbar burst fractures: A systematic review and meta-analysis. Annals of Translational Medicine. 2022;**10**(6):309. DOI: 10.21037/atm-22-903

[9] Li K-C, Li AF-Y, Hsieh C-H, Chen H-H. Transpedicle body augmenter in painful osteoporotic compression fractures. European Spine Journal. 2007; **16**:589-598. DOI: 10.1007/s00586-006-0197-6

[10] Li K-C, Hsieh C-H, Lee C-Y, Chen T-H. Transpedicle body augmenter: A further step in treating burst fractures. Clinical Orthopaedics and Related Research (1976–2007). 2005;**436**: 119-125. DOI: 10.1097/01.blo.0000158316.89886.63

[11] Li K-C, Li AF, Hsieh C-H, Liao T-H, Chen C-H. Another option to treat Kümmell's disease with cord compression. European Spine Journal. 2007;**16**:1479-1487. DOI: 10.1007/s00586-006-0094-z

[12] Li K-C, Yu S-W, Li A, Hsieh C-H, Liao T-H, Chen J-H, et al. Subpedicle

decompression and vertebral reconstruction for thoracolumbar Magerl incomplete burst fractures via a minimally invasive method. Spine. 2014; **39**(5):433-442. DOI: 10.1097/BRS.0000000000000186

[13] Su Y, Ren D, Zou Y, Lu J, Wang P. A retrospective study evaluating the correlation between the severity of intervertebral disc injury and the anteroposterior type of thoracolumbar vertebral fractures. Clinics. 2016;**71**: 297-301

[14] Pumberger M, Fuchs M, Engelhard N, Hermann KG, Putzier M, Makowski MR, et al. Disk injury in patients with vertebral fractures—A prospective diagnostic accuracy study using dual-energy computed tomography. European Radiology. 2019; **29**:4495-4502

[15] Mi J, Sun X-j, Zhang K, Zhao C-Q, Zhao J. Prediction of MRI findings including disc injury and posterior ligamentous complex injury in neurologically intact thoracolumbar burst fractures by the parameters of vertebral body damage on CT scan. Injury. 2018;**49**(2):272-278

[16] Kawakyu-O'Connor D, Bordia R, Nicola R. Magnetic resonance imaging of spinal emergencies. Magnetic Resonance Imaging Clinics. 2016;**24**(2):325-344. DOI: 10.1016/j.mric.2015.11.004

[17] Lee KY, Kim M-W, Seok SY, Kim DR, Im CS. The relationship between superior disc-endplate complex injury and correction loss in young adult patients with thoracolumbar stable burst fracture. Clinics in Orthopedic Surgery. 2017;**9**(4):465-471

[18] Aono H, Ishii K, Takenaka S, Tobimatsu H, Nagamoto Y, Horii C, et al. Risk factors for a kyphosis recurrence after short-segment temporary posterior fixation for thoracolumbar burst fractures. Journal of Clinical Neuroscience. 2019;**66**:138-143. DOI: 10.1016/j.jocn.2019.04.035

[19] Peng Z, Cui Z, Kuang X, Yu C, Ruan Y, Li C, et al. Intervertebral disc injury is the mainspring for the postoperative increase in cobb angle after thoracolumbar burst fracture. Journal of Orthopaedic Surgery. 2022; **30**(2):10225536221088753

[20] Oner FC, van der Rijt RR, Ramos LM, Dhert WJ, Verbout AJ. Changes in the disc space after fractures of the thoracolumbar spine. The Journal of Bone and Joint Surgery British. 1998; **80**(5):833-839. DOI: 10.1302/0301-620X.80B5.0800833

[21] Wang J, Zhou Y, Zhang ZF, Li CQ, Zheng WJ, Liu J. Radiological study on disc degeneration of thoracolumbar burst fractures treated by percutaneous pedicle screw fixation. European Spine Journal. 2013;**22**:489-494

[22] Verlaan J-J, Dhert WJ, Oner FC. Intervertebral disc viability after burst fractures of the thoracic and lumbar spine treated with pedicle screw fixation and direct end-plate restoration. The Spine Journal. 2013;**13**(3):217-221. DOI: 10.1016/j.spinee.2012.02.032

[23] Fredrickson B, Edwards W, Rauschning W, Bayley J, Yuan H. 1992 Volvo award in experimental studies vertebral burst fractures: An experimental, morphologic, and radiographic study. Spine. 1992;**17**(9): 1012-1021. DOI: 10.1097/00007632-199209000-00002

[24] Fredrickson BE, Mann KA, Yuan HA, Lubicky JP. Reduction of the intracanal fragment in experimental burst fractures. Spine. 1988;**13**(3):

267-271. DOI: 10.1097/00007632-198803000-00008

[25] Frankel H, Hancock D, Hyslop G, Melzak J, Michaelis L, Ungar G, et al. The value of postural reduction in the initial management of closed injuries of the spine with paraplegia and tetraplegia. Spinal Cord. 1969;7(3):179-192

[26] Li K-C, Hsieh C-H, P68. Pedicle augmenter in treating burst fracture. The Spine Journal. 2003;**3**(5):148. DOI: 10.1016/S1529-9430(03)00351-6

[27] Li K-C, Wong T-U, Kung F-C, Li A, Hsieh C-H. Staging of Kümmell's disease. Journal of Musculoskeletal Research. 2004;**8**(01):43-55. DOI: 10.1142/S0218957704001181

[28] Tropiano P, Huang RC, Louis CA, Poitout DG, Louis RP. Functional and radiographic outcome of thoracolumbar and lumbar burst fractures managed by closed orthopaedic reduction and casting. Spine. 2003;**28**(21):2459-2465. DOI: 10.1097/01.BRS.0000090834.36061.DD

[29] Carlo P, Francesco C. Preoperative manual on-table-traction for the reduction of thoracolumbar burst fractures: A technical note. Journal of Craniovertebral Junction & Spine. 2018;**9**(1):73. DOI: 10.4103/jcvjs.JCVJS_3_18

[30] Li Y, Du Y, Ji A, Wang Q, Li L, Wu X, et al. The clinical effect of manual reduction combined with internal fixation through Wiltse Paraspinal approach in the treatment of thoracolumbar fracture. Orthopaedic Surgery. 2021;**13**(8):2206-2215. DOI: 10.1111/os.13090

[31] Khan MR, Mirdad TM. Ipsilateral dislocation of the shoulder and elbow. Saudi Medical Journal. 2001;**22**(11):1019-1021

[32] Bohlman HH, Ducker TB. Spine and spine cord injuries. In: Herkowitz HN, Garfin SR, Balderston RA, et al., editors. Rothman-Simeone The Spine. 4th ed. Vol. 2. Philadelphia: WB Saunders Company; 1999. pp. 889-1002

[33] Harrington R, Budorick T, Hoyt J, Anderson P, Tencer A. Biomechanics of indirect reduction of bone retropulsed into the spinal canal in vertebral fracture. Spine. 1993;**18**(6):692-699. DOI: 10.1097/00007632-199305000-00003

[34] Lin RM, Panjabi MM, Oxland TR. Functional radiographs of acute thoracolumbar burst fractures. A biomechanical study. Spine. 1993;**18**(16):2431-2437. DOI: 10.1097/00007632-199312000-00011

[35] Mumford J, Weinstein JN, Spratt KF, Goel VK. Thoracolumbar burst fractures: The clinical efficacy and outcome of nonoperative management. Spine. 1993;**18**(8):955-970

[36] Deramond H, Depriester C, Galibert P, Le Gars D. Percutaneous vertebroplasty with polymethylmethacrylate: Technique, indications, and results. Radiologic Clinics of North America. 1998;**36**(3):533-546. DOI: 10.1016/S0033-8389(05)70042-7

[37] Lindsey RW, Dick W. The fixateur interne in the reduction and stabilization of thoracolumbar spine fractures in patients with neurologic deficit. Spine. 1991;**16**(3 Suppl):S140-S145. DOI: 10.1097/00007632-199103001-00020

[38] Chen H-H, Wang W-K, Li K-C, Chen T-H. Biomechanical effects of the body augmenter for reconstruction of the vertebral body. Spine. 2004;**29**(18):E382-E3E7. DOI: 10.1097/01.brs.0000139308.65813.70

[39] Li K-C, Chen H-H, Li A, Hsien C-H. Safe zone for application of transpedicle body augmenter. Journal of Orthopaedic Surgery Taiwan. 2004;**21**(3):125-133

[40] Van Eenenaam DP, Georges Y. Delayed post-traumatic vertebral collapse (Kummell's disease): Case report with serial radiographs, computed tomographic scans, and bone scans. Spine. 1993;**18**(9):1236-1241

[41] Golimbu C, Firooznia H, Rafii M. The intravertebral vacuum sign. Spine. 1986;**11**(10):1040-1043

[42] Osterhouse MD, Kettner NW. Delayed posttraumatic vertebral collapse with intravertebral vacuum cleft. Journal of Manipulative and Physiological Therapeutics. 2002;**25**(4):270-275. DOI: 10.1067/mmt.2002.123164

[43] Garfin SR, Yuan HA, Reiley MA. New technologies in spine: Kyphoplasty and vertebroplasty for the treatment of painful osteoporotic compression fractures. Spine. 2001;**26**(14):1511-1515

[44] Hiwatashi A, Moritani T, Numaguchi Y, Westesson P-L. Increase in vertebral body height after vertebroplasty. American Journal of Neuroradiology. 2003;**24**(2):185-189

[45] McKiernan F, Jensen R, Faciszewski T. The dynamic mobility of vertebral compression fractures. Journal of Bone and Mineral Research. 2003; **18**(1):24-29. DOI: 10.1359/jbmr.2003.18.1.24

[46] Fukuta S, Miyamoto K, Masuda T, Hosoe H, Kodama H, Nishimoto H, et al. Two-stage (posterior and anterior) surgical treatment using posterior spinal instrumentation for pyogenic and tuberculotic spondylitis. Spine. 2003; **28**(15):E302-E3E8. DOI: 10.1097/01.BRS.0000083318.40123.5E

[47] Perrin RG, McBroom RJ. Spinal fixation after anterior decompression for symptomatic spinal metastasis. Neurosurgery. 1988;**22**(2):324-327

[48] Walker MP, Yaszemski MJ, Kim CW, Talac R, Currier BL. Metastatic disease of the spine: Evaluation and treatment. Clinical Orthopaedics and Related Research (1976-2007). 2003;415: S165-SS75. DOI: 10.1097/01.blo.0000092977.12414.f9

[49] Roberson JR, Whitesides TE Jr. Surgical reconstruction of late post-traumatic thoracolumbar kyphosis. Spine. 1985;**10**(4):307, 12. DOI: 10.1097/00007632-198505000-00003

[50] Daniaux HS, Genelin P, Lang A, T. Kathrein A. Application of posterior plating and modifications in thoracolumbar spine injuries: Indication, techniques, and results. Spine. 1991; **16**(3):S125-SS33

[51] Chen IH, Chien J-T, Yu T-C. Transpedicular wedge osteotomy for correction of thoracolumbar kyphosis in ankylosing spondylitis: Experience with 78 patients. Spine. 2001;**26**(16):E354-EE60

[52] Lehmer SM, Keppler L, Biscup RS, Enker P, Miller SD, Steffee AD. Posterior transvertebral osteotomy for adult thoracolumbar kyphosis. Spine. 1994; **19**(18):2060-2067. DOI: 10.1097/00007632-199409150-00009

[53] Magerl F, Aebi M, Gertzbein S, Harms J, Nazarian S. A comprehensive classification of thoracic and lumbar injuries. European Spine Journal. 1994;**3**: 184-201. DOI: 10.1007/BF02221591

[54] Gaines RW, Satterlee CC, Groh GI. Experimental evaluation of seven different spinal fracture internal fixation devices using nonfailure stability testing:

The load-sharing and unstable-mechanism concepts. Spine. 1991;**16**(8):902-909

[55] Kuklo TR, Polly DW Jr, Owens BD, Zeidman SM, Chang AS, Klemme WR. Measurement of thoracic and lumbar fracture kyphosis: Evaluation of intraobserver, interobserver, and technique variability. Spine. 2001; **26**(1):61-66

[56] Oner F, Van Gils A, Dhert W, Verbout A. MRI findings of thoracolumbar spine fractures: A categorisation based on MRI examinations of 100 fractures. Skeletal Radiology. 1999;**28**:433-443. DOI: 10.1007/s002560050542

[57] Che Y-J, Hou J-J, Guo J-B, Liang T, Zhang W, Lu Y, et al. Low energy extracorporeal shock wave therapy combined with low tension traction can better reshape the microenvironment in degenerated intervertebral disc regeneration and repair. The Spine Journal. 2021;**21**(1):160-177. DOI: 10.1016/j.spinee.2020.08.004

[58] Beekmans SV, Emanuel KS, Smit TH, Iannuzzi D. Stiffening of the nucleus pulposus upon axial loading of the intervertebral disc: An experimental in situ study. JOR Spine. 2018;**1**(1):e1005. DOI: 10.1002/jsp2.1005

[59] Duclos SE, Michalek AJ. Residual strains in the intervertebral disc annulus fibrosus suggest complex tissue remodeling in response to in-vivo loading. Journal of the Mechanical Behavior of Biomedical Materials. 2017; **68**:232-238. DOI: 10.1016/j.jmbbm.2017.02.010

[60] Tschoeke SK, Hellmuth M, Hostmann A, Robinson Y, Ertel W, Oberholzer A, et al. Apoptosis of human intervertebral discs after trauma compares to degenerated discs involving both receptor-mediated and mitochondrial-dependent pathways. Journal of Orthopaedic Research. 2008; **26**(7):999-1006. DOI: 10.1002/jor.20601

[61] Korres DS, Babis GC, Paraskevakou H, Stamos K, Tsarouchas J, Lykomitros V. Spontaneous interbody fusion after controlled injuries to the spine: An experimental study in rabbits. Clinical Spine Surgery. 2000;**13**(1):31-35

[62] Akeda K, Yamada T, Inoue N, Nishimura A, Sudo A. Risk factors for lumbar intervertebral disc height narrowing: A population-based longitudinal study in the elderly. BMC Musculoskeletal Disorders. 2015;**16**:1-9. DOI: 10.1186/s12891-015-0798-5

[63] Chen J-X, Xu D-L, Sheng S-R, Goswami A, Xuan J, Jin H-M, et al. Risk factors of kyphosis recurrence after implant removal in thoracolumbar burst fractures following posterior short-segment fixation. International Oorthopaedics. 2016;**40**:1253-1260. DOI: 10.1007/s00264-016-3180-9

[64] Huang W, Chang Z, Zhang J, Song R, Yu X. Interspinous process stabilization with rocker via unilateral approach versus X-stop via bilateral approach for lumbar spinal stenosis: A comparative study. BMC Musculoskeletal Disorders. 2015;**16**:1-8. DOI: 10.1186/s12891-015-0786-9

[65] Shen H, Fogel GR, Zhu J, Liao Z, Liu W. Biomechanical analysis of lumbar fusion with proximal interspinous process device implantation. International Journal for Numerical Methods in Biomedical Engineering. 2021;**37**(8):e3498. DOI: 10.1002/cnm.3498

[66] Li K-C, Hsieh C-H, Liao T-H. Cement lumbar interbody fusion (CLIF)

for lowgrade degenerative spondylolisthesis with minimum 10-year follow-up. Journal of Surgery. 2022;**7**(16):1-9. DOI: 10.29011/2575-9760.001691

[67] Li K-C, Hsieh C-H, Liao T-H. Clinical outcome-supported advance of cement lumber interbody fusion for degenerative lumbar scoliosis. Journal of Surgery. 2023;**8**(1):1-8. DOI: 10.29011/2575-9760.001697

Chapter 9

Motor Recovery in Different Types of Brachial Plexus Injury Surgeries

Armando Armas-Salazar, Fátima Ximena Cid-Rodríguez, José Luis Navarro-Olvera, Edgar Abarca-Rojano, Noé Tellez-León, María de la Luz Montes-Castillo, Ana Isabel García-Jerónimo and José Damián Carrillo-Ruiz

Abstract

Brachial plexus injuries (BPI) affect mostly the young population. The management of these injuries is complex and there are many surgical options for treatment. To evaluate the patient motor component, the British Medical Research Council motor grading scale (BMRC), range-of-motion (ROM), disability of the arm, shoulder, and hand questionnaire (DASH), and push and pull dynamometer are the main clinical assessment tools that provide information about the clinical status regarding motor function. The purpose of this chapter is to show the motor recovery on interventions that are available as surgical alternatives for the management of BPI, through a systematic review of the literature.

Keywords: brachial plexus injury, peripheral nerve surgery, clinical outcome, motor recovery, systematic review

1. Introduction

Brachial plexus injuries (BPI) are highly disabling [1]. The functional restoration of these injuries tends to focus on motor recovery, this being reported in 94% of the articles published on brachial plexus surgery, displacing the evaluation of other fundamental aspects such as sensory, pain, quality of life, functional impact, and psychosocial context [2, 3]. However, motor recovery is directly related to improvement in quality of life [4]. Motor recovery can be evaluated in various ways, using clinimetric scales and assessment tools to measure strength such as the British Medical Research Council motor grading scale (BMRC) [5], active/passive range-of-motion (ROM) [6], and tools that allow us to quantitatively measure strength (push-and-pull dynamometer) [7]. Being the BMRC the most standardized, reliable, and valid measurement tool for evaluating muscle strength in patients with BPI [8]. Brachial plexus surgery has different objectives, where relative to motor recovery elbow flexion and shoulder abduction and stability are prioritized due to the greater chance for success [9]. However, we recognize the importance of considering other functions of the upper limb such as the motor functions of the hand, and some authors even mention the importance of restoring elbow extension [10].

2. Surgical techniques on brachial plexus surgery

The management of BPI is complex and there is more than one way of approaching it surgically. The alternatives for treatment include surgical neurolysis, end-to-end sutures, nerve grafting, nerve transfers, muscle/tendon transfers, and a combination of them (multiple interventions) [7]. Surgical success depends on several factors such as the patient's age, patterns of injury, severity of injury, timing of surgery, surgical technique, quality of the donor nerves, and length of nerve grafts, among others [11, 12]. Prospective, randomized controlled clinical trials that compared all the surgical repair strategies for BPI and their clinical outcomes have not been performed. Therefore, some considerations continue to generate uncertainty in surgical decision-making. For this reason, we consider it appropriate to evaluate if the current perception of effectiveness in terms of motor recovery of all surgical techniques is correct and guide the development of new studies on the subject.

The surgical treatment of BPI is based on a combination of evidence-based practice, feasibility, and the personal experience of the surgeon [12]. Prominent surgeons around the world have proposed different treatment algorithms that are likely based on multiple factors that include things such as patient populations, body mass index, insurance status, socioeconomic status, mechanisms of injury, injury patterns, location, and severity, among other relevant factors [13, 14].

2.1 Surgical Neurolysis

Surgical neurolysis is a technique that began to be used in the World War by exploration of the wound and wide debridement of the affected nerve [15]. The purpose of surgical neurolysis is to decompress the affected nerve structures. Neurolysis consists of making multiple longitudinal cuts along the epineurium and dissecting the connective tissue that surrounds the injured nerve structures, lysing the adhesions formed in the compartment [16].

In 1996, Clarke et al. [17] reported a study without a control group where they determined that neurolysis did not represent significant clinical changes compared to spontaneous recovery. It was a transcendent study because it ended up defining neurolysis as an ineffective technique for the management of BPI, this argument added to the popularization of nerve transfer and nerve graft, led to the abandonment of surgical neurolysis and decreasing the number of clinical studies carried out on this technique. However, Morgan R. et al. (2020) recently reported the results of a study using surgical neurolysis for 21 adult patients with post-traumatic BPI, observing that some patients achieved a BMRC rating score > 3 in elbow flexion after surgery [18]. The mechanism of symptomatology in the patients included in the study of Morgan R. is probably explained by the connective tissue that surrounds the nerve structures, generating a compressive phenomenon that causes strangulation of the nerve [19, 20]. Therefore, we can assume that surgical neurolysis can be effective in some specific cases. The results shown by this study and the results showed by Morgan R. support the need to reevaluate neurolysis alone as a surgical technique for the functional restorations of patients with BPI, through a well-controlled study, where it seems to be useful for those patients with post-traumatic compressive neuropathy.

2.2 End-to-end suture

End-to-end suture is a surgical technique that consists of directly confronting the free edges of the transected nerve structure by using a suture to conserve continuity. This alternative is useful in cases of neural transaction when it is possible to face the limits without causing tension (<1–2 cm) [21]. The material commonly used to repair the damage is a monofilament like interrupted nylon or polypropylene suture (6–0 to 8–0) [22]. It is imperative that the surgeon must perform the suture taking into consideration the anatomical alignment of the nerve bundles [22]. Other possible applications according to Kim et al. for transected nerves when there is no nerve action potential and the procedure is to dissect sharply the proximal and distal stumps, with adequate cross-sections approach the nerve endings avoiding excessive tension in the suture site. In acute partial lacerations (72 hours) end to end improved functional outcomes in 73% over a population of 22 patients with 16 patients that achieve grade 3 function as a primary repair [22].

2.3 Nerve graft and nerve transfer

Nerve grafts and nerve transfer are other surgical alternatives that surgeons often use to treat BPI. A systematic review published by Garg et al. shows that the data strongly favors nerve transfer over traditional nerve grafting for the restoration of improved shoulder and elbow function in patients with complete traumatic upper BPI [23]. However, several articles show uncertain results. Hardcastle et al. published a systematic review where they compared nerve graft versus nerve transfer for the restoration of the shoulder abduction in traumatic brachial plexus palsy, observing that the proportion of functional recovery of shoulder function for nerve transfer was not statistically significant (OR 1.34, 95% CI: 0.27–6.72) compared with nerve transfer, establishing that nerve transfer and grafting are similarly effective in terms of shoulder abduction [24]. Other studies show controversial results in pediatric and adult populations [25, 26]. Therefore, the choice of the best treatment modality is still controversial. The evidence suggests that in upper trunk BPI in adults, the Oberlin procedure and other nerve transfer techniques are the more successful approaches to restoring elbow flexion and shoulder abduction compared with nerve grafting [27]. The decision between performing nerve graft versus nerve transfer is controversial in this context, a prospective, randomized; controlled trial would be necessary to evaluate the factors involved in clinical outcomes such as the pattern and location of injury.

2.4 Muscle and tendon transfer

The muscle/tendon transfer is more complex technique with higher morbidity, these types of techniques are usually indicated for patients with long-term evolution after injury (>6–12 months). The time interval between the injury and the surgical intervention is relevant because after 12–18 months of injury, the nerve regeneration is reduced [28]. Moreover, atrophy and fibrosis of muscles innervated by the affected nervous structure result in poor outcomes [29]. Therefore, muscle/tendon transfer should be considered for patients who have large evolution or patients without recovery after a primary intervention. Possibly the muscle/tendon transfers are the surgical techniques that have the best motor outcomes in severe injuries [30]. It is necessary to carry out new studies to evaluate whether this technique is adequate in patients with a recent injury (< 6 months), comparing its effectiveness and morbidity with other conventional techniques.

3. Materials and methods

3.1 Systematic review

This systematic review was carried out according to the Preferred Reporting Items for Systematic Reviews and Meta-Analyses (PRISMA) guidelines (PROSPERO ID: CRD42022296184) [31]. The selection criteria, search, and data extraction are summarized in **Figure 1**. The main objective of this search is to establish the magnitude of changes in motor status after surgical intervention in adult patients with BPI according to the type of intervention. A focused question was developed by the Patient population, Intervention, Control, Outcome (PICO) method: Do adult patients with BPI (patient population) undergoing surgery (intervention) have motor recovery (outcome), according to the type of surgical intervention (comparison)?

3.1.1 Eligibility criteria

According to prospectively deposited eligibility criteria, we included any reports of adult patients with a diagnosis of post-traumatic BPI who underwent primary surgical intervention in studies that reported pre- and post-operative motor clinical

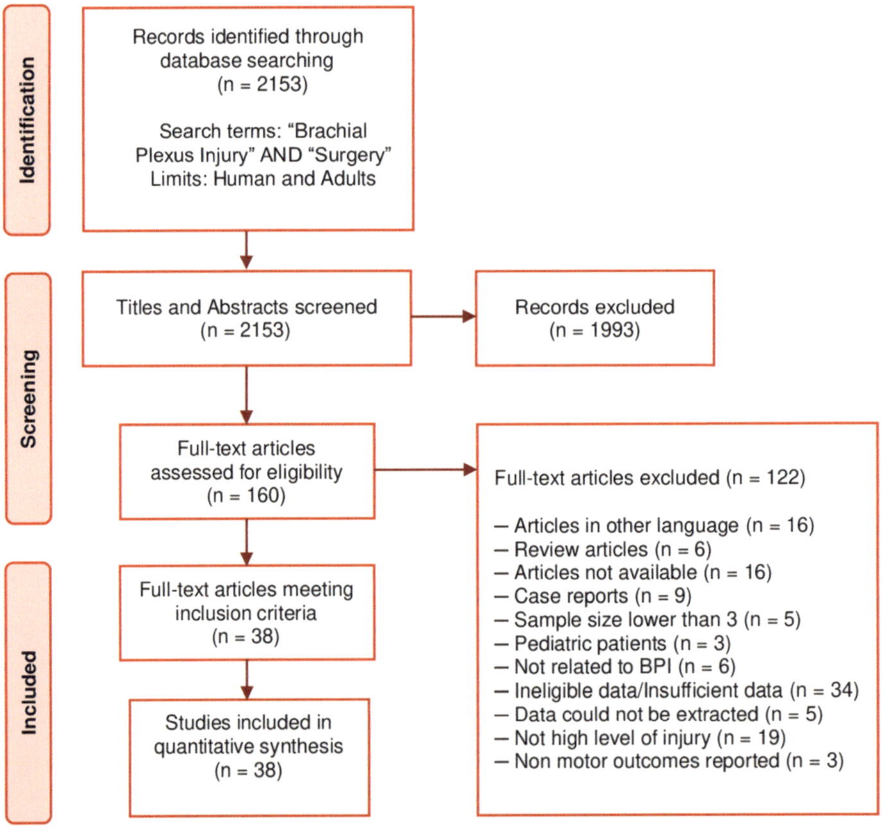

Figure 1.
Flow diagram according to PRISMA guidelines. Brachial plexus injury.

assessment. Conversely, we excluded pediatric populations (obstetric brachial plexus palsy), BPI with the intermediate or low location of injury (distal arm, elbow, forearm, wrist, and hand), case reports, publications with a population of n < 3, basic science research, article reviews, and publications written in other languages than English.

3.1.2 Search strategy

Studies were identified using the advanced search in PubMed with the Mesh terms "Brachial Plexus Injury" as the main topic and "Surgery" as a subtopic. We added "Humans" and "Adults" to avoid animal models and obstetric brachial plexus palsies (pediatric populations). For the "title" and "abstract" fields, 2153 total articles published between 1968 and 2021 were found. No constraints on study design, year of publication, or publication status were imposed. From the 2153 unique records identified by this search, screening for relevance by title and abstract resulted in 1993 articles being excluded. Of the remaining 160 articles selected for full-text evaluation, a total of 122 were excluded (**Figure 1**).

3.1.3 Data extraction

The final dataset consisted of 38 studies (**Table 1**) and was analyzed to extract specific parameters to be used for all subsequent analyses. During the first and second phases of the systematic review, the titles and abstracts were screened by two reviewers. If a clinic outcome was not mentioned in the abstracts, articles were excluded (A.S.A and G.J.A.I). During the last phase, full-text articles were evaluated by another author (C.R.J.D) and checked by two different reviewers (A.S.A and G.J.A.I). Disagreement between observers regarding the inclusion of publications was resolved through a consensus between different observers. The data extraction was focused on collecting data regarding the location of the injury, demographic (mean age and proportion of males), procedural (mean follow-up and interval injury-surgery), and motor status (pre- and postoperative).

Study (Author & Year)	Sample size (n)	Type of surgery	Type of Study*
Altaf F (2012) [32]	13	SN; MI	CS
Azab A (2017) [33]	13	MTT	CS
Baltzer H (2016) [34]	29	NG; NT	PS
Baltzer H (2016) [35]	51	NT	RS
Bertelli J (2016) [36]	13	NG	RS
Cambon A (2012) [37]	7	MTT	CS
Cambon A (2018) [38]	11	NT	RS
Coene L (1992) [39]	57	MI	RS
Cho A (2015) [40]	19	NT	RS
Dolan R (2011) [1]	21	NT	PS
Dubuisson A (2002) [41]	134	EE; SN; NT	RS
Elkwood A (2011) [42]	8	MTT	CS
Friedman A (1990) [43]	3	NG	CS

Study (Author & Year)	Sample size (n)	Type of surgery	Type of Study*
Frueh F (2016) [44]	6	NT	CS
Gao K (2013) [45]	22	NT	RS
Garcia A (2014) [46]	6	NT	CS
Gousheh J (1995) [21]	217	EE; NG; SN	RS
Gutkowska O (2017) [47]	33	SN	CS
Haninec P (2012) [48]	21	EE	CS
Jerome J (2012) [49]	15	NT	PS
Kachrama. C (2017) [50]	15	MTT	RS
Kim D (2003) [22]	42	EE; NG; SN	RS
Khalifa H (2012) [51]	24	NG; NT	RS
Laubscher M (2015) [52]	27	EE	RS
Lee Y (2008) [53]	6	NG	CS
Li G (2019) [11]	465	EE; MTT; NG; SN; NT	RS
Malessy M (1998) [54]	25	NT	CS
Maldonado A (2017) [55]	65	MTT:MI	RS
Moor B (2010) [56]	12	NG	PS
Nicoson M (2016) [57]	13	MTT	RS
Roganovic Z (2004) [58]	131	NG	RS
Roganovic Z (2005) [59]	81	NG	RS
Roganovic Z (2007) [60]	9	NG	RS
Sallam A (2017) [61]	52	NG; NT	RS
Soldado F (2016) [28]	8	NT	RS
Stewart M (2001) [62]	59	NG; SN	RS
Stockinger T (2008) [63]	6	NT	RS
Wolfe S (2014) [64]	10	NG	RS

**The studies included were non-controlled, non-randomized before and after studies (quasi-experimental studies). SN: Surgical neurolysis. EE: End-to-end suture. NG: Nerve graft. NT: Nerve transfer. MTT: Muscle/tendon transfer. MI: Multiple interventions (different surgical approaches performed on the same patient). CS: Case series. RS: Retrospective study. PS: Prospective study.*

Table 1.
Studies included.

3.1.4 Quality assessment

All articles included in this work were graded independently by two reviewers (A.S.A and G.J.A.I) and subsequently reviewed by the same authors in a consensus meeting using the Newcastle Ottawa Quality assessment tool [65, 66], for assessing the quality of the included studies and was adapted for the evaluation of motor recovery in BPI. The following characteristics were considered for the evaluation: representativeness of the study, mechanism of injury, injury location, surgical technique description, preoperative motor status, postoperative motor outcome, motor evaluation according to BMRC, follow-up, mortality/morbidity. Three subjective qualitative categories were used to define quality, no concerns (NC), unclear (U), and many concerns (MC). Disagreements were resolved by consensus.

3.1.5 Outcomes

Motor recovery was collected using the British Medical Research Council (BMRC) motor rating scale, considering the results reported in the included studies before and after the intervention using this tool. Brachial plexus surgery focuses on elbow flexion recovery and shoulder abduction, depending on the characteristics of the injury. Therefore, the data from the evaluation of two muscle structures were collected mainly, the biceps brachii and the deltoid, wherein those cases in which both outcomes were reported, elbow flexion was prioritized to define the outcome of the patient. Effective motor recovery was established in any patient who showed a BMRC ≥3 after the intervention. It was decided to defer the evaluation of ROM because it is intended to establish that surgical techniques have a more significant impact on the exclusive recovery of strength, regardless of joint stability. In order to increase the sample size of sub-groups, those articles that reported different types of surgical interventions (mixed studies), were divided into subgroups according to the type of surgical intervention performed (nerve transfer, nerve graft, muscle/tendon transfer, end-to-end suture, surgical neurolysis, and multiple interventions (different surgical techniques performed in the same patient)).

3.1.6 Data analysis

Statistical analyses were conducted using SPSS 25.0 for Windows software (SPSS, Inc., Chicago, IL). There are no complete clinical trials (controlled, randomized, and blinded) reported about each of the surgical techniques included in the analysis. For this reason, it was decided to include noncontrolled studies, where despite being studies that do not have a control group, they are valid for the analysis because the patients are being considered a self-control group, evaluating themselves before and after the surgical intervention. To calculate the effect size, contingency tables were created using two variables for motor outcome according to BMRC: motor recovery (≥M3), and absence of motor recovery (<M2), considering these variables for the group of patients before and after surgery. The effect size measure used was relative risk (RR). To define whether there was a statistically significant association between motor recovery and surgery, a 95% confidence interval (CI) was calculated for each effect size, this analysis was done for each article/subgroup and the results were graphed in a Forrest plot using the Review Manager Software from Cochrane (V.5.4.1) [67]. A p-value <0.05 was considered statistically significant.

3.2 Results

Table 1 provides a summary of the characteristics of the 38 articles that were included in the quantitative analysis. There were 34 retrospective studies (including 11 case series) and four prospective noncontrolled, nonrandomized studies. Regarding demographic and procedural factors these were the results: mean age 29.95 ± 5.27, percentage of males 88.1%, mean follow-up in months 33.31 ± 17.17, and mean interval injury-surgery in months 7.23 ± 4.5. Relative to the analysis of the quality of the publications, the following results were obtained are shown in **Figure 2**. Location of the injuries was represented to be mostly infraclavicular in 70.86% of the cases affecting

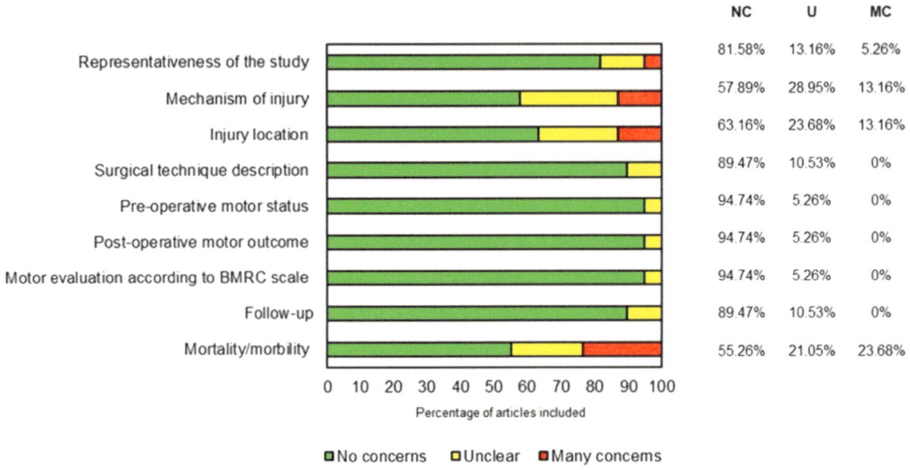

Figure 2.
Overall quality of included studies.

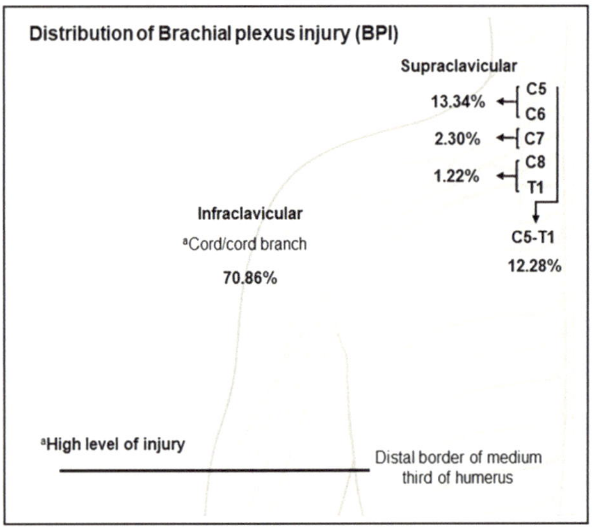

Figure 3.
Patterns of injury of the brachial plexus injuries included in the analysis.

cords or terminal branches of the brachial plexus at high level of injury (**Figure 3**). **Table 2** shows the demographic and procedural characteristics of the included studies according to the type of intervention.

3.2.1 Motor recovery

The priority in BPI motor recovery is commonly focused on restoring elbow flexion. According to the search for functional results in surgical management, the main therapeutic objective of the included studies was the re-establishment of elbow flexion of 31.58%, followed by shoulder abduction (28.95%), global motor recovery

Factor	Nerve Transfer Mean ± SD (n = 501)	Nerve Graft Mean ± SD (n = 566)	Muscle/ tendon transfer Mean ± SD (n = 118)	End-to-end suture Mean ± SD (n = 216)	Surgical Neurolysis Mean ± SD (n = 251)	*Multiple interventions Mean ± SD (n = 97)
Age (yrs)	30.58 ± 5.76	30.33 ± 4.59	29.92 ± 3.87	27.41 ± 4.5	29.81 ± 9.2	31.6 ± 3.55
Number of males	85.91 ± 11.83	89.13 ± 12.71	89.19 ± 7.8	87.71 ± 7.12	89.75 ± 8.85	90 ± 10
Length of follow-up (mos)	34.36 ± 3.54	33.66 ± 15.75	33.56 ± 19.77	33.71 ± 19.09	36.54 ± 21.07	18.33 ± 17.38
Injury-to-surgery period (mos)	7.36 ± 4.18	6.98 ± 4.08	10.23 ± 7.77	4.43 ± 2.98	6.18 ± 1.84	6.6 ± 1.9

**Multiple interventions: Different surgical techniques performed in the same patient.*

Table 2.
Demographic and procedural factors from BPI surgical groups.

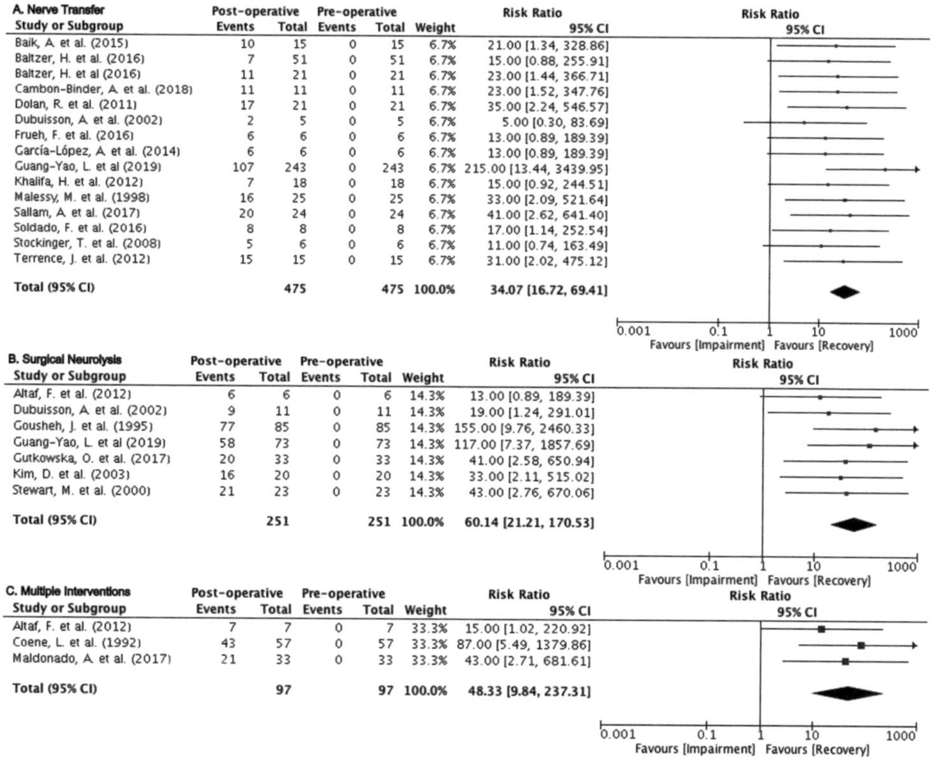

Figure 4.
Forrest plot of motor outcomes for patients with BPI after different types of surgical techniques. Proportions of patients reaching British Medical Research Council grade 3 (BMRC) or higher (≥M3) and corresponding 95 percent confidence intervals (CI); black diamonds represent the pooled proportions (PP) and corresponding 95 percent intervals, where those effect measures that are closer to zero represent the types of surgical intervention that most favors the motor recovery (≥M3) after the intervention. A. Nerve transfer PP (RR: 34.07 (CI: 16.72–69.41)). B. Surgical neurolysis PP (RR: 60.14 (CI: 21.21–170.53)). C. Multiple interventions PP (RR: 48.33 (CI: 9.84–170.53)).

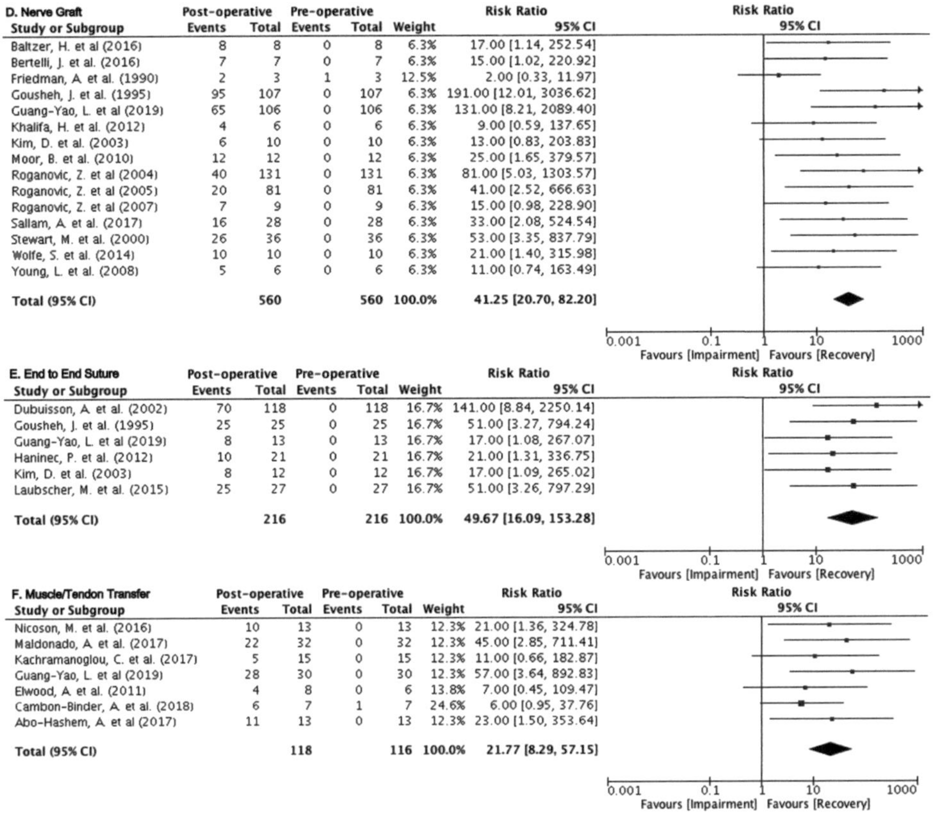

Figure 5.
Forrest plot of outcomes for patients with BPI after different types of surgical techniques. Proportions of patients reaching British Medical Research Council grade 3 (BMRC) or higher (≥M3) and corresponding 95 percent confidence intervals (CI); black diamonds represent the pooled proportions (PP) and corresponding 95 percent intervals, where those effect measures that are closer to zero represent the types of surgical intervention that most favors the motor recovery (≥M3) after the intervention. D. Nerve graft PP (RR: 41.25 (CI: 20.70–82.20)). E. End-to-end PP (RR: 49.67 (CI: 16.09–153.28)). F. Muscle/tendon transfer PP (RR: 21.77 (CI: 8.29–57.15)).

(23.68%), handgrip (15.79%), external rotation (2.63%), and elbow extension (2.63%). Regarding the outcome variable defined as motor recovery, this was defined as any patient who showed a recovery of strength after surgery ≥M3 according to BMRC. **Figures 4** and **5** shows the effect sizes (RR) and CI of the different articles and subgroups according to the type of surgical intervention. The results according to the type of surgery are the following: surgical neurolysis group (RR: 60.14 (CI: 21.21–170.53)), end-to-end suture (RR: 49.67 (CI: 16.09–153.28)), multiple interventions (RR: 48.33 (CI: 9.84–237.31)), nerve graft (RR: 41.25 (CI: 20.70–82.20)), nerve transfer (RR: 34.07 (CI: 16.72–69.41)) and muscle/tendon transfer (RR: 21.77 (CI: 8.29–57.15)).

4. Discussion

According to the information presented in this chapter, we conclude that all the surgical technics improve motor recovery in brachial plexus injuries. However, the clinical aspects, the time of lesion and the surgeon's abilities and expertise are the keys to decision-making. Our experience in this field allows us to define that the surgical management of BPI should be carried out progressively, starting with simple interventions (surgical neurolysis and end-to-end suture) and making them increasingly complex according to the severity and location of the injury (nerve graft, nerve transfer, and muscle/tendon transfer).

The surgery should follow the next principles: surgical neurolysis should be performed in some patients with preservation of nerve continuity and conduction that presents compressive neuropathy. End-to-end suture is preferred if the defect is too large to be anastomosed without tension directly. In large defects, nerve grafts should be performed, with direct intraplexal repair. If necessary, utilize the sural nerve, radial nerve (superficial branch), or the medial cutaneous nerve. After 6–12 months postinjury, the nerve regenerative capacity is reduced, and thus, the muscle fibrosis and degeneration. For this reason, muscle/tendon transfer should be considered in order to use a healthy muscle and fresh nerve transfer.

The main limitation of this study is that no heterogeneity tests were performed to assess which of the different surgical techniques have a greater motor recovery. However, a meta-analysis requires other fundamental factors needed to be involved in the data synthesis (demographic, socioeconomic, surgical injury interval, severity, pattern of the lesion, location, and extent of the injury, among others). Unfortunately, this was not possible in this study because many of the articles on the subject were reported in a nonstandardized way omitting some data, so it was impossible to include all of them. Second, the articles considered were case series and some nonrandomized and noncontrolled studies (Level of evidence III-IV). According with the last paragraph we highlight the need to develop a study that contains the methodological and demographical information mentioned before. There are a few clinical trials on brachial plexus surgery with a lack of high methodological rigor, highlighting the need to increase the level of scientific evidence in the production related to this topic [7, 16].

Čebron U. et al. (2021) evaluated the most frequently cited articles according to the type of surgery relative to adult BPI, observing that in the last 30 years, the most cited articles are related to nerve transfer, nerve graft, and muscle/tendon transfer [68]. For that reason, in recent years, the study of techniques such as surgical neurolysis and end-to-end suture has been abandoned considerably. Accordingly, our study highlights the need to retake the study of these techniques by comparing them with current trends in surgical management, because these displaced techniques show effective results in terms of motor recovery.

5. Conclusion

This study, beyond comparing the effectiveness of the different techniques, shows that they are all effective for motor recovery. Therefore, it is necessary to reassess those that have been displaced over time (surgical neurolysis and end-to-end suture), added to the popularization of new techniques (nerve transfer and muscle/tendon transfer). Conversely, these results highlight the need to increase the level of evidence and methodological rigor in the literature related to brachial plexus surgery, carrying out well-powered, well-controlled, and well-randomized studies to have clearer knowledge about the precise indications of each one of these surgical alternatives in the management of BPI.

Conflict of interest

The authors declare no conflict of interest.

Permissions

The permission to use the images/materials included in this study has been obtained.

Acronyms and abbreviations

BMRC	British Medical Research Council motor grading scale
BPI	Brachial Plexus Injury
DASH	Disability of the Arm Shoulder and Hand questionnaire
MC	Many Concerns
NC	Not Clear
PICO	Patient population, Intervention, Control, Outcome
PRISMA	Preferred Reporting Items for Systematic Reviews and Meta-Analyses
ROM	Range of Motion
U	Unclear

Author details

Armando Armas-Salazar[1,2], Fátima Ximena Cid-Rodríguez[2,3], José Luis Navarro-Olvera[2], Edgar Abarca-Rojano[1], Noé Tellez-León[4], María de la Luz Montes-Castillo[4], Ana Isabel García-Jerónimo[5] and José Damián Carrillo-Ruiz[2,6,7]*

1 Postgraduate Department, School of Higher Education in Medicine, National Polytechnic Institute, Mexico City, Mexico

2 Functional and Stereotactic Neurosurgery and Radiosurgery Service, General Hospital of Mexico, Mexico City, Mexico

3 Faculty of Medicine, Popular Autonomous University of the State of Puebla, Puebla, Mexico

4 Physical Medicine and Rehabilitation Service of the General Hospital of Mexico, Mexico City, Mexico

5 Epidemiology Service of the General Hospital of Mexico, Mexico City, Mexico

6 Research Direction of the General Hospital of Mexico, Mexico City, Mexico

7 Faculty of Health Sciences, Direction of Anahuac University Mexico, Mexico City, Mexico

*Address all correspondence to: josecarrilloruiz@yahoo.com

References

[1] Dolan RT, Butler JS, Murphy SM, Hynes D, Cronin KJ. Health-related quality of life and functional outcomes following nerve transfers for traumatic upper brachial plexus injuries. The Journal of Hand Surgery: European Volume. 2011;**37**(7):642-651. DOI: 10.1177/1753193411432706

[2] Armas-Salazar A, García-Jerónimo AI, Villegas-López FA, Navarro-Olvera JL, Carrillo-Ruiz JD. Clinical outcomes report in different brachial plexus injury surgeries: a systematic review. Neurosurgical Review. 2022;**45**(1):411-419. DOI: 10.1007/s10143-021-01574-6

[3] Dy CJ, Garg R, Lee SK, Tow P, Mancuso CA, Wolfe SW. A systematic review of outcomes reporting for brachial plexus reconstruction. The Journal of Hand Surgery. 2015;**40**(2):308-313. DOI: 10.1016/j.jhsa.2014.10.033

[4] Holdenries M, Schenck TL, Akpaloo J, Muller-Felber W, Holzbach T, Giunta RE. Quality of life after brachial plexus lesions in adults. Handchirurgie, Mikrochirurgie, Plastische Chirurgie. 2013;**45**:229-234. DOI: 10.1055/s-0033-1353161

[5] James MA. Use of the Medical Research Council muscle strength grading system in the upper extremity. The Journal of Hand Surgery. 2007;**32**(2):154-156. DOI: 10.1016/j.jhsa.2006.11.008

[6] Lea RD, Gerhardt JJ. Range-of-motion measurements. The Journal of Bone and Joint Surgery. American Volume. 1995;**77**(5):784-798. DOI: 10.2106/00004623-199505000-00017

[7] Martins RS, Siqueira MG, Heise CO, Foroni L, Teixeira MJ. A prospective study comparing single and double fascicular transfer to restore elbow flexion after brachial plexus injury. Neurosurgery. 2013;**72**(5):709-715. DOI: 10.1227/NEU.0b013e318285c3f6

[8] Paternostro-Sluga T, Grim-Stieger M, Posch M, Schuhfried O, Vacariu G, Mittermaier C, et al. Reliability and validity of the Medical Research Council (MRC) scale and a modified scale for testing muscle strength in patients with radial palsy. Journal of Rehabilitation Medicine. 2008;**40**(8):665-671. DOI: 10.2340/16501977-0235

[9] Brophy RH, Wolfe SW. Planning brachial plexus surgery: Treatment options and priorities. Hand Clinics. 2005;**21**(1):47-54. DOI: 10.1016/j.hcl.2004.09.007

[10] Gribble PL, Mullin LI, Cothros N, Mattar A. Role of cocontraction in arm movement accuracy. Journal of Neurophysiology. 2003;**89**(5):2396-2405. DOI: 10.1152/jn.01020.2002

[11] Li GY, Xue MQ, Wang JW, Zeng XY, Qin J, Sha K. Traumatic brachial plexus injury: A study of 510 surgical cases from multicenter services in Guangxi, China. Acta Neurochirurgica. 2019;**161**(5):899-906. DOI: 10.1007/s00701-019-03871-y

[12] Limthongthang R, Bachoura A, Songcharoen P, Osterman AL. Adult brachial plexus injury: Evaluation and management. The Orthopedic Clinics of North America. 2013;**44**(4):591-603. DOI: 10.1016/j.ocl.2013.06.011

[13] Kliot M, Socolovsky M, Rasulic L, Midha R, Garozzo D. Manual of peripheral nerve surgery: From the basics to complex procedures. Acta Neurochirurgica. 2018;**160**(3):663. DOI: 10.1007/s00701-017-3450-3

[14] Shin AY, Socolovsky M, Desai K, Fox M, Wang S, Spinner RJ. Differences in management and treatment of traumatic adult pan brachial plexus injuries: a global perspective regarding continental variations. The Journal of Hand Surgery: European Volume. 2022;**47**(1):40-51. DOI: 10.1177/17531934211039677

[15] Midha R, Grochmal J. Surgery for nerve injury: Current and future perspectives. Journal of Neurosurgery. 2019;**130**(3):675-685. DOI: 10.3171/2018.11.JNS181520

[16] Andrisevic E, Taniguchi M, Partington MD, Agel J, Van Heest AE. Neurolysis alone as the treatment for neuroma-in-continuity with more than 50% conduction in infants with upper trunk brachial plexus birth palsy. Journal of Neurosurgery. Pediatrics. 2014;**13**(2):229-237. DOI: 10.3171/2013.10.PEDS1345

[17] Clarke HM, Al-Qattan MM, Curtis CG, Zuker RM. Obstetrical brachial plexus palsy: Results following neurolysis of conducting neuromas-in-continuity. Plastic and Reconstructive Surgery. 1996;**97**(5):974-982. DOI: 10.1097/00006534-199604001-00014

[18] Morgan R, Elliot I, Banala V, Dy C, Harris B, Ouellette EA. Pain relief after surgical decompression of the distal brachial plexus. Journal of Brachial Plexus and Peripheral Nerve Injury. 2020;**15**(1):22-32. DOI: 10.1055/s-0040-1716718

[19] Quintão NL, Santos AR, Campos MM, Calixto JB. The role of neurotrophic factors in genesis and maintenance of mechanical hypernociception after brachial plexus avulsion in mice. Pain. 2008;**136**(1-2):125-133. DOI: 10.1016/j.pain.2007.06.027

[20] Sikandar S, Minett MS, Millet Q, Santana-Varela S, Lau J, Wood JN, et al. Brain-derived neurotrophic factor derived from sensory neurons plays a critical role in chronic pain. Brain. 2018;**141**(4):1028-1039. DOI: 10.1093/brain/awy009

[21] Gousheh J. The treatment of war injuries of the brachial plexus. The Journal of Hand Surgery. 1995;**20**(3):68-76. DOI: 10.1016/s0363-5023(95)80173-1

[22] Kim DH, Han K, Tiel RL, Murovic JA, Kline DG. Surgical outcomes of 654 ulnar nerve lesions. Journal of Neurosurgery. 2003;**98**(5):993-1004. DOI: 10.3171/jns.2003.98.5.0993

[23] Garg R, Merrell GA, Hillstrom HJ, Wolfe SW. Comparison of nerve transfers and nerve grafting for traumatic upper plexus palsy: A systematic review and analysis. The Journal of Bone and Joint Surgery. American Volume. 2011;**93**(9):819-829. DOI: 10.2106/JBJS.I.01602

[24] Hardcastle N, Texakalidis P, Nagarajan P, Tora MS, Boulis NM. Recovery of shoulder abduction in traumatic brachial plexus palsy: A systematic review and meta-analysis of nerve transfer versus nerve graft. Neurosurgical Review. 2020;**43**(3):951-956. DOI: 10.1007/s10143-019-01100-9

[25] Simic V, Savic A, Jovanovic M, Vitosevic F, Djurovic B, Milosevic C, et al. Nerve grafting versus common Infraclavicular Intraplexal nerve transfer in elbow flexion restoration. Turkish Neurosurgery. 2018;**28**(4):636-644. DOI: 10.5137/1019-5149.JTN.20296-17.2

[26] Tora MS, Hardcastle N, Texakalidis P, Wetzel J, Chern JJ. Elbow flexion in neonatal brachial plexus palsy: A meta-analysis of graft versus transfer. Child's Nervous System. 2019;**35**(6):929-935

[27] Ali ZS, Heuer GG, Faught RW, Kaneriya SH, Sheikh UA, Syed IS, et al. Upper brachial plexus injury in adults: Comparative effectiveness of different repair techniques. Journal of Neurosurgery. 2015;**122**(1):195-201. DOI: 10.1007/s00381-019-04133-z

[28] Soldado F, Ghizoni MF, Bertelli J. Thoracodorsal nerve transfer for triceps reinnervation in partial brachial plexus injuries. Microsurgery. 2015;**36**(3):191-197. DOI: 10.1002/micr.22386

[29] Gordon T, Tyreman N, Raji MA. The basis for diminished functional recovery after delayed peripheral nerve repair. The Journal of Neuroscience. 2011;**31**:5325-5334. DOI: 10.1523/JNEUROSCI.6156-10.2011

[30] Hoang D, Chen VW, Seruya M. Recovery of elbow flexion after nerve reconstruction versus free functional muscle transfer for late, traumatic brachial plexus palsy: A systematic review. Plastic and Reconstructive Surgery. 2018;**141**:949-959. DOI: 10.1097/PRS.0000000000004229

[31] McInnes MDF, Moher D, Thombs BD, McGrath TA. Bossuyt PM; and the PRISMA-DTA group, Clifford T, et al. preferred reporting items for a systematic review and meta-analysis of diagnostic test accuracy studies: The PRISMA-DTA statement. JAMA. 2018;**319**(4):388-396. DOI: 10.1001/jama.2017.19163

[32] Altaf F, Mannan K, Bharania P, Sewell MD, Di Mascio L, Sinisi M. Severe brachial plexus injuries in rugby. Injury. 2012;**43**(3):272-273. DOI: 10.1016/j.injury.2011.04.001

[33] Azab A, A-H, Alsabbahi MS. Bipolar transfer of latissimus Dorsi Myocutaneous flap for restoration of elbow flexion in late traumatic brachial plexus injury. Annals of Plastic Surgery. 2017;**78**(2):198-201. DOI: 10.1097/SAP.0000000000000907

[34] Baltzer HL, Kircher MF, Spinner RJ, Bishop AT, Shin AY. A comparison of outcomes of triceps motor branch–to–axillary nerve transfer or sural nerve Interpositional grafting for isolated axillary nerve injury. Plastic and Reconstructive Surgery. 2016;**138**(2):256-264. DOI: 10.1097/PRS.0000000000002368

[35] Baltzer HL, Wagner ER, Kircher MF, Spinner RJ, Bishop AT, Shin AY. Evaluation of infraspinatus reinnervation and function following spinal accessory nerve to suprascapular nerve transfer in adult traumatic brachial plexus injuries. Microsurgery. 2016;**37**(5):365-370. DOI: 10.1002/micr.30070

[36] Bertelli JA, Ghizoni MF. Results of nerve grafting in radial nerve injuries occurring proximal to the humerus, including those within the posterior cord. Journal of Neurosurgery. 2016;**1**:179-185. DOI: 10.3171/2014.12.JNS141944.test

[37] Cambon-Binder A, Belkheyar Z, Durand S, Rantissi M, Oberlin C. Elbow flexion restoration using pedicled latissimus dorsi transfer in seven cases. Chirurgie de la Main. 2012;**31**(6):324-330. DOI: 10.1016/j.main.2012.10.169

[38] Cambon-Binder A, Preure L, Dubert-Khalifa H, Marcheix PS, Belkheyar Z. Spinal accessory nerve repair using a direct nerve transfer from the upper trunk: Results with 2 years follow-up. The Journal of Hand Surgery: European Volume. 2018;**43**(6):589-595. DOI: 10.1177/1753193418755618

[39] Coene LNJEM, Narakas AO. Operative management of lesions of the axillary nerve, isolated or combined with

other nerve lesions. Clinical Neurology and Neurosurgery. 1992;**94**:64-66. DOI: 10.1016/0303-8467(92)90025-x

[40] Cho AB, Iamaguchi RB, Bersani Silva G, Paulos RG, Kiyohara LY, Sorrenti L, et al. Intercostal nerve transfer to the biceps motor branch in complete traumatic brachial plexus injuries. Microsurgery. 2015;**35**(6):428-431. DOI: 10.1002/micr.22453

[41] Dubuisson AS, Kline DG. Brachial plexus injury: A survey of 100 consecutive cases from a single service. Neurosurgery. 2002;**51**(3):673-683. DOI: 10.1227/01.NEU.0000023600.59365.41

[42] Elkwood AI, Holland NR, Arbes SM, Rose MI, Kaufman MR, Ashinoff RL, et al. Nerve allograft transplantation for functional restoration of the upper extremity: Case series. The Journal of Spinal Cord Medicine. 2011;**34**(2):241-247. DOI: 10.1179/107902611X12972448729521

[43] Friedman AH, Nunley JA, Urbaniak JR, Goldner RD. Repair of isolated axillary nerve lesions after infraclavicular brachial plexus injuries. Neurosurgery. 1990;**27**(3):403-407. DOI: 10.1097/00006123-199009000-00010

[44] Frueh FS, Ho M, Schiller A, Ducommun P, Manoliu A, Andreisek G, et al. Magnetic resonance Neurographic and clinical long-term results after Oberlin's transfer for adult brachial plexus injuries. Annals of Plastic Surgery. 2017;**78**(1):67-72. DOI: 10.1097/SAP.0000000000000924

[45] Gao K, Lao J, Zhao X, Gu Y. Outcome of contralateral C7 transfer to two recipient nerves in 22 patients with the total brachial plexus avulsion injury. Microsurgery. 2013;**33**(8):605-611. DOI: 10.1002/micr.22137

[46] García-López A, Navarro R, Martinez F, Rojas A. Nerve transfers from branches to the flexor carpi Radialis and pronator Teres to reconstruct the radial nerve. The Journal of Hand Surgery. 2014;**39**(1):50-56. DOI: 10.1016/j.jhsa.2013.10.011

[47] Gutkowska O, Martynkiewicz J, Mizia S, Bąk M, Gosk J. Results of operative treatment of brachial plexus injury resulting from shoulder dislocation: A study with A long-term follow-up. World Neurosurgery. 2017;**105**:623-631. DOI: 10.1016/j.wneu.2017.06.059

[48] Haninec P, Kaiser R. The end-to-side Neurorrhaphy in axillary nerve reconstruction in patients with brachial plexus palsy. Plastic and Reconstructive Surgery. 2012;**129**(5):882-883. DOI: 10.1097/PRS.0b013e31824b2a5b

[49] Jerome JTJ, Rajmohan B. Axillary nerve neurotization with the anterior deltopectoral approach in brachial plexus injuries. Microsurgery. 2012;**32**(6):445-451. DOI: 10.1002/micr.21973

[50] Kachramanoglou C, Carlstedt T, Koltzenburg M, Choi D. Long-term outcome of brachial plexus Reimplantation after complete brachial plexus avulsion injury. World Neurosurgery. 2017;**103**:28-36. DOI: 10.1016/j.wneu.2017.03.052

[51] Khalifa H, Belkheyar Z, Diverrez JP, Oberlin C. Results of 24 nerve repairs at more than one year post-injury. Chirurgie de la Main. 2012;**31**(6):318-323. DOI: 10.1016/j.main.2012.09.001

[52] Laubscher M, Held M, Maree M, Solomons M. Radial nerve lacerations --the outcome of end-to-end repairs in penetrating trauma. Hand Surgery. 2015;**20**(1):67-72. DOI: 10.1142/S0218810415500094

[53] Lee YH, Chung MS, Gong HS, Chung JY, Park JH, Baek GH. Sural nerve autografts for high radial nerve injury with nine centimeter or greater defects. The Journal of Hand Surgery. 2008;**33**(1):83-86. DOI: 10.1016/j.jhsa.2007.10.004

[54] Malessy MJA, Thomeer RTWM. Evaluation of intercostal to musculocutaneous nerve transfer in reconstructive brachial plexus surgery. Journal of Neurosurgery. 1998;**88**(2):266-271. DOI: 10.3171/jns.1998.88.2.0266

[55] Maldonado AA, Kircher MF, Spinner RJ, Bishop AT, Shin AY. Free functioning Gracilis muscle transfer with and without simultaneous intercostal nerve transfer to musculocutaneous nerve for restoration of elbow flexion after traumatic adult brachial pan-plexus injury. The Journal of Hand Surgery. 2017;**42**(4):293. DOI: 10.1016/j.jhsa.2017.01.014

[56] Moor BK, Haefeli M, Bouaicha S, Nagy L. Results after delayed axillary nerve reconstruction with interposition of sural nerve grafts. Journal of Shoulder and Elbow Surgery. 2010;**19**(3):461-466. DOI: 10.1016/j.jse.2009.07.011

[57] Nicoson MC, Franco MJ, Tung TH. Donor nerve sources in free functional gracilis muscle transfer for elbow flexion in adult brachial plexus injury. Microsurgery. 2016;**37**(5):377-382. DOI: 10.1002/micr.30120

[58] Roganovic Z, Petkovic S. Missile severances of the radial nerve. Results of 131 repairs. Acta Neurochirurgica. 2004;**146**(11):1185-1192. DOI: 10.1007/s00701-004-0361-x

[59] Roganovic Z. Missile-caused median nerve injuries: Results of 81 repairs. Surgical Neurology. 2005;**63**(5):410-418. DOI: 10.1016/j.surneu.2004.08.007

[60] Roganovic Z, Ilic S, Savic M. Radial nerve repair using an autologous denatured muscle graft: Comparison with outcomes of nerve graft repair. Acta Neurochirurgica. 2007;**149**(10):1033-1039. DOI: 10.1007/s00701-007-1269-z

[61] Sallam AA, El-Deeb MS, Imam MA. Nerve transfer versus nerve graft for reconstruction of high ulnar nerve injuries. The Journal of Hand Surgery. 2017;**42**(4):265-273. DOI: 10.1016/j.jhsa.2017.01.027

[62] Stewart MPM, Birch R. Penetrating missile injuries of the brachial plexus. Journal of Bone and Joint Surgery. British Volume (London). 2001;**83**(4):517-524. DOI: 10.1302/0301-620x.83b4.11583

[63] Stockinger T, Aszmann OC, Frey M. Clinical application of pectoral nerve transfers in the treatment of traumatic brachial plexus injuries. The Journal of Hand Surgery. 2008;**33**(7):1100-1107. DOI: 10.1016/j.jhsa.2008.03.010

[64] Wolfe SW, Johnsen PH, Lee SK, Feinberg JH. Long-nerve grafts and nerve transfers demonstrate comparable outcomes for axillary nerve injuries. The Journal of Hand Surgery. 2014;**39**(7):1351-1357. DOI: 10.1016/j.jhsa.2014.02.032

[65] Sneiders D, Bulstra LF, Hundepool CA, Treling WJ, Hovius SER, Shin AY. Outcomes of single versus double fascicular nerve transfers for restoration of elbow flexion in patients with brachial plexus injuries: A systematic review and meta-analysis. Plastic and Reconstructive Surgery. 2019;**144**(1):155-166. DOI: 10.1097/PRS.0000000000005720

[66] Zeng X, Zhang Y, Kwong JS, Zhang C, Li S, Sun F, et al. The methodological quality assessment tools for preclinical and clinical studies,

systematic review and meta-analysis, and clinical practice guideline: A systematic review. Journal of Evidence-Based Medicine. 2015;**8**(1):2-10. DOI: 10.1111/jebm.12141

[67] Review Manager (RevMan) [Computer program]. Version 5.4. The Cochrane Collaboration. 2020

[68] Čebron U, Mayer JA, Lu C, Daigeler A, Prahm C, Kolbenschlag J. Treatment trends of adult brachial plexus injury: A bibliometric analysis. Plastic and Reconstructive Surgery. Global Open. 2021;**9**(9):3803. DOI: 10.1097/GOX.0000000000003803

Chapter 10

Nerve Transfers in Adult Brachial Plexus Injuries

Raj Kumar Manas

Abstract

Brachial plexus injuries are semi-emergency conditions that require early intervention. Nerve transfers in adult brachial plexus injuries have become the standard treatment that gives reasonably good results if performed before the degeneration of muscle end plates. A clinical diagnosis based on clinical examinations supported by radiological and electrophysiological investigations is required that guides the specific procedures to be chosen. The surgeons must prioritize the objectives of reconstruction and keeping the different lifeboats for the use in future before choosing a specific nerve transfer. Also, it is important to be familiar with different nerve transfers so that one can select and perform a specific one based on pre-operative examinations and intraoperative findings of nerve stimulations. The author aims to describe the approach for exploring and dissecting the brachial plexus and different surgical techniques of nerve transfers used for different muscle reinnervations in different scenarios.

Keywords: nerve transfer, adult brachial plexus injury, brachial plexus exploration, nerve transfer for shoulder and elbow function, reconstruction in brachial plexus

1. Introduction

Brachial plexus injury is one of the most devastating conditions which (if not treated on time), can cause irreversible loss of functions of the upper limb.

Historically, the outcome of surgical interventions in brachial plexus injuries was not very promising until Millesi described the concept of nerve grafting and found that when a nerve is injured, a useful recovery can be achieved by microsurgery if the two ends of the nerve are repaired or reconstructed by nerve graft [1]. Later on, Narakas also showed better results supported by many other brachial plexus surgeons across the world [2]. The surgical management of the brachial plexus has improved over the past few decades due to advancements in microsurgery, a better understanding of nerve regeneration, and nerve coaptation techniques with nerve glue. Although Nerve grafting revolutionized the treatment of brachial plexus injury, this may not be always possible especially when there is root avulsion injury and when the gap between two cut ends of nerves is more.

Nerve transfers in the form of neurotizing the injured nerve or part of the brachial plexus with the healthy, uninjured nerve either intraplexal or extraplexal can give reasonably better results if performed on time. Various nerve surgeons described and evolved various nerve transfers which have become the standard of care in brachial plexus injuries. An earlier description of Neurotization or nerve transfer was described by A. Lurje in 1948 who identified several neurotizers as n. phrenicus, n. thoracalis longus, nn. thoracales anterior can be used to neurotize injured brachial plexus segments [3].

Oberlin in 1994 described using Flexor carpi ulnaris fascicle to neurotize the muscular branch of the musculocutaneous nerve to reinnervate the biceps and found M4 recovery [4]. Later on, it was modified to perform double innervations by coapting median nerve fascicles to the brachialis, the idea originally described by McKinnon [5]. Somsak Leechavengvongs in 2003 described transferring nerve to the long head of triceps to deltoid muscles in upper brachial plexus palsy which has shown excellent recovery of M4 power [6]. Although, the techniques described are simpler, replicable, and often give good results has received worldwide acceptance. But before planning a nerve transfer surgery for the brachial plexus, it is important to understand the integrity of which nerve is lost and which is preserved before planning for neurotization.

2. Nerve transfer

2.1 Prerequisite for successful nerve transfer

- The donor nerve or its fascicle to be transferred should be expandable [7, 8].
- The coaptation of the nerves from the donor to the recipient should be tension free and any nerve graft should be used selectively and avoided if possible
- The transfer should be close to the target muscles
- The transferred nerve should be pure motor if the aim of transfer is for motor recovery
- Donor nerve should have a maximum number of axons
- Early transfer gives better recovery
- There should be a complete passive range of motion across the joints before planning the nerve transfer.

2.2 Objective

A complete examination of the brachial plexus, understanding the relevant anatomy (**Figure 1**) with documentation is important that involves 58 muscles supplied by different nerves of the brachial plexus. Apart from the examination of the brachial plexus proper, it is important to evaluate what are the priorities of reconstruction (**Table 1**), available donors, and recipient's nerves to be neurotized to define aims and objectives for nerve transfers (**Table 2**).

2.3 Brachial plexus exploration

Brachial plexus is explored *under* general anesthesia [8, 9]. The surgeons must discuss with the anesthetist the duration of prolonged surgery, and the requirement of intraoperative nerve monitoring (in which case muscle relaxant is to be avoided or

DOI: http://dx.doi.org/10.5772/intechopen.110711

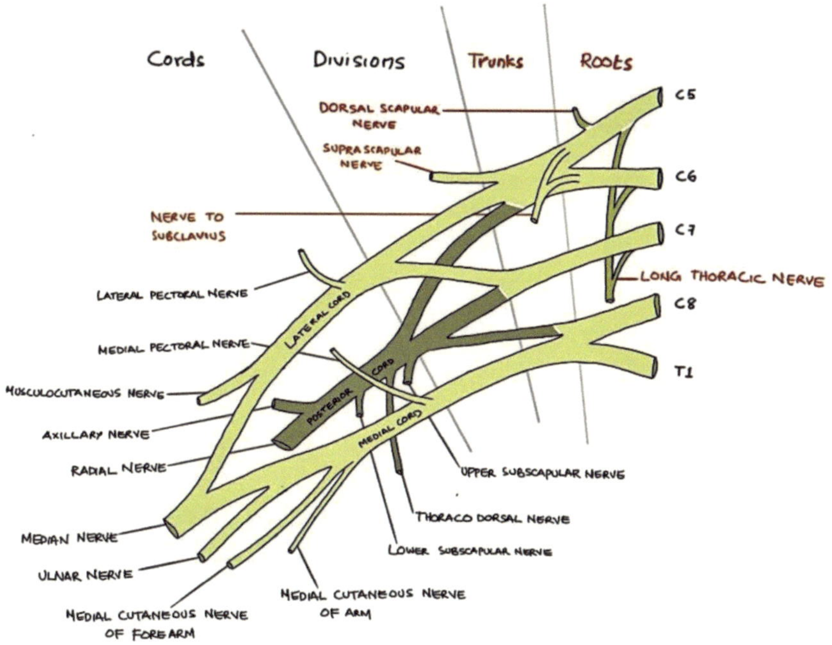

Figure 1.
Schematic diagram of Brachial Plexus (Sketched by Dr Jishnu).

Elbow flexion
Shoulder stability with shoulder abduction and external rotation
Hand and wrist flexion
Sensation of the hand
Elbow extension
Wrist & fingers extension
Recovery of Intrinsic muscles of hand

Table 1.
Objective of reconstruction (In decreasing order) [9].

is given in low dose only at the time of induction). Foleys catheterization is performed if one expects a longer duration of surgery.

The patient is *positioned* supine for supraclavicular brachial plexus exploration and a shoulder bag beneath the affected shoulder is placed. The entire upper limb is painted and exposed to see the muscle contraction. If one is planning to perform intercostal nerve or contralateral C7 nerve transfer, it is desired to prepare the chest and contralateral neck also. Same way, both legs are prepared for nerve graft if required.

2.4 Marking

Suprasternal notch, posterior border of the sternocleidomastoid, and if possible prominence of external jugular vein is marked **Figure 2**. Supraclavicular brachial plexus can be explored through either a transverse incision or a V-shaped incision.

For Shoulder		For Elbow		For Hand		For Sensation	
Donor	**Recipient**	**Donor**	**Recipient**	**Donor**	**Recipient**	**Donor**	**Recipients**
• SAN • Long head of triceps	• SSN • Axillary nerve	• Fascicle of Ulnar nerve • Fascicle of median nerve • ICN • SAN	• Biceps branch of MCN • Brachialis branch of MCN	CC7	Median nerve C8,T1	ICN, Intercosto-brachial nerve, Sensory branch of ICN	Lateral contribution of median nerve

SAN, Spinal accessory nerve; SSN, suprascapular nerve; ICN, intercostal nerve; MCN, musculocutaneous nerve; CC7, contralateral C7 nerve.

Table 2.
The different nerve transfers.

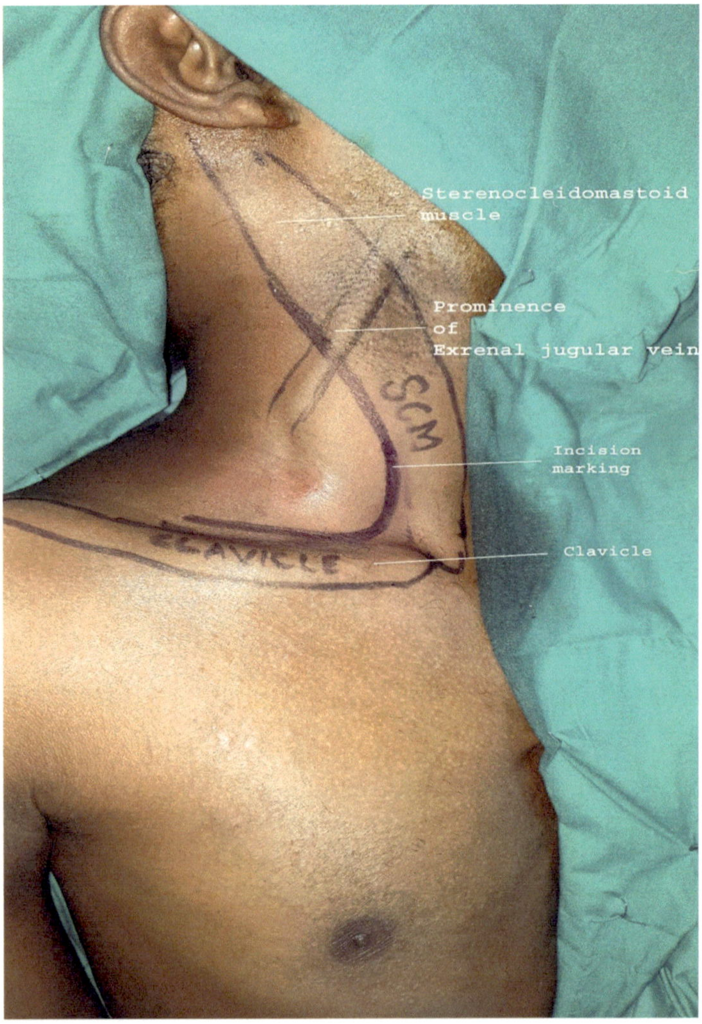

Figure 2.
Marking for exploration of brachial plexus.

DOI: http://dx.doi.org/10.5772/intechopen.110711

One limb of V is marked at the posterior border of the sternocleidomastoid, whereas the other is marked 1 cm above and parallel to the clavicle.

The marked incision line is infiltrated with 1:2 lakh adrenaline with saline. Once the incision is made over the marked line, the skin and platysma flap are elevated. In the upper portion of the incision, one will find the external jugular vein which is ligated. In the upper part of the neck, one will encounter several branches of the cervical plexus that may be confused with the spinal accessory nerve (**Figure 3**).

The spinal accessory nerve arises from the posterior border of the sterno-cleidomastoid, runs obliquely, and supplies to the trapezius giving multiple branches. In the lower parts, one gets a layer of fatty tissue which is raised as a triangular flap and is sutured back while closing the neck wound to reduce the dead space (**Figure 4**).

The transverse cervical artery is encountered in the lower part which can be preserved or clipped (**Figure 5**).

The Omohyoid muscle that runs transversely is divided and the first trunk of the brachial plexus is visualized that is upper trunk or the Erb's point. From the upper trunk, a suprascapular nerve will arise and the upper trunk further divides into anterior and posterior divisions.

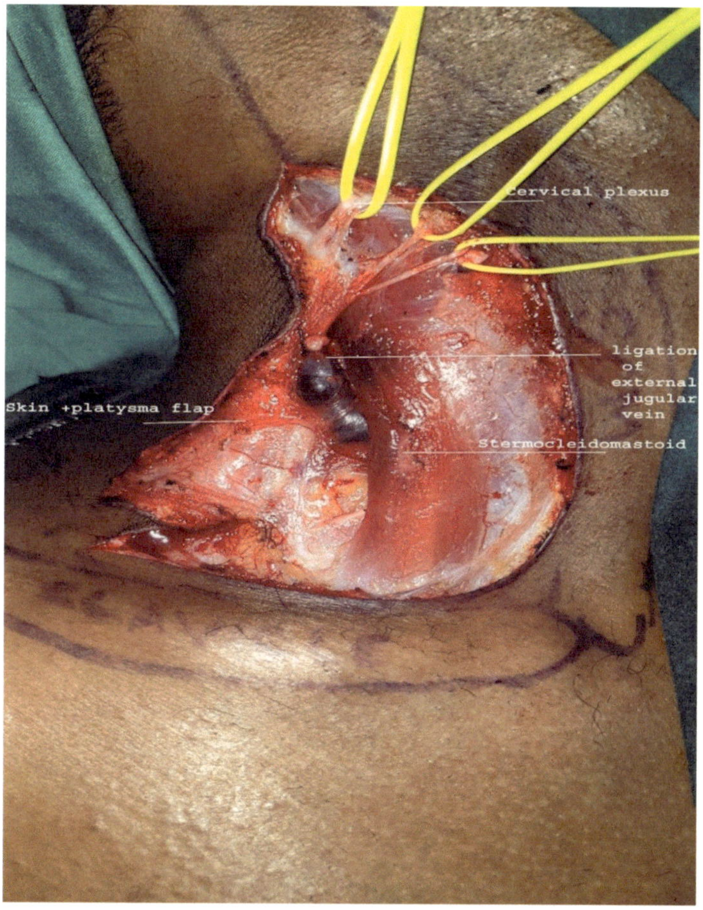

Figure 3.
Raising of skin platysma flap and preservation of cervical plexus.

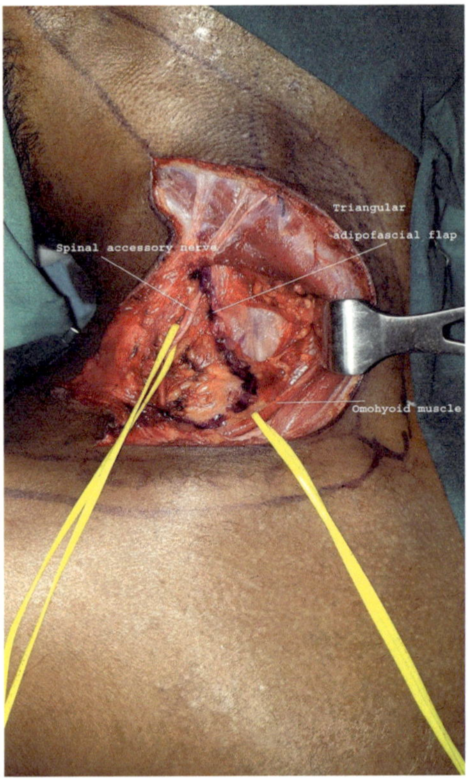

Figure 4.
marking for the adipo-fascial flap, dissection of spinal accessory nerve, and omohyoid muscle in the lower part.

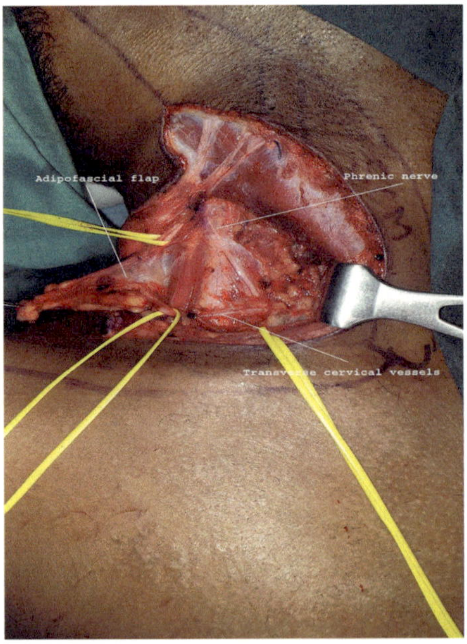

Figure 5.
raising of the adipo-fascial flap, dissecting phrenic nerve and transverse cervical vessels.

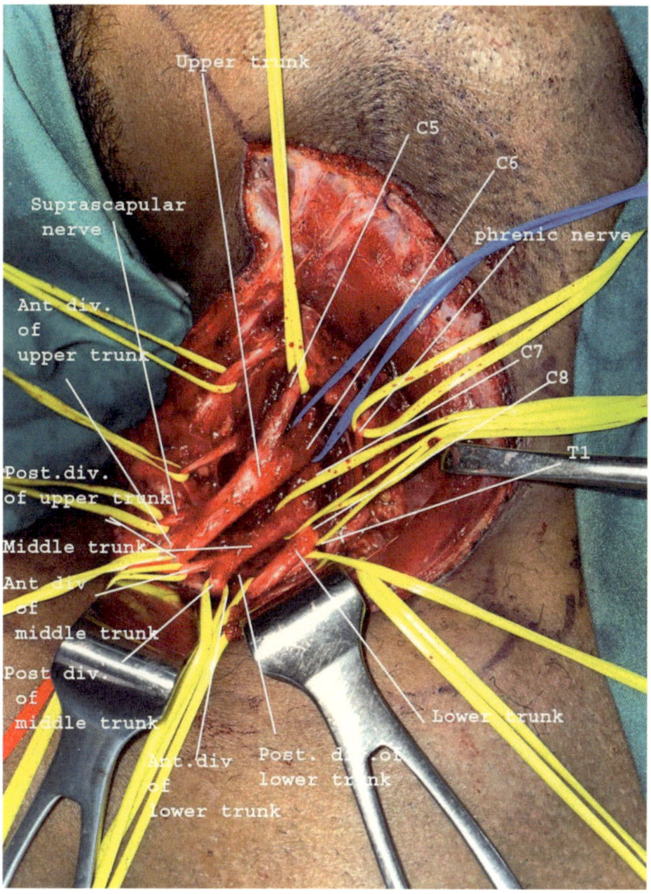

Figure 6.
Supraclavicular brachial plexus with roots, trunk & division.

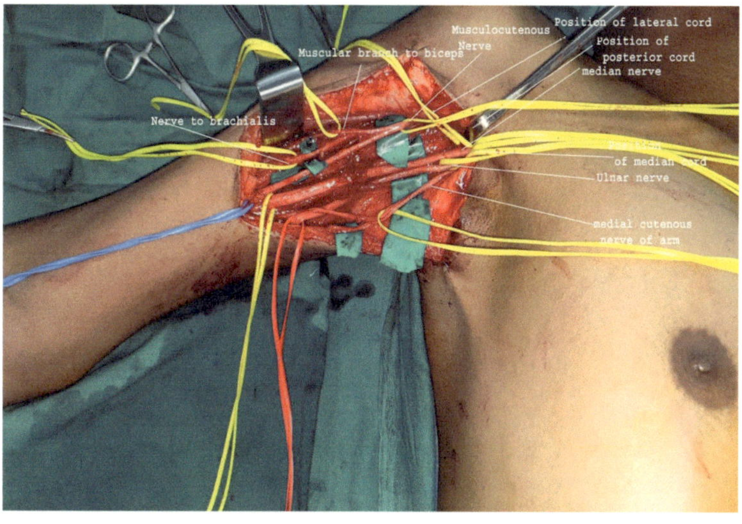

Figure 7.
Infraclavicular brachial plexus with its terminal branches.

On the medial side one can easily identify and dissect the phrenic nerve which runs longitudinally and pierces into the diaphragm, the strong contraction of the diaphragm can be felt when stimulating it. C7 which continues to form the middle trunk is further divided into anterior and posterior divisions. The lower trunk which is formed by roots from C8, T1 which is usually just closer to the subclavian artery also divided into two divisions. The roots, trunks, and divisions lie in supraclavicular regions (**Figure 6**).

All the cords are in the infraclavicular region and are named according to their relation with the axillary artery.

The posterior division of all trunks forms the posterior cord which lies posterior to the axillary artery. The anterior division of the upper and middle trunk forms the lateral cord. The anterior division of the lower trunk forms the medial cords. These cords further divided into terminal branches (**Figure 7**).

3. Specific nerve transfer

3.1 For shoulder abduction and stability

3.1.1 Spinal accessory to supra-scapular nerve transfer

3.1.1.1 Relevant anatomy

Spinal accessory nerve is not a part of the brachial plexus and arises from the cranial fossa, it emerges in the proximal part of the sternocleidomastoid and supplies it, then runs in an oblique course and gives several branches to the trapezius.

Whereas suprascapular arises from the upper trunk at Erb's point, going posteriorly, laterally, and inferiorly to supply supraspinatus and infraspinatus.

3.1.1.2 Exploration and transfer

Spinal accessory nerve transfer can be done during supraclavicular brachial plexus exploration by an anterior approach or via a posterior approach. Each approach has its advantages and disadvantages.

3.1.2 Anterior approach

3.1.2.1 Advantages

- No separate incision is required.
- Easy to dissect.

3.1.2.2 Disadvantages

- In severe injury mainly in case of avulsion or rupture of the upper trunk and C5, and C6 roots of the brachial plexus, the suprascapular nerve displaces more distally and lies below the clavicle where it is difficult to dissect. Also, in case of severe fibrosis of the upper trunk, the suprascapular nerve is either injured or fibrosed, in that case, the posterior approach is preferred. Also, it provides a large future scar on the neck in exploration via the anterior approach.

- Many surgeons do not routinely explore the brachial plexus and directly go for distal nerve transfer; in that case, accidental injury to proximal branches of the trapezius can be avoided.

3.1.2.3 Technique

Spinal accessory nerve is identified & dissected in the upper part of the neck during supraclavicular exploration of the brachial plexus. It runs obliquely to give several branches to the trapezius. Branches in the upper part are usually preserved to save the function of the trapezius. A larger, terminal branch is usually selected, cut, and prepared for transfer in the supraclavicular region. The spinal accessory nerve can be confused with branches of the cervical plexus which can be confirmed by electric stimulation of the nerve which causes good contraction of the trapezius in the case of the spinal accessory nerve.

The suprascapular nerve which usually arises at Erb's point (C5, C6 upper trunk) runs lateral & posteriorly to supply the supraspinatus and infraspinatus muscles. It can be easily identified by rolling the index finger over the nerve and entering into the suprascapular notch. It is cut from its origin and its distal cut end is coapted with the proximal cut end of the spinal accessory nerve with fibrin glue or sutures.

3.1.3 Posterior approach

3.1.3.1 Advantages

- A relatively virgin area on the back that is away from the zone of trauma where donor and recipient nerves can be easily dissected [9, 10].

- Neurotization is close to the neuromuscular junction of the supraspinatus, so less time to be traveled by axons for regeneration and reinnervation of muscle.

3.1.3.2 Disadvantages

- The number of axons of the donor 'spinal accessory nerve' decreases as it travels distally

- Difficult dissection

- The patient's position has to be changed to prone or lateral decubitus during the surgery.

3.1.3.3 Technique

The patient is positioned prone and bony landmarks of the acromion process; the spine of the scapula and midline of the back are marked. The points are joined. The spinal accessory nerve is found at 40% of the distance from the posterior midline and acromion process. The suprascapular nerve is found at the midpoint of the line joining the superior angle of the scapula medially and acromion laterally.

A skin incision is made parallel to the spine of the scapula and the skin flap is raised on both sides. A plane is dissected in between the trapezius and supraspinatus which is delineated by a layer of fatty tissue. Just below the trapezius muscle, the spinal accessory nerve can be identified as supplying it with its branches. It is dissected as far as possible and is cut distally to prepare it for transfer.

The suprascapular nerve is dissected which lies beneath the superior transverse ligament and requires to be divided. Once the ligament is divided, the suprascapular nerve can be dissected and the proximal portion of it is cut which is coapted with a distal portion of the spinal accessory nerve.

3.2 Somsak transfer

Leechavengvongs [6] first reported transferring the nerve to the long heads of the triceps branch of the radial nerve to the anterior branch of the axillary nerve through the posterior approach in 7 patients and achieved M4 power in all patients with an average shoulder abduction of 124 degrees. Later on, it became a reliable procedure addressing the shoulder by reinnervating the deltoid, especially in C5 & C6 brachial plexus injuries with intact C7 roots supplying the triceps. It is done in conditions where the suprascapular nerve is either functional so that deltoid function is superadded with suprascapular nerve or it is combined with SAN to SSN (spinal accessory nerve to suprascapular nerve transfer) transfer for shoulder abduction. Also, it can be done in cases of isolated C5 injury or axillary nerve injury.

3.2.1 Techniques

Somsak transfer is either done in the supine position or a lateral position. The posterior border of the deltoid is marked and a longitudinal incision is made over the posterior aspect of the upper arm. Once the posterior border of the deltoid is delineated it is lifted upward and we get the two divisions of the axillary nerve supplying the deltoid. The axillary nerve arises from the posterior cord, comes out of quadrangular space, and supplies the deltoid. Usually, the anterior division of the deltoid is selected for reinnervation, however, the axillary nerve proper can be used too as the recipient nerve.

Just below the deltoid, triceps muscles will be visualized, the innervations of which can be dissected by lifting one head of the triceps or in between the two heads of the triceps (long and lateral heads). Once we identify the nerve supplying the long head of the triceps, we stimulate it to confirm the contraction of the triceps and isolate it. It is cut distally and is mobilized proximally to coapt with the axillary nerve.

3.2.1.1 Key points (Somsak Transfer)

Indication: C5 injury C5, C6 injury Isolated axillary nerve injury
• Patients with C7 injury or triceps weakness are not candidates for this transfer
• It is important to stimulate the nerve supplying the long head of the triceps intraoperatively to confirm the presence of a strong contraction
• The sensory branch of the axillary nerve can be confused with one of the divisions of the axillary nerve. It is used as a guide to trace the main nerve. Intraoperative stimulation helps in identifying the motor branch.
• Palpating the posterior border of the deltoid pre-operatively helps in marking our incision

3.2.1.2 Other nerve transfers for shoulder stability

- Thoracodorsal nerve to long thoracic nerve (in patients with winging of the scapula)

- Intercostal nerve to anterior branch of axillary nerve or long thoracic nerve

- Phrenic nerve to suprascapular nerve transfer

- Phrenic nerve to axillary nerve (with nerve graft)

3.3 Elbow flexion

3.3.1 Oberlin transfer

Christopher Oberlin first described the technique of transfer of ulnar nerve fascicle to branch to the musculocutaneous nerve in 1994 in the case of C5, C6 avulsion injury [4]. The simplicity of this procedure and reasonably good results has made this procedure popular and it can be easily replicated by any peripheral nerve surgeon. However, he described choosing any fascicles of the ulnar nerve for transfer. Since at the arm level, the ulnar nerve is usually mixed, so transferring the ulnar nerve fascicle (10%) will result in transferring some motor fibers (10). Later on, other groups suggested fascicles of the nerve supplying the flexor carpi ulnaris which are generally located poster medially to be selected for transfer to a muscular branch of the musculocutaneous nerve (3).

McKinnon [5] described the double fascicular transfer of the FCU fascicle of the ulnar nerve and motor fascicle of the median nerve to the biceps and brachialis of the musculocutaneous. Oberlin included double innervations by coapting the median nerve fascicle to the muscular branch of the brachialis (4). Few people also named it as Oberlin I & 2 transfer (5).

3.3.1.1 Indications

C5 &C6 injury with intact C8 &T1.

3.3.1.2 Technique

Oberlin transfer is performed by making an incision on the medial side of the upper arm which is usually made in the groove that is palpable just below the inferior border of the biceps muscle [4, 5, 9].

Once the skin flap is raised and the medial border of the biceps is delineated, the biceps is elevated. Just below the biceps, we can identify the **musculocutaneous nerve** which gives a muscular branch to the biceps and brachialis and continues as a lateral anti-brachial cutaneous nerve.

The biceps branch usually arises 10–12 cm distal to the acromion [4].

The musculocutaneous nerve travels forward and in the lower parts, it supplies the brachialis muscle by giving a muscular branch to the brachialis before it continues as LABC.

On the more medial side, the ulnar nerve travels anterior to the triceps; intrafascicular dissection is done under microscope magnification in the proximal aspect

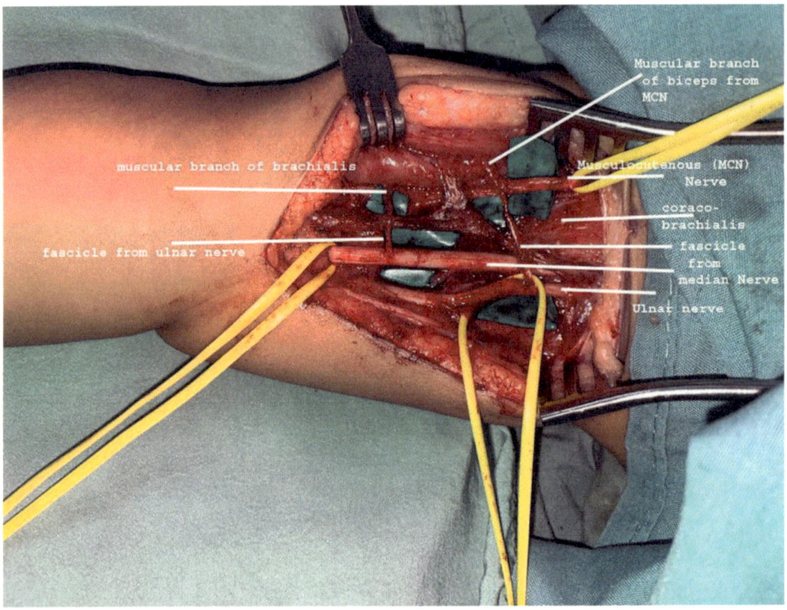

Figure 8.
Oberlin transfer (median nerve fascicle to muscular branch of biceps (from MCN- Musculocutaneous nerve) transfer and Ulnar nerve fascicle to muscular branch of brachialis transfer).

slightly lower level than the muscular branch to the biceps. Once donor fascicle (FCU) is identified, which is on the posteromedial aspect toward the surgeon and selected. It is confirmed by intraoperative nerve stimulation. The fascicle is dissected and divided distally and coapted with the biceps muscular branch.

The Brachialis branch arises from the musculocutaneous nerve several centimeters below the acromion before it becomes and to be continued as LABC (LABC is usually superficial and larger, whereas the brachialis branch enters into the muscles).

Just medial to the MCN, **the median nerve** runs just anterior to the brachial artery. While stimulating the median nerve, we perform intrafascicular dissection to select the fascicle (motor) to be coapted with a muscular branch to the brachialis.

In a similar way, the fascicle of the median nerve (either FCR or FDS) is dissected & identified, stimulated by a nerve stimulator, confirmed, and coapted with the muscular branch to the brachialis (**Figure 8**).

3.3.1.3 Key points (Oberlin Transfer)

• C8 &T1 functions should be preserved.
• Choosing the posteromedial fascicle of the ulnar nerve that supplies the forearm muscles esp. FCU
• Motor fascicles in the median nerve are located on the medial aspect, whereas the sensory component is on the lateral aspect of the median nerve
• Nerve transfer is to be done close to the biceps and brachialis muscles to decrease the time taken to regenerate the axons.

3.3.2 Intercostal nerve transfer

Intercostal nerve transfer has been used for neurotization of the musculocutaneous nerve as it is out of the zone of the trauma of the brachial plexus (extra plexus) and is frequently available as a donor nerve that is expandable [9]. Apart from neurotizing the musculocutaneous nerve, it can also be used to neurotize the triceps, and deltoid, as a donor for FFMT (Free functioning muscle transfer) or to provide sensation to the hand. It can be used even in cases with a history of rib fracture although one should be cautious in patients with a history of rib fracture, hemothorax, thoracotomy, or phrenic nerve palsy before selecting intercostal nerves as a donor. The commonly used donor is ICN 3,4,5 although from 2nd to 6th ICN can be used.

Relevant anatomy: intercostal nerve runs in the intercostal space on the inferior aspect of the ribs.

3.3.2.1 Technique

The intercostal nerve can be explored through a curvilinear inframammary incision made over the anterior chest wall. This incision is usually connected with the incision in the arm for exploration of the musculocutaneous nerve or incision for the infraclavicular brachial plexus. Once the skin flap is raised, the pectoralis major muscle is retracted and ribs and intercostal muscles are exposed. An incision is made on the anterior surface of the ribs parallel to the upper and lower border with the elevation of the periosteum causing the intercostal nerve to come into the intercostal space which usually lies along the inferior border. It can also be identified by dissecting the sensory branch which lies along the anterior axillary line Careful dissection of intercostal muscles helps in separating the intercostal nerve. It is dissected till the costochondral joint to gain sufficient length to reach

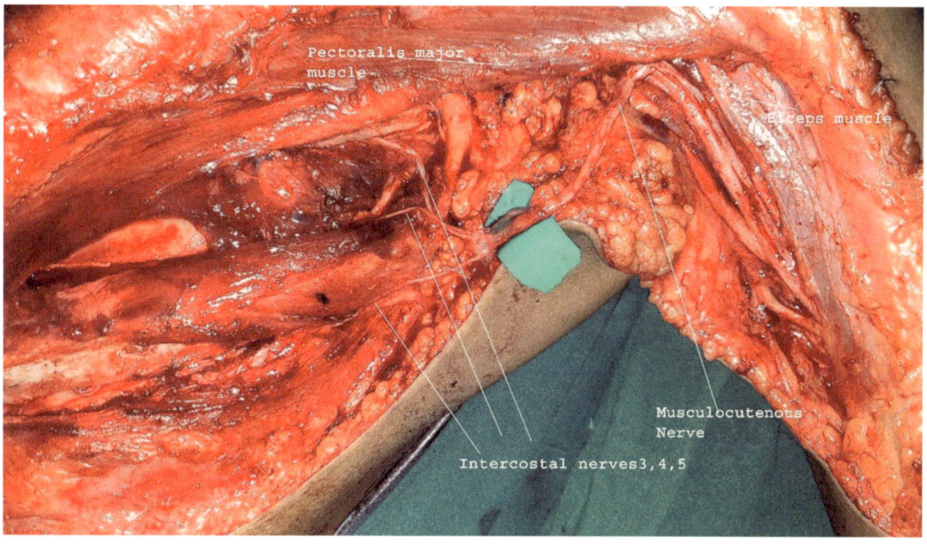

Figure 9.
Intercostal nerve to musculocutaneous nerve transfer.

the musculocutaneous nerve easily for coaptation without tension. The repair is performed in an abduction position of the shoulder so that there is less risk of its rupture of coaptation during the postoperative period. Care is taken not to injure the pleura during dissection.

Once 2 or 3 intercostal nerves are dissected, they are brought together and connected with the musculocutaneous nerve (**Figure 9**). Bhandari et al. have described the splint & weld technique [11, 12] for gluing the intercostals nerves.

3.3.2.2 Key points (intercostal nerve to MCN transfer)

• It is ideal to take three ICN to match with a diameter of MCN
• Care should be taken to avoid injury to the pleura.
• Nerve coaptations are done without tension.
• Nerve coaptation is done in the position of abduction of the shoulder so that during the postoperative period, repair should not be stretched.
• Fibrin glue simplifies the coaptation of the nerve due to technical difficulty in suture repair
• To gain extra-length of MCN, one can dissect it from its origin at the lateral cord that can be approached in the deltopectoral region. Once it is cut from its origin, it is retrieved through the arm and brought into the axilla for tensionless anastomosis.
• The arm is strapped and immobilized with the chest for a period of 3 weeks, then passive mobilization is started gradually.
• Chest physiotherapy is to be performed regularly
• Post-operative reinnervation of the biceps can be elicited by pinching the biceps and the presence of chest pain by the patient.
• Preoperatively, a Pulmonary function test can be performed to assess lung function in case of phrenic nerve palsy or when planning both the intercostal & phrenic nerves as a donor.

4. Hand functions

4.1 Contralateral C7 nerve transfer

Contra lateral C7 nerve transfer originally described by Gu [10] in 1989 has been a topic of debate because of many reasons like its route of transfer, relative post-operative weakness of donor's nerve, and the risk associated with variable outcomes [13, 14]. However, with many studies published with good outcomes, it has been proven to be a safe and useful donor which is expandable because of contributions coming from many spinal roots. Sometimes it is the only option left for addressing hand function especially in pan brachial plexus palsy or for recipient nerve for FFMT.

4.1.1 Technique

The contralateral brachial plexus is explored conventionally on the unaffected side and the C7 nerve root is dissected up to its branches as anterior and posterior divisions. The posterior division is commonly used is divided distally to be transferred as it has more motor axons compared to the anterior division. Half of the C7 nerve fascicles causing pectoralis major contraction are usually chosen and transferred

DOI: http://dx.doi.org/10.5772/intechopen.110711

to the ipsilateral side. If we find contraction of hand muscles during intraoperative stimulation, one should not use C7.

After division, a subcutaneous tunnel is created and either a non-vascularized nerve graft (sural nerve) or vascularized ulnar nerve graft (VUNG based on superior ulnar collateral artery & vein) is bridged connecting the cut proximal end of the C7 nerve to another end of the median nerve, suprascapular nerve or musculocutaneous nerve depending upon the reconstruction planned.

The posterior division of contralateral C7 can be brought to the ipsilateral side either with a pre-spinal route, retro-esophageal route, or subcutaneous route to reduce the time taken for axonal regeneration.

4.1.2 Key points (contralateral C7 nerve transfer)

- It is better to select the posterior division of Contralateral C7 as it has a greater number of motor axons.
- It is decided intraoperatively while stimulating the nerve and sees any significant hand muscle contraction before dividing C7 when there is a plan to take entire C7
- The ulnar nerve can be used as a free ulnar nerve graft by anastomosing its vascular pedicle in the neck with a thoracodorsal artery or transverse cervical artery

5. Conclusion

Nerve transfer in the brachial plexus has revolutionized the treatment and has become the standard of care to restore useful recovery of upper limb functions in the majority of brachial plexus injuries patients.

The nerve transfers described for shoulder abduction and stability are spinal accessory nerve to supra-scapular nerve transfer which can be superadded with Somsak transfer (using the long head of the triceps branch to the axillary nerve) depending upon the involvement of the C7 root. If hand functions are good, ulnar and median nerve fascicles can be used to neurotize muscular branches of the musculocutaneous nerve to restore elbow flexion. Although intercostal nerves equally give comparable results when used to reinnervate the musculocutaneous nerve, the Spinal accessory nerve or Phrenic nerve are other options that can be considered to neurotize the musculocutaneous nerve. For hand, either contra lateral C7 nerve is used esp. in pan brachial plexus or distal nerve transfer should be considered depending upon the availability of other expandable nerves.

A thorough pre-operative clinical examination, documentation with planning followed by careful intraoperative dissection, microscopic coaptation of nerves, and understanding the regenerating processes of axons with post-operative physiotherapy are keys to the recovery of a good nerve transfer in brachial plexus injuries.

Author details

Raj Kumar Manas
All India Institute of Medical Sciences, New Delhi, India

*Address all correspondence to: rajmanas007@rediffmail.com

References

[1] Millesi H. Surgical management of brachial plexus injuries. The Journal of Hand Surgery. 1977;**2**(5):367-378. DOI: 10.1016/s0363-5023(77)80046-4

[2] Narakas AO. The treatment of brachial plexus injuries. International Orthopaedics. 1985;**9**(1):29-36. DOI: 10.1007/BF00267034

[3] Lurje A. Concerning surgical treatment of traumatic injury to the upper division of the brachial plexus (Erb's type). Annals of Surgery. 1948;**127**(2):317-326

[4] Oberlin C, Béal D, Leechavengvongs S, Salon A, Dauge M, Sarcy J. Nerve transfer to biceps muscle using a part of tulnar nerve for C5–C6 avulsion of the brachial plexus: Anatomical study and report of four cases. The Journal of Hand Surgery. 1994;**19**(2):232-237. DOI: 10.1016/0363-5023(94)90011-6

[5] Mackinnon SE, Novak CB, Myckatyn TM, Tung TH. Results of reinnervation of the biceps and brachialis muscles with a double fascicular transfer for elbow flexion. The Journal of Hand Surgery. 2005;**30**(5):978-985. DOI: 10.1016/j.jhsa.2005.05.014

[6] Leechavengvongs S, Witoonchart K, Uerpairojkit C, Thuvasethakul P. Nerve transfer to deltoid muscle using the nerve to the long head of the triceps, part II: A report of 7 cases. The Journal of Hand Surgery. 2003;**28**(4):633-638. DOI: 10.1016/s0363-5023(03)00199-0

[7] Sinha S, Sharma R, Khani M, Mansari N. Adult brachial plexus injuries: Surgical strategies. In: Mahapatra AK, Midha R, Sinha S, editors. Surgery of Brachial Plexus. Noida, India: Thieme; 2016. pp. 1-12, Chapter 1

[8] Bhandari P, Bhatoe H, Mukherjee M, Deb P. Management strategy in post traumatic brachial plexus injuries. The Indian Journal of Neurotrauma. 2012;**9**(1):19-29. DOI: 10.1016/j.ijnt.2012.04.010

[9] Spinner RJ, Shin AY, Hebert-Blouin M-N, Elhassan BT, Bishop AT. Traumatic brachial plexus injury. In: Wolfe SW, Hotchkiss RN, Pederson WC, Kozin SH, editors. Green's Operative Hand Surgery. 6th ed. Philadelphia: Elsevier. pp. 1235-1291, chapter 38

[10] Bhandari PS, Deb P. Posterior approach for both spinal accessory nerve to suprascapular nerve and triceps branch to axillary nerve for upper plexus injuries. The Journal of Hand Surgery. 2013;**38**(1):168-172

[11] Bhandari PS. A novel technique in fibrin gluing of intercostal nerves: Splint and weld. Indian Journal of Plastic Surgery: Official Publication of the Association of Plastic Surgeons of India. 2020;**53**(2):298-300. DOI: 10.1055/s-0040-1716430

[12] Bhandari PS. Use of fibrin glue in the repair of brachial plexus and peripheral nerve injuries. The Indian Journal of Neurotrauma. 2013;**10**:30-32. DOI: 10.1016/j.ijnt.2013.05.008

[13] Gu YD. Cervical nerve root transfer from the healthy side in the treatment of brachial plexus root avulsion. Zhonghua Yi Xue Za Zhi. 1989;**69**(10):563-565 38. Chinese

[14] Gu YD, Zhang GM, Chen DS, Yan JG, Cheng XM, Chen L. Seventh cervical nerve root transfer from the contralateral healthy side for treatment of brachial plexus root avulsion. The Journal of Hand Surgery. 1992;**17**(5):518-521. DOI: 10.1016/s0266-7681(05)80235-9

Chapter 11

Orthotic and Prosthetic Management in Brachial Plexus Injury: Recent Trends

Om Prasad Biswal, Smita Nayak and Rajesh Kumar Das

Abstract

The brachial plexus is a network of intertwined nerve that controls movement and sensation in arm and hand. Any injury to the brachial plexus can result in partial or complete damage of arm and hand. The surgery is a common indicative procedure in brachial plexus injury in case of non-spontaneous recovery. The loss of function of hand due to injury can be replaced by using body powered or externally powered devices. Recent development in treatment protocol of prosthetic and orthotic science using artificial intelligence helps in rehabilitating the persons with brachial plexus injury to regain his confidence and perform daily activities. Combination of advancement in surgical procedure along with artificially intelligent devices opens a new array to rehabilitate the person with brachial plexus injury.

Keywords: grasp, artificial intelligence, neural network, assistive technology, external powered device

1. Introduction

Brachial plexus injury (BPI) is one of the common and an unfortunate injury from the patient's perspective, which mostly results from high energy trauma to the neck and upper limbs. Patients with brachial plexus injuries clinically represent devastating injuries and complications with unpredictable outcomes. Stress on the clavicle and adjacent structures including the brachial plexus and subclavian vasa may lead to effectively crippling function in one or rarely both upper limbs. As clavicle is the strongest link in the shoulder area, sudden movements or stress due to trauma can result in the clavicle fracture. Then, all the tensile forces are transferred from the medulla to the neurovascular fibers and nerve roots, which can in turn lead to the upper limb muscle weakness innervated by nerve roots of C5, C6, C7, C8, and T1.

In adults, prevalence of brachial plexus injury shows 89% for male predominantly with a mean age of 29 years and median age of 25 years [1, 2]. Traumatic injuries, such as motorcycle collisions, have the majority in epidemiology of BPI, approximately 44–70% [3, 4]. The most common cause of BPI in children is obstetric brachial plexus palsy (OBPP), with a prevalence rate between 0.38 and 4.6 per 1000 live births [5–7].

Other possible causes for brachial plexus palsy may include iatrogenic injuries, such radiation therapy and as well as those that can occur during surgical and anesthesia procedures.

Patient loses his significant functional ability to perform activity of daily livings (ADL) as well as potential functions in his/her occupation. It is important that this valuable segment of our population should be functionally restored as early as possible to the best of our ability. With modern technology in hand and microsurgery, this is very much feasible provided that the patient is treated in time. There are also treatment techniques available for late clinical referrals, but early treatment brings up a huge difference to the eventual outcome.

The results of brachial plexus injury treatment have considerably improved with the introduction of advanced diagnostic modalities, microsurgical techniques, and magnification. Few years back it was considered a difficult or impossible task to restore a functioning limb in many of the patients with brachial plexus injuries, which just recently microsurgical techniques in neurolysis, nerve repair, nerve grafting, and nerve transfer have made it possible.

This article explains the various orthotic and prosthetic managements, current developments and trends for brachial plexus injuries based on a substantial survey of published peer-reviewed literature, and the insights gained by the author in treating several cases of brachial plexus injuries.

2. Clinical anatomy of brachial plexus complex

The brachial plexus is a supersystem network of nerve fibers that supplies the skin and musculature of the upper extremities. It begins in the root of the neck, passes through the axilla, and runs through the entire upper extremity, usually composed of five roots, three stems, six strands, and three bundles. The brachial plexus is divided into five parts—roots, trunks, divisions, cords, and branches. This complex network is formed by the anterior rami (divisions) of cervical spinal nerves from C5 to C8 and the first thoracic spinal nerve, T_1 (**Figure 1**). The roots of the brachial plexus converge to form three trunks at the back of the neck. A combination of C5 and C6 roots form superior trunk, middle trunk is continuation of C7, and inferior trunk is the combination of C8 and T1 roots. The trunks pass over laterally, crossing the posterior triangle of the neck. Each trunk divides into two branches within the posterior triangle of the neck or above or behind the clavicle. One of them moves anteriorly and the other posteriorly; thus, they are known as the anterior and posterior divisions.

Once both the divisions enter the axilla, they combine to form three cords, named by their positions with respect to the axillary artery. The cords give rise to the major branches of the brachial plexus which mainly control the sensory and motor functions of the upper limbs, shoulder, and chest. The lateral cord is formed by the anterior division of the superior trunk and the anterior division of the middle trunk, and the lateral root of median nerve, musculocutaneous nerve, and lateral pectoral nerve are the main nerve branches. The posterior cord is formed by the posterior division of the superior trunk, the posterior division of the middle trunk, and the posterior division of the inferior trunk, and the subscapular nerve, thoracodorsal nerve, axillary nerve, and radial nerve are the main nerve branches. The medial cord is formed by the anterior division of the inferior trunk, and the main nerve branches are the medial antebrachial cutaneous nerve, ulnar nerve, and medial root of median nerve.

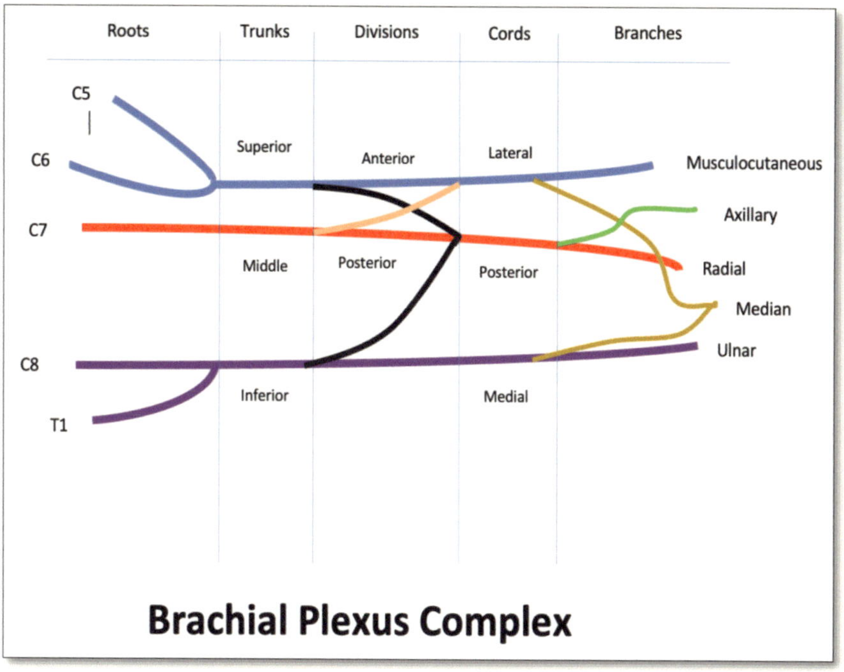

Figure 1.
Diagrammatic representation of course of the brachial plexus.

3. Clinical relevance of brachial plexus injury

Generally, BPI can be divided into partial (upper or lower) and complete. The damage of different nerve branches often leads to the dysfunction of corresponding corridor. The clinical representations of upper brachial plexus injury widely referred as Erb's palsy. The forearm is positioned in pronation due to the weakness of biceps brachii. The wrist is weakly flexed due to the weakened wrist extensors, while the wrist flexors are in normal tone. The major characteristics are lack of shoulder abduction, elbow flexion, and an internal and external rotation of the upper extremity, which is often termed as "waiter's tip deformity" [8]. Lower root of the brachial plexus (C8-T1) injury leads to claw hand deformity. Complete injury damages both sensory and motor functions of the limb.

3.1 Manifestations in nerve regeneration after brachial plexus injury

Complete avulsion of the nerve proximal to the dorsal root ganglion or complete avulsion of the nerve root from the spinal cord occurs, and it falls under preganglionic injuries. Injury to the nerve distal to the dorsal root ganglion within the trunk, division, cord, or terminal nerve branches is known as postganglionic injuries. Both preganglionic and postganglionic injury have different yet significant prognostic and therapeutic implications. Preganglionic injuries generally lead to complications such as complete loss of motor and sensation in the distribution of the involved root and denervation of the deep paraspinal muscles of the neck. In postganglionic injuries, i.e., distal to the spinal ganglia, the cell bodies are intact and have more favorable prognosis than is associated with preganglionic injuries. Developments of regenerative microenvironment around the injury, the reinnervation of nerve to target tissue, and axon regeneration are related to the repair process of BPI. At the distal end of the injury, the axons and myelin sheath degenerate and disintegrate into nerve debris. Autophagy reaction is produced by Schwann cells (SCs) followed by Wallerian degeneration at the end of the nerve involved. In the early stage of injury to clear degenerative myelin debris, Schwann cells assist macrophages and also plays a vital role in formation of basement membranes to promote growth and provide channels by secreting laminin, which can guide axons to grow rapidly in the right direction. The proliferating Schwann cells form a solid cell cord (band of Büngner) in the nerve basal lamina enclosed by the basement membrane. This band Büngner has a good guiding effect on the growth of nerve axons, and in addition it not only produces related molecules that promote axon regeneration, but also helps to separate molecules that inhibit regeneration in the endoneurial tube, by which the regeneration and repair of injured nerve can be accelerated [9–11].

Schwann cells, nerve axons, fibroblasts, etc., produce mainly three types of neurotrophic factors (NTFs), which bind with specific receptors on the surface of target cells [12]. In the regeneration and repair of injured brachial plexus, these NTFs play different roles. Neurotrophin, one of the NTF, includes nerve growth factor (NGF) and brain-derived neurotrophin factor (BDNF). NGF can promote the transduction of intracellular signal in damaged nerve, which is an important factor in the acceleration of the growth of axons and the recovery of nerve function. BDNF and its tyrosine kinase receptor B (TrkB) mRNA assist in restoration of neural pathways and enhance regeneration of axons and reconnection of injured muscles. Another NTF neurocytokinin includes ciliary neurotrophic factor (CNTF). Fibroblast growth factor (FGF) and other NTFs such as glial cell line-derived neurotrophic factor (GDNF), insulin-like growth factor (IGF) can enhance and proliferate the axons and Schwann cells of mature spinal cord [13]. Some previous studies have already explained that NTFs can improve regeneration of nerve cell and can accelerate motor nerve conduction velocity [11, 14]. The formation and regeneration of microenvironment is an important factor that not only affects the repair of brachial plexus injury, and in long-term objectives, it is also responsible for resurrection of motor and sensory functions in upper extremity.

4. History of orthotic and prosthetic managements in brachial plexus injury

BPI leads to weakness in upper extremity muscles, hyporeflexia and is commonly associated with upper limb pain. The general principles of upper extremity orthotic and prosthetic managements in BPI are to prevent shoulder joint pain prevent contractures, improve function, e.g., enable positioning of hand in space to allow two handed activities, improve cosmesis and body image, to support the weight of the upper limb, and thus ease the traction forces on the shoulder, and secondarily, such support may assist in edema control.

One of the key goals in rehabilitation and orthotic prescription after BPI is to support the shoulder to prevent subluxation, as impaired innervation to the shoulder girdle leads to inherent instability of the glenohumeral joint, combined with weakening of the shoulder girdle, which in turn causes glenohumeral subluxation. Treatment and prevention of shoulder pain and subluxation is also a common rehabilitative goal in brachial plexus injury patients. **Table 1** represents the orthotic and prosthetic management of brachial plexus injury patients depending on their level of injuries, motor deficits, and functional needs.

Level	Motor deficit	Functional need	Orthotic and prosthetic prescription
C5-C6	Shoulder abduction Shoulder flexion Elbow flexion Wrist extension	Shoulder support Prevent shoulder subluxation Elbow flexion	Wilmer carrying shoulder-elbow-wrist support orthosis, Aeroplane splint, Gunslinger splint, Steeper Stanmore flail arm orthosis, Humeral cuff
C5, C6, C7	Shoulder flexion Shoulder abduction Elbow flexion Elbow extension weakness Wrist extension Finger extension Thumb extension weakness	Shoulder support Prevent shoulder subluxation Elbow flexion Wrist support Finger extension Wrist support Finger extension 1st extension	Wilmer carrying orthosis with arm trough, Functional arm orthosis (FAO), Aeroplane splint, Gunslinger splint
C8, T1	Wrist flexors Finger flexors Thumb flexors Finger extensors Thumb extensors	Wrist stabilization Finger flexion Some amount of finger extension Intrinsics of hand	Static or dynamic wrist hand orthosis, Elbow or wrist driven, tenodesis splint, Knuckle bender splint
C5-T1	Entire ipsilateral upper limb May include scapular motion	Shoulder support Prevent shoulder subluxation Edema control Normal function	Slings, Hemi arm slings, Functional arm orthosis (FAO), Wilmer carrying orthosis with hand support

Table 1.
Orthotic and prosthetic management for BPI depending on the level of injury, motor deficits, and functional needs.

Management of C5, C6, C7 level of injury, a standard shoulder sling can be a simple orthotic aid, which is readily available to support the shoulder, but the concern is the potential development of elbow flexion and shoulder adduction or internal rotation contractures. Even with the return of motor function, the developed contracture may limit functional use of the limb. Other commercially available slings are Bobath sling, static shoulder–elbow sling, Roylan hemi arm sling and humeral cuff (Patterson Medical Holdings, Inc.), etc. Another option that can possibly reduce subluxation and maintain appropriate positioning of the flaccid upper extremity, particularly in patients who are ambulatory, is GivMohr Sling (GivMohr Corporation) [15]. Standard shoulder sling exerts additional upward force from the elbow joint to control shoulder subluxation. An upward force is transferred through the shoulder sling along the length of the forearm, wrist, and hand. The downward weight of the hand and distal forearm pushes the elbow and humerus upward and provides an efficient transmission of force by creating a fulcrum point at the level of the proximal forearm [16]. The shoulder cap fits snugly over the acromioclavicular joint region and applies the fulcrum to the proximal forearm from above, which is a better refinement of preventing shoulder subluxation and shoulder pain compared to slings and hemislings [2, 16, 17]. But the concern is unilaterally functional patients may have difficulty while donning and doffing, because it has more straps and adjustments. Newer design concepts such as Steeper Stanmore flail-arm orthosis have rectified this problem with fewer straps and an adjustable locking device at the elbow. The hemisling and the shoulder caps have certain differentiation in advantages such as hemislings and are commercially available at lower cost with ease of donning and doffing, whereas the shoulder caps have the advantages of greater stability and comfort with respect to hemislings.

Patients with C5-C6 injury clinically represent with weakness of the shoulder girdle musculature as well as the elbow joint flexion more often than the extension, while because of the relative weakness of the external rotators and abductors, shoulders are internally rotated or adducted. Shoulder internal rotation contractures are found to be the most common. Almost 50–70% of patients may be found with a complications of internal rotation contractures in obstetric brachial plexus palsy [18–20]. In later stages, weakness of the shoulder girdle may have the possibility to cause joint dysplasia over the period and increased glenohumeral instability and subluxation. The patient retains control of hand and wrist movements and some amount of elbow extension as of triceps, if the lower trunk or lower nerve roots (C7, C8, and T1) are preserved. These patients need support of the shoulder and elbow without impeding the wrist and hand movements [21].

Ratchet shoulder abduction orthotic (SAO) devices such as Wilmer carrying orthosis with shoulder-elbow-wrist support, or a Wilmer carrying elbow-wrist-hand orthosis, aero plane splints, gunslinger splints can be indicated, in which shoulder and elbow can be locked in different positions and can be placed in position either by the opposite arm or by leveraging it against a table or other object. A cable-powered device like shoulder-driven elbow-wrist-fingers tenodesis splint or even a myoelectric exoskeletal device, which can be functional by slide input controls by potentiometers, are also prescribed [21, 22]. A cable-controlled elbow functions very similar to control of elbow unit in above-elbow prosthesis by protraction and retraction of the contralateral shoulder. Allowing the elbow movement may lead to loss of control of the glenohumeral joint, and the shoulder may remain subluxed with the additional weight of the orthosis. Mobile arm supports can also be the options for individuals with brachial plexus injury.

C5-T1 injury or the complete brachial plexus injury causes a complete flail arm with both profound hypotonia and hyporeflexia. Orthotic prescription for flail arm is required for potential support and protection for the arm and providing some function to the arm. Essentially, orthoses that immobilize and protect the arm are Wilmer carrying orthosis, gunslinger splint, etc., which are composed of a shoulder support, elbow ratchet, forearm support, and distal trough that can accommodate functional devices. Extending the trough of the shoulder cap all the way to the fingertips also helps to control edema and provides protection to the weak upper extremity. Currently, orthotic management in brachial plexus injury is adding function to the weakened limb. A functional arm orthosis (FAO) can be interpreted to borrow the power from an intact trapezius muscle shrug or from the opposite arm.

Patients with C8-T1 nerve injury or the lower trunk of the brachial plexus injury (Klumpke's palsy) may have shoulder and elbow function preserved with loss of wrist and hand motor control. So, these patients often require orthoses such as the tenodesis splint or dynamic wrist hand orthosis with MCP assist to stabilize the wrist and restore grip and pinch functions rather supporting the shoulder and enhancing the function.

In most severe forms of brachial complex injuries, authors have suggested a more controversial yet functional approach of management that involves immediate prosthetic fitting followed by amputation of the affected extremity above or below the elbow. However, still it is been referred as a controversial approach as the amputation must take place soon after the initial injury to ensure compliance with the prosthesis. But the concern is that the amputation of involved limb is an irreversible procedure, and as we must conduct this early after the injury, the less conservative treatment time and opportunity is available for assessing for any possible neurologic recovery. Therefore, the decision regarding amputation must be made before adequate assessment of any possible recovery of motor and sensory function [23–25].

5. Recent trends in orthotic management of BPI

5.1 Neuromuscular electrical stimulation (NMES) in rehabilitative orthotic devices

NMES is often referred as muscle stimulation that uses an electrical current to produce muscle contractions for the purpose of restoring motor functions in individuals who have muscle weakness or paralysis. NMES creates an electrical field near motor axons of peripheral nerves that is of sufficient strength to depolarize the axonal membranes, and thus, it operates by depolarizing motor axons rather than muscle fibers directly, eliciting action potentials and, consequently, muscle contractions. Neuromuscular electrical stimulation is a modality that involves the application of electrodes connected to a device that provides electrical current to a partially or completely denervated muscle with the goal of promoting functional recovery. NMES has been used in the rehabilitation of multiple central neurological conditions, including stroke, cerebral palsy, traumatic brain injury, multiple sclerosis, and spinal cord injury, with demonstrable success [26]. There have been very less evidence for its effectiveness in peripheral nerve injury and central nervous system injuries. In a randomized study comprising patients with severe median nerve compression, the group treated with postoperative electrical stimulation demonstrated improvements in functional outcomes as compared to the control group [27]. According to Denise Justice et al. [26], NMES studies in the treatment of neonatal brachial plexus palsy did not report loss of motor function, there were reports of improvement in function, and thus, NMES in peripheral nerve therapy was considered reasonable. These results show that there is mixed evidence regarding NMES being associated with improvement in muscle strength, while it can be a vital modality for improving muscle tone [26]. NMES can be applied with surface electrodes on the skin over the targeted muscles or nerves. NMES stimulators range from being capable of delivering a range of a single channel of electrical current to delivering seven to eight independent channels of stimulation. NMES current waveforms are typically characterized by a hierarchy of monophasic or biphasic current pulses. The pulse wave frequency, amplitude, and width or duration of the pulses determine the strength of the muscle contractions elicited. Stimulators are equipped with pattern controllers that allow the patient or clinician to set or adjust some of these stimulation parameters like pulse width, pulse frequency, and the duration and coordination of muscle contractions. Many sophisticated commercially available NMES systems have controllers that receive real-time input from patients, which enables them to adjust the stimulation and elicit subsequent muscle contractions and movements produced. User interfaces with such controllers range from buttons and switches to external or implanted sensors or biopotential recording electrodes [28].

5.1.1 Theory of application of NMES stimulations in brachial plexus injury

Many studies suggest that, by inciting depolarization of cell membrane and opening voltage-gated calcium channels, electrical stimulation can increase intracellular Ca^{2+} transients level, and the increase of Ca^{2+} influx can improve the expression of nerve growth factor (NGF), brain-derived neurotrophin factor (BDNF), and its tyrosine kinase receptor B (TrkB) mRNA, which are the closest transducers for motor neuron regeneration [29], which can also be referred as creating artificial neural network (ANN). Electrical stimulation has also been found effective in promoting reconnection of axons and muscles, accelerate nerve conduction speed, enhance muscle fiber vitality, and followed by restore damaged nerve function. Many research studies show that the main objective of electrical stimulation in downstream pathways is inducing synthetic reactions, so that the use of low frequency stimulation can increase cyclic adenosine monophosphate (cAMP) level in nerve cells and then cAMP can be induced to activate phosphokinase A (PKA).As long as a short electrical stimulation can cause a series of closed loop reactions, it promotes the growth of dorsal root ganglion (DRG) by regulating cell growth-related proteins, cAMP response element binding protein (CREB), and cytoskeleton proteins [30], which in turn activate downstream pathways and increase the expression of BDNF. By inhibiting phosphodiesterase, cAMP can be enhanced and maintained at a certain level, and it elevates BDNF [31].

5.1.2 Patterns of stimulations in NMES stimulator devices

There are three categories of NMES available currently, i.e., cyclic NMES, EMG-triggered NMES, and proportionally controlled NMES. In cyclic NMES, electrodes are placed on the skin over muscle bellies that are targeted for activation. The wrist, finger, and thumb extensors are targeted for the activation of stimulation. A single pair of electrodes may be adequate to produce hand opening and wrist extension. In some patients, elbow extensors or shoulder muscles may also be targeted. Cyclic NMES is considered to be most simple, commercially available, and the most used NMES administering method [32, 33]. Some of the examples of commercially available cyclic NMES units are Myoplus 2 pro (NeuroTrac®), Intelect NMES (DJO Global, Inc.), etc. These units often have two channels. The intensity of stimulation can be adjusted and delivered from each channel to a level that produces comfortable muscle contractions and the desired movement, e.g., hand opening. Stimulation is delivered according to an on–off control pattern, with the timing of the cycle, the number of repetitions, and the maximum intensity of stimulation preset by a therapist. When the pulse stimulation begins, stimulation frequency and duration elicit repeated muscle contractions, therefore arm and hand movement happen, followed by relaxation duration. Cyclic NMES requires no input from the patient. The patient can simply relax his/her limb during the stimulation duration, and let the stimulator activate the muscles, and sometimes patients are also instructed to move the arm or hand in synchrony with the stimulation. Research studies related to cyclic NMES show regimens ranging from 1.5 to 2.5 hours per day for 6–12 weeks [33, 34].

5.1.3 Assistive stimulation control and task-practice training using NMES devices

As the patient is prompted to produce his/her own effort to prompt the movement, EMG-triggered NMES may be more effective in promoting neurologic changes leading to better recovery. Triggered NMES system, e.g., Neuromove, Zynex, etc., elicits repetitive muscle contractions through the EMG-triggered stimulators. As the EMG signal exceeds a preset threshold, the stimulator turns on, and a preset frequency of stimulation is delivered to the target muscle for a preset duration, which is known as stimulation width. After the stimulation turns off, the cycle repeats [35, 36]. NMES is effective when it is used to assist goal-oriented task practice may lead to better outcomes than might be achieved with NMES modalities like cyclic NMES or EMG-triggered NMES, which can be challenging to use in task practice because the timing of the stimulation pattern is preprogrammed [37]. Sensors worn on the body can provide alternative methods of triggering stimulation. A force sensitive resistor on the arm has been used to trigger NMES to the motor points of corresponding muscle when the patient achieves some threshold degree of joint movement while attempting to complete the task [38]. Switch-triggered NMES systems (e.g., NESS H200, Bioness, Inc.) use push buttons to trigger stimulation (**Figure 2**). The push buttons may be operated by a therapist or by the patient. Push buttons give the therapist or patient control of the initiation and duration of stimulation, which makes it more feasible to incorporate NMES into task practice [40, 41].

In proportionally controlled NMES stimulation such as Myoplus 2 pro, NeuroTrac® (**Figure 3**), the intensity of the NMES is not preset, but the patient can regulate intensity by a control strategy that translates his/her desired movement into stimulation intensities, which is being regulated in real time. Thus, proportionally controlled NMES can be differentiated from cyclic and triggered NMES methods.

5.2 Functional electrical stimulation (FES) in orthotic devices

Contralaterally controlled functional electric stimulation (CCFES) is one of the advance functional rehabilitation protocols that can be implemented to enhance the recovery of paretic limb after brachial plexus injury [34, 42]. It uses current pulse width from the contralateral side (non-paretic) upper limb to regulate the intensity of electrical stimulation delivered to the motor unit of the affected upper limb. CCFES treatment is a goal-oriented task practice which can either be in repetitive practice which is self-administered or therapist-guided. The current pulse width stimulation intensity delivered to the affected side is proportional to the degree of respective range of motion of the normal side. It was initially developed at the Cleveland Functional Electrical Stimulation (FES) Center and is a proportionally controlled NMES approach in which the intensity of stimulation to the paretic finger and thumb extensors is proportionally controlled by an instrumented glove worn on the opposite (contralateral) hand (**Figure 4**). CCFES device consists of an instrumented glove, stimulator, and surface electrodes. Up to seven monopolar channels of biphasic current can be delivered by the he stimulator. With the glove, the patient can control the degree of opening of the affected hand and can practice using it in task-oriented therapy. The stimulation intensity can be modulated and delivered as with input from surface electrode, so that each channel can be programmed individually. Also, the individual channel can be programmed automatically by interpreting cyclic stimulation. Pulse duration can be adjusted for specific stimulus channel, so that patterns of stimulation can be customized according to the change in stimulus intensity, which in turn is related either to the function of the input signal from instrumented glove or to the cyclic stimulation pattern. The patient can open their hands (Hand CCFES) or simultaneous reach with hand opening (Arm + Hand CCFES) repeatedly over a midline activities of daily living (ADL) exercise

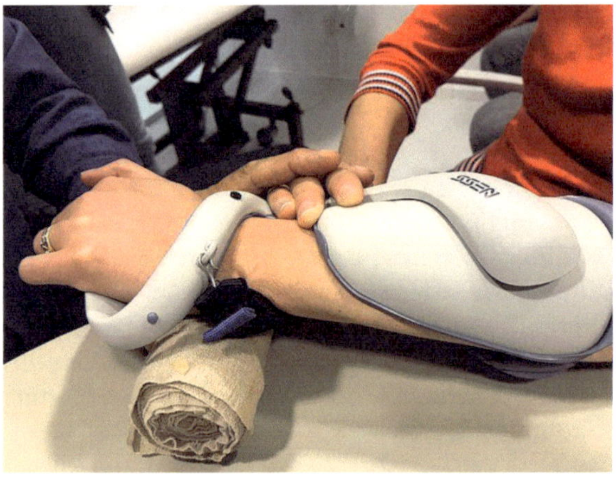

Figure 2.
Switch triggered stimulation in NESS H200, Bioness, Inc. [39].

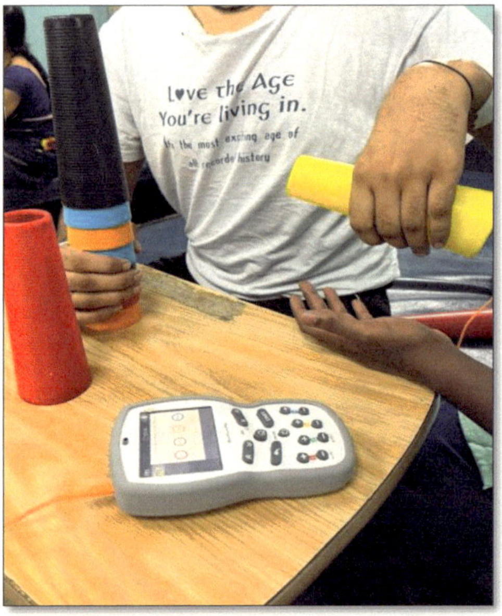

Figure 3.
Goal-oriented task practice training of BPI patient by NMES stimulation using Myoplus 2 pro, NeuroTrac®.

session of selectable duration by prompting the sound and light ques. MATLAB R2022b can be used to program the stimulator. EMG signals can also be used from the impaired upper limb to deliver proportionally controlled NMES in accordance with the patient's motor intention. In proportionally controlled NMES, the approach capitalizes on the principle of intention-driven movement, linking the patient's motor commands to the stimulated movement and the resulting proprioceptive feedback to the brain.

This pattern of artificial reinstatement of the sensorimotor integration may have the possibilities to enhance Hebbian-type neuroplasticity (i.e., connections between neurons that are simultaneously active and are strengthened), which may

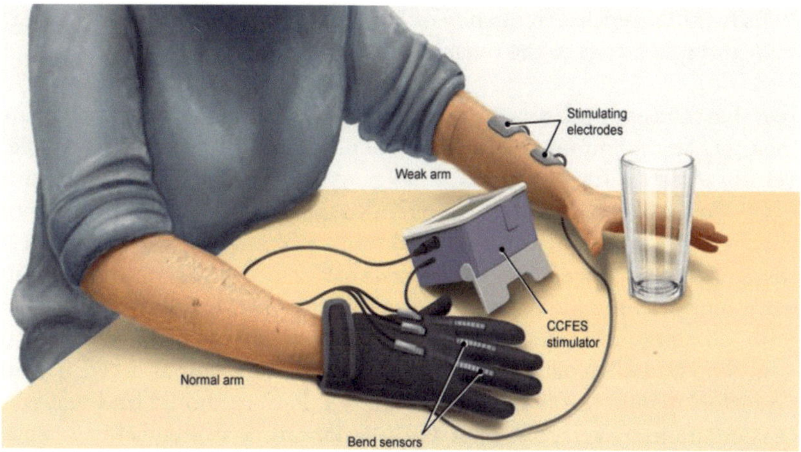

Figure 4.
Illustration of contralaterally controlled functional electrical stimulation (CCFES) [43].

lead to better motor recovery. Hence, proportionally controlled NMES may be more effective than other NMES stimulations [44]. The command hand glove generally consists of three bend sensors, which are placed on dorsal aspect of 2nd, 3rd, and 4th digits. These use pre-gelled surface electrodes to target small and large muscles in the forearm, hand, etc., which are commercially available in various sizes.

5.2.1 Pattern of stimulation in FES stimulator devices

Cyclic stimulation is generally given at the motor points of individual muscles for gaining the muscle tone and conduction by cyclic pattern involving interrupted galvanic current. Rehastim (Hasomed GmbH, Magdeburg, Germany) is a 8-channel stimulator may be used into the training environment with two bipolar, self-adhesive electrodes (diameter: 40 mm), and applied biphasic square pulse frequency 30 Hz to 50 Hz, pulse width ranging from 300 μs–500 μs. The stimulation of this integrated neuroprosthesis can be updated in a closed-loop, real-time iteration at 50 Hz–60 Hz via a controller area network/universal serial bus (CAN/USB) port using an algorithm. Whenever the brain–machine interface (BMI) classifier output will be positive, NMES can be applied for 5–7 s to the motor points of individual muscles at a joint during respective movement [45]. For example, in Erb's palsy, three fibers of deltoid muscle (anterior, lateral, and posterior) or its motor points. In elbow, stimulation is given to motor point of brachialis muscle and triceps muscle on the anterior aspect and posterior aspect, respectively, just above the elbow region. Thus, for wrist and fingers movements, stimulations are given at the motor points of the flexor and extension muscle groups. Hence, each motor point is stimulated from proximal to distal as one complete stimulation cycle. Each motor point may be stimulated for 10–15 contractions. This cyclic stimulation can be given from 4 to 6 weeks depending on the severity of the injury. As the muscle tone starts to improve, muscle strength also begins to recover, followed by improvement of the conduction. After muscle strength gains approximately 1 or 1+ grade alongside improvement in conduction, the stimulation is shifted from interrupted galvanic current to faradic current to stimulate the muscle in groups, which is otherwise known as faradism. It stimulates for a short duration through interrupted direct current with a pulse width ranging from 300 μs to 500 μs with a frequency of 50–100 Hz. Faradism produces tetanic contraction and relaxation of the muscle, and the pulse frequency and duration can be adjusted [46].

Implantable microstimulator or multichannel implantable pulse stimulation approaches may be recommended for brachial plexus injury patients who have been carefully screened for hypotonia. Emerging technology that uses implanted nerve cuff electrodes to deliver high-frequency stimulus waveforms to nerves may prove capable of generating nerve pulse. Adding such pulse stimulation to an NMES neuroprosthesis could conceivably improve its effect and widen its applicability. Implementing upper limb neuroprostheses in brachial plexus injured patients has been a major challenge over the years, while another major challenge is developing an intuitive method by which patients control stimulation to their affected arm and hand without interfering with the task being attempted. Patient should find neuroprosthesis is easier and more effective than any compensatory strategy already attempted before, and thus, it can be successful [47, 48].

5.3 Implementation of brain-machine interface (BMI) in hybrid neuroprosthesis exoskeleton

Armeo Spring, Hocoma, Volketswil, Switzerland is a commercially available 3D workspace rehabilitation exoskeleton for shoulder, elbow, and wrist joints. It comes with seven degrees of freedom to provide antigravity support for the paretic arm and to provide movement kinematics and grip force. Gravity compensation adjustment is also incorporated into the device, so that patients with severe impairments can perform task-oriented practice with a virtual augmentative environment. There are two springs that are incorporated into the device, by which the unweighing can be realized. The real-time sensor data may be used to display a three-dimensional multi-joint visualization of the user's arm and exoskeleton in virtual reality (**Figure** 5) [49].

To capture the angles of all arm joints and the grip force from a shared memory block, a file mapping communication may be used. The virtual arm software can be programmed in HMD (Kaiser XL50) and SPS framework. Skeletal meshes can be made up of a set of polygons designed to make up the surface of the Skeletal Mesh, VertexBone and VertexSkin engines, etc., or a hierarchy of interconnected bones and joint segments which can be used to animate the vertices of the polygons in the three-dimensional real-time visualization software. The 3D models, rigging, and animations are created in an external modeling and animation application (Unreal engine 4, 3DSMax, Maya, Softimage, etc.) and are then imported into skeletal mesh engines. The bone vertices of the meshed model may be modified according to the degree of freedoms the user can provide in online closed-loop feedback. This can be designed measuring the joint angles and grip forces of the device. The joint angles of the exoskeleton can be directly represented in virtual reality, whereas the grip forces can be augmented to feedback real-time hand function.

Prior to each session, patients must be instructed to perform a natural wrist movement during the assigned tasks aiming at maximum movements, respectively. For an example, the ROM of wrist and elbow movements are calculated as the sum of maximum extension and flexion and can be computed as the mean of each session. The three-dimensional visualization of the fingers and wrist in real-time virtual augmentation software should be applied during each task as implicit online feedback of the respective joint movement. Patient needs to be trained with two exoskeleton sessions: with and

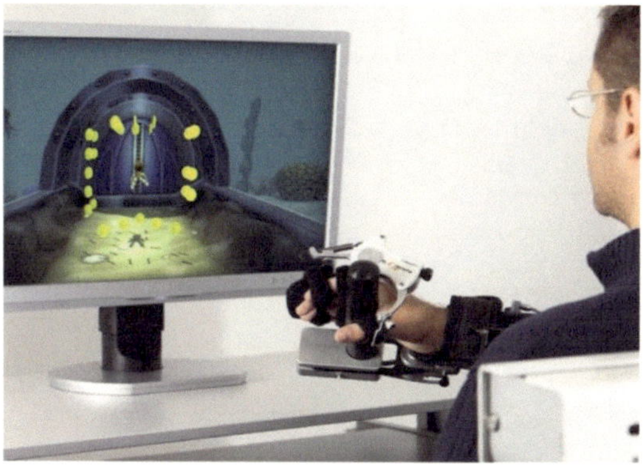

Figure 5.
Integrated neuroprosthesis with a gravity-compensating, seven degree-of-freedom exoskeleton, Armeo Spring exoskleteon, Hocoma, and virtual environment feedback attached to the paretic arm [50].

without BMI-controlled NMES. Both the exoskeleton and the maximum pulse stimulation intensity (S_{max}) are calibrated individually. The exoskeleton is adjusted to provide required gravity compensation for every joint and unrestricted joint movements in three-dimensional space. The S_{max} for individual muscle or each muscle group is determined as the output current approaching the motor threshold but that is still perceived as comfortable. In brachial plexus injury, depending on the severity of upper limb impairment, prolonged supra-motor threshold stimulation may be perceived as painful and was therefore the stimulation intensity and is thus set according to patient's comfort level.

5.3.1 Electroencephalographic (EEG) signal acquisition

Since many years, any brain disorders can be easily diagnosed by visual inspection of EEG signals. In healthy adults, the amplitudes and frequencies of such signals change from one state to another of the human, such as simple situations like wakefulness and sleep. The characteristics and amplitudes of the waves also change in accordance with age. Five major brain waves have been distinguished into five bandpass by their different frequency ranges, from low to high frequencies, respectively, are called alpha (α), theta (θ), beta (β), delta (δ), and gamma (γ). In 1929, Berger introduced the alpha and beta waves. In 1938, Jasper and Andrews used the term "gamma" for the waves of above 30 Hz. The delta refers to all low frequency waves below the alpha range and the theta waves as those having frequencies within the range of 4–7.5 Hz [51]. A beta wave rhythm varies within the range of 14–26 Hz, while amplitude normally under 30 μV and is found in normal adults (**Figure 6**). Usual waking rhythm of the brain like active thinking, active attention, solving concrete problems, etc., is associated with beta rhythm, and when a person is in a panic state, the corresponding rhythm may be acquired. Mainly over the frontal and central regions of the brain, beta wave rhythm can be encountered. A central beta rhythm is related to the Rolandic alpha or sensory-motor rhythm (SMR) and can be influenced by motor activity or tactile stimulation [52]. The gamma rhythm, often referred as fast beta wave, has frequencies above 30–45 Hz. The gamma wave band has also been proved to be a good indication of event-related synchronization (ERS) of the brain, and the gamma wave has been considered to be a good indication [53].

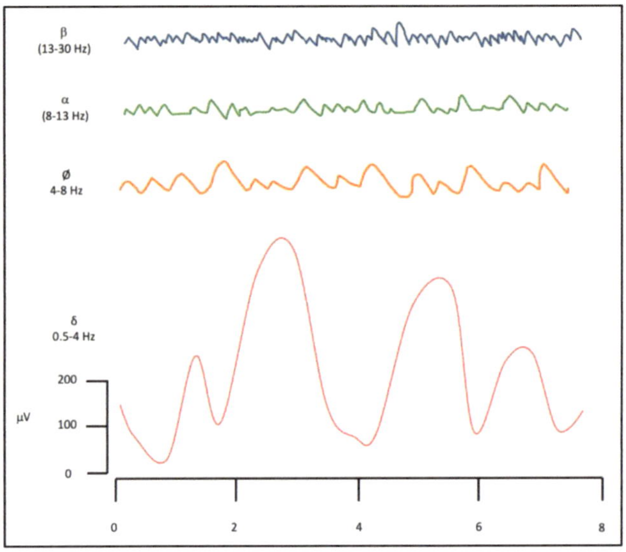

Figure 6.
Normal beta (β), alpha (α), theta (θ), and delta (δ) rhythms in order of high to low frequencies.

5.3.2 Classification and feature extraction of recorded EEG signals

Electroencephalographic (EEG) signals can be recorded with Cerebair (Nihon Kohden, Japan), Sienna Ultimate (EMS Biomedical, Austria), BrainAmp DC amplifiers, and anti-aliasing filter (BrainProducts, Munich, Germany) from approximately 21 Ag/AgCl scalp disposable gel-less and pre-gelled type electrodes over central and frontal regions of the brain. Each signal is sampled with up to 16 bits and is very popular in many commercially available EEG recording systems. Therefore, it is essential to store the archived signal masses in memory volumes. However, the memory size for archiving the EEG signals is often much lesser than that used for archiving radiological images.

A calculation procedure indicates that for a 1 hour recording from disposable electrodes (gel-less, and pre-gelled types) with an amplification rate of 1000 Hz in accordance with international 10–20 system.

$$N_E x \text{ seconds } x \text{ minutes } xfx\, b \approx \text{GB}. \tag{1}$$

GB = memory size, N_E = numbers of electrodes, f = frequency of amplification rate, b = bits.

Thus, a memory size of 21 × 60 × 60 × 1000 × 16 ≈ 1.20 Gbits ≈ 0.15 Gbyte is required. In today's technology of SSDs, hard drives, optical disks, CDs, and zip disks, there should be enough storage facilities for a large group of patients. EEG reading formats can easily be converted to spreadsheets that will be readable by most signal processing software packages such as MATLAB for different EEG machines.

Since electrode impedance often exceeds the frequency range of the physiological signals, ambient noise may compromise the recordings. Therefore, the high frequency noise must be avoided during this period so that all potential sources of electrical noise from the sampling environment can be removed and aliasing error can be avoided [54–59].

Since EMG may contaminate via compensatory movements with EEG, it may implicit artifacts that can compromise EEG-based BMI training [60]. In order to avoid or minimize these artifacts, the patients must be instructed to avoid blinking, chewing, and any head and body movements other than the joint movements. Also, the clinician should conduct visual inspection and feedback so that alternative BMI control can be prevented. After receiving the raw EEG signal, the data is filtered through bandpass, and DC notch filters and then spanning for visual artifact rejection are performed. Using EEGLAB-Toolbox (MATLAB Central, MathWorks), each session of event-related spectral perturbation (ERSP) of the feedback electrodes is calculated [49].

Surface electromyography (EMG) of the individual muscle or each muscle group is to be recorded with a Butterworth high bandpass filter and a sampling rate of 500–1000 Hz. An individual EMG threshold is set to calibrate the EMG classifier. The activity of the bipolarized EMG channels is measured and analyzed followed by discrimination between movement, and rest need to be performed.

The waveform length (λ)

$$\lambda(t_1) = P_t \left| x(t_o + 1) - x(t_o) \right| \tag{2}$$

$$\text{whereas } P_t = t_1 + t_o \tag{3}$$

$$t_o = t_1 - w + 1 \tag{4}$$

is calculated for each bipolarized EMG channel within a sliding window of w (ms). To correct for a delayed response of the subject to the cues, we calculated the cross- correlation of a vector L = $\lambda(t_1)$ containing the waveform length feature with a vector P = $P_{(t1)}$ which encodes the trial phase, where $P_{(t1)} = 1$ if t1 is part of the movement phase, otherwise $P_{(t1)} = 0$.

To improve the assignment of the waveform length to the movement or rest class (M_λ or R_λ, respectively), latency of the maximum of the cross-correlation sequence can be used as an offset. With a receiver operating characteristic (ROC) analysis, the threshold for the discrimination between the two distributions M_λ and R_λ is set. The criterion for threshold selection may be set as such that the false-positive rate must be lower than 5% to ensure high specificity of the classifier.

5.3.3 Desynchronization of BMI and NMES classifiers

As event-related desynchronization (ERD) is correlated to movement in the beta (β) band gets detected by EEG in the ipsilateral hemisphere of the brain (**Figure 7**). The brain-machine interface (BMI) environment stimulates EMG recordings of patient's joint during the movement [58, 61]. Once both the EMG and EEG classifier gives a positive output, NMES stimulation may be triggered. The same EMG filtering and feature extraction procedure can be used during the NMES session. Then, the samples of each data packet from these channels can be joined together to form a wavelength, which is to be computed, summed up for bipolar channels, and compared to the threshold for movement detection. As soon as it crosses the threshold, the EMG classifier will give a positive output.

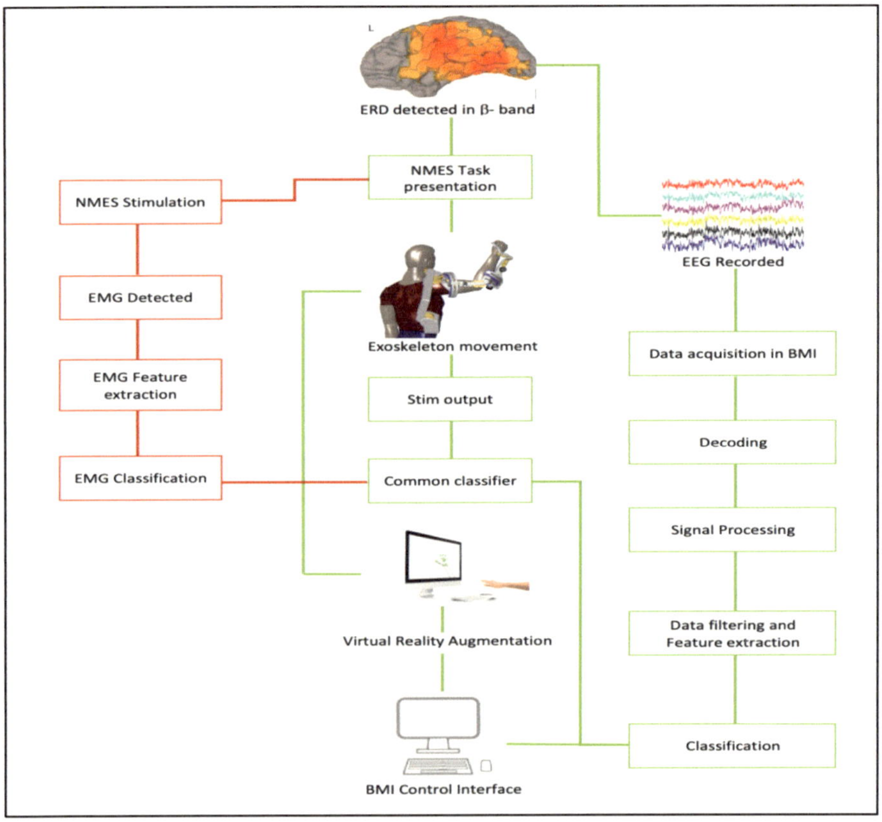

Figure 7.
Illustration of the flowchart of closed loop environment for hybrid brain-machine interface.

The sensitivity and specificity of the classifier of a linear discriminant analysis (LDA) are indicated by the true-positive rate (T_p) and the true-negative rate (T_n), respectively, while N is the total number of sample blocks in either during the movement or rest period. The positively and negatively classified sample blocks are $_pN$ and $_nN$, respectively.

$$\text{The false} - \text{positive rate}\left(F_p\right) = 1 - T_n.$$

TPR and TNR are calculated by

$$T_p = \frac{pNm}{Nm} \tag{5}$$

$$T_n = \frac{pNr}{Nr} \tag{6}$$

For the different classifier modalities, i.e., EEG, EMG, and hybrid EEG/EMG, the classification accuracy (X) of a BMI system is computed by

$$X = \left(\frac{Tp + Tn}{2}\right) x100 \tag{7}$$

The correct response rate (C_R) is calculated by the ratio between the number of BMI-controlled NMES assistance (N_{NMES}) and the number of trials (N_t).

$$CR = \frac{Nnmes}{Nt} \text{x 100} \tag{8}$$

The feasibility of integrating a hybrid BMI approach based on EEG/EMG into an integrated neuroprosthesis exoskeleton followed by neurofeedback training by stimulating NMES involving virtual environment increases the stability of classification and data extraction and can be expected that using BMI + NMES with neuroprosthesis exoskeleton can be more effective on ROM and ERD than the implementation of exoskeleton alone [62].

6. Recent trends in prosthetic management of BPI

6.1 Surface electromyographic (sEMG) virtual reality augmentative biofeedback in prosthetic (bionic) hand reconstruction

Hand reconstruction has seen many new approaches to replace the non-functioning plexus limb. The bionic hand/myoelectric/hybrid prosthetic hand uses the myoelectric signal from the electrical voltage generated during muscle contraction to control some movement. In patients with brachial plexus injury, this type of prosthesis uses the rest of the human body's neuromuscular system to control flexion/extension of the elbow, supination/pronation of forearm (rotation), or inhibiting functional grasps [2].

Bionic reconstruction can be recommended for patients with failed surgical treatment alternatives (i.e., nerve repair, nerve transfers, and secondary reconstructions resulting in futile upper limb function). Patients with simultaneous central nervous system injury, unstable fractures of the affected limb, untreated or resilient mental health problems, lack of compliance and commitment to adhere to a long-lasting rehabilitation program cannot be adequate candidates for a biofeedback training in bionic hand reconstruction. Tinel signs are suggested to be eliminated along the neural axis of the major peripheral nerves indicating the presence of viable axons suitable for nerve transfer surgery. Multidisciplinary team consisting of experienced prosthetists, reconstructive surgeons, orthopedic surgeons, physiatrists, psychologists, and physiotherapists should be formed for the assessment of the patients whether they are fit into the reconstruction procedure and explain to the patient that the functionality of a myoelectric prosthesis. Other interventions, such as psychological support, posture training, and/or strengthening of the remaining muscles, are also indicated [25].

Surface electromyographic signals (sEMG) electrodes are generally used on the exact skin position, where muscle contraction can be palpated with the finger, e.g., 5 cm distal to the elbow joint on the dorsal extensor compartment when the patient is asked to think of extending his/her wrist and fingers. While the sEMG electrode is moved to the volar aspect of the forearm, placing it on the pronator teres muscle, ask the patient to attempt pronating his/her forearm. Patient's movements can be assessed and evaluated while the signal being observed on the computer screen. When the patient thinks of this movement, the amplitude repeatedly increases [63]. In some cases, sEMG signals are not found. In these cases, nerve and muscle transfer need to be performed to establish new EMG signal sites, which delay signal training for 6–9 months. At least two separate EMG signal sites are needed for dexterous control of prosthetic hand.

As soon as two or more EMG signals have been identified, sEMG-guided signal training should be given to patient to get acquainted with adjustment of the voltage gain of each signal independently to achieve a similar signal amplitude threshold for all signals during training, which will make signal separation and comprehension easier during the training of the patient. But during training phase relaxation should be allowed as muscle strength may decrease faster in patients with complex nerve injuries and faint myoactivity. Depending on the number of available EMG signals and the degrees of freedom of the bionic hand, it is necessary to use methods for switching between these degrees of freedom through pattern recognition software. One frequently used method of switching between degrees of freedom is via the simultaneous contraction of two muscles, also known as co-contraction.

Hybrid hand fitting and prosthetic training are needed to be given with individually tailored socket onto or below the functionless plexus hand (**Figure 8**). Strength training for elbow flexors and shoulder muscles should be performed, if co-activation of the muscles used for prosthetic control is observed while lifting the arm. Simple grasping tasks, such as picking up manipulating small objects, boxes, signal independency should be improved through strength training, simple tasks of daily living, and co-activation of signal amplitude training. As the patient must lift the weight of his/her own hand in addition to the hybrid prosthetic hand, the device might feel rather heavy.

It should be noted that many tasks might be restricted since the paralyzed hand gets in the way and phase relaxation should be allowed in-between. Direct visualization of this muscle activity is vital for patient as it allows him/her to mentally grasp the pattern of myoelectric hand control and follow the training progress more consciously.

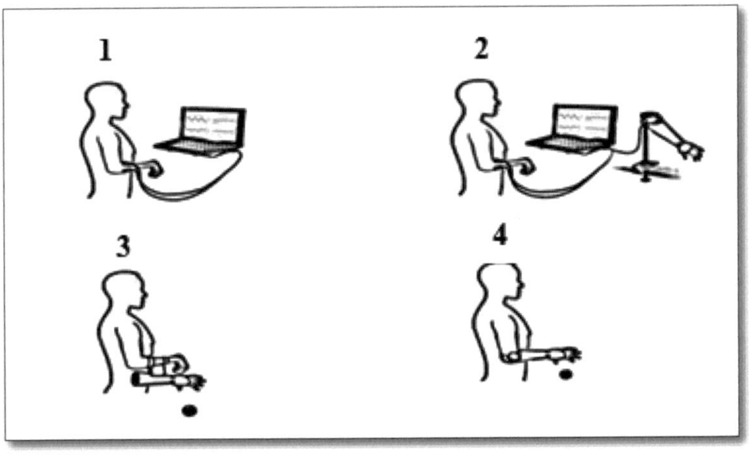

Figure 8.
(1) To identify the highest EMG amplitude over a specific target muscle, several motor commands may be attempted with virtual augmentation, and different signal positions can also be compared. (2) The EMG activity in a patient's arm is directly translated into prosthetic function after using a tabletop prosthesis. (3) Patient can visualize and embrace the use of future prosthetic hand, after the fitting and training with a hybrid prosthetic hand. (4) EMG signals can be trained and optimized either with sEMG biofeedback or with the prosthetic hand itself, after prosthetic reconstruction [64].

6.1.1 Elective amputation of affected limb and prosthetic hand replacement

Depending on the availability of site of the various EMG signals, the level of amputation (transradial, transhumeral, or, in rare cases, glenohumeral) should be precisely planned by the multidisciplinary team consisting of the patient's psychologist, prosthetist, physiotherapist, and the surgeon responsible for the amputation so that patient's expectations can be familiarized with everyone and unresolved questions regarding the planned amputation and clear communication regarding decision of amputation can be made; otherwise, it will result in irreversible and life-altering surgery. Elective amputation is to be performed as described previously followed by post-operative wound healing, and patient should be trained adjacent joints for improved upper limb mobility. The EMG signal training and selection of EMG electrodes' site should be followed up after 4–6 weeks of post-operative wound healing. These electrode positions and motor commands might differ slightly from the ones found before amputation. The prosthetist must design the prosthesis which may consist of prosthetic socket, hook/hand, silicone liner, and sEMG electrodes depending on the sites of EMG signals and co-contraction of muscles. Then, the procedure must follow post-prosthetic training from open/close the prosthetic hand without any co-contraction with weight of the prosthetic device being supported, followed by prosthetic movements on different arm positions such as the elbow flexion or extension. Patient should be trained for simple grasping tasks simultaneously with activities of daily living training staring with rather simple tasks as opening a door to slowly adding complexity and tasks that the patient considers relevant for his/her specific life adaptation or function.

7. Conclusion

Brachial plexus injuries have shown an upward trend in recent years with the frequent occurrence of accidental injuries such as car accidents, fall from heights, and external force pulling. Over the years it is been an absolute challenge for the prosthetists and orthotists to facilitate functions in BPI patients. Advancement in the field of brain–machine interface, artificial intelligence and replication of anatomical movements with prosthetic arm have emerged as excellent and effective treatment protocols for BPI. The interpretation of BMI with neuromuscular stimulation with exoskeleton assistive device has shown impressive effects on ROM, cortical modulation, and pain. In the future, novel restorative framework may be implemented while retaining their voluntary effort in BMI-NMES training goal-oriented training sessions. Additionally, due to the reduced neuromuscular interface in BPI affected patients, it is not clear whether currently commercially available prosthetic arm systems designed for otherwise healthy amputees can significantly enhance the prosthetic function in patients with brachial plexus injury, and hence, novel technologies for prosthetic control may be explored in future. Future studies should evaluate the applicability and benefits of the listed novel technologies as controlled trials with higher patient numbers will demonstrate the positive effects of the current rehabilitation protocols of patients with severe brachial plexus injuries.

Acknowledgements

The completion of this chapter is attributed to and supported by many people's support and encouragement. We thank our colleagues from Prosthetics and Orthotics

Services, Department of Physiotherapy and Department of Occupational Therapy, Institute of Rehabilitation, Christian Medical College (CMC), who provided their insights and expertise that greatly assisted us successfully completing the chapter.

Conflict of interest

The authors declare no conflict of interest.

Nomenclature

BPI	brachial plexus injury
OBPP	obstetric brachial plexus palsy
ADL	activities of daily living
SCs	Schwann cells
NTF	neurotrophic factors
NGF	nerve growth factor
BDNF	brain-derived neurotrophin factor
TrkB	tyrosine kinase receptors
mRNA	messenger ribonucleic acid
CNTF	ciliary neurotrophic factor
FGF	fibroblast growth factor
GDNF	glial cell line-derived neurotrophic factor
IGF	insulin-like growth factor
LMN	lower motor neuron
SAO	shoulder abduction orthosis
FAO	functional arm orthosis
NMES	neuromuscular electrical stimulation
ANN	artificial neural network
cAMP	cyclic adenosine monophosphate
PKA	protein kinase A
DRG	dorsal root ganglion
CREB	cyclic-AMP response binding protein
EMG	electromyographic
CCFES	contralaterally controlled functional electrical stimulation
FES	functional electrical stimulation
BMI	brain-machine interface
EEG	electroencephalogram
ERD	event-related desynchronization
sEMG	surface electromyographic

Author details

Om Prasad Biswal[1], Smita Nayak[2]* and Rajesh Kumar Das[3]

1 Prosthetics and Orthotics Services, PMR Department, Christian Medical College (CMC), Vellore, Tamilnadu, India

2 Pt. Deendayal National Institute for the Persons with Physical Disabilities (Divyangjan), New Delhi, India

3 Artificial Limbs Manufacturing Corporation of India, Kanpur, India

*Address all correspondence to: smitank7@gmail.com

References

[1] Midha R. Epidemiology of brachial plexus injuries in a multitrauma population. Neurosurgery. 1997;**40**:1182-1189. DOI: 10.1097/00006123-199706000-00014

[2] Sumarwoto T, Suroto H, Mahyudin F, Utomo DN, Hadinoto SA, Abdulhamid M, et al. Brachial plexus injury: Recent diagnosis and management. Open Access Macedonian Journal of Medical Sciences. 2021;**9**:13-24. DOI: 10.3889/oamjms.2021.5578

[3] Kouyoumdjian JA. Peripheral nerve injuries: A retrospective survey of 456 cases. Muscle & Nerve. 2006;**34**:785-788. DOI: 10.1002/mus.20624

[4] Eser F, Aktekin L, Bodur H, Atan C. Etiological factors of traumatic peripheral nerve injuries. Neurology India. 2009;**57**:434. DOI: 10.4103/0028-3886.55614

[5] Coroneos CJ, Voineskos SH, Christakis MK, Thoma A, Bain JR, Brouwers MC. Obstetrical brachial plexus injury (OBPI): Canada's national clinical practice guideline. BMJ Open. 2017;7:e014141. DOI: 10.1136/bmjopen-2016-014141

[6] Maillet M, Romana C. Complete obstetric brachial plexus palsy: Surgical improvement to recover a functional hand. Journal of Children's Orthopaedics. 2009;**3**:101-108. DOI: 10.1007/s11832-009-0161-1

[7] Thatte M, Mehta R. Obstetric brachial plexus injury. Indian Journal of Plastic Surgery. 2011;**44**:380. DOI: 10.4103/0970-0358.90805

[8] Chater M, Camfield P, Camfield C. Erb's palsy—Who is to blame and what will happen? Paediatrics & Child Health. 2004;**9**:556-560. DOI: 10.1093/pch/9.8.556

[9] Chen S, Chen Z-G, Dai H, Ding J, Guo J, Han N, et al. Repair, protection and regeneration of peripheral nerve injury. Neural Regeneration Research. 2015;**10**:1777. DOI: 10.4103/1673-5374.170301

[10] Jang SY, Shin YK, Park SY, Park JY, Lee HJ, Yoo YH, et al. Autophagic myelin destruction by schwann cells during wallerian degeneration and segmental demyelination: Autophagy in demyelination. Glia. 2016;**64**:730-742. DOI: 10.1002/glia.22957

[11] Barton M, John J, Clarke M, Wright A, Ekberg J. The glia response after peripheral nerve injury: A comparison between Schwann cells and olfactory Ensheathing cells and their uses for neural regenerative therapies. International Journal of Molecular Sciences. 2017;**18**:287. DOI: 10.3390/ijms18020287

[12] Chao MV. Neurotrophins and their receptors: A convergence point for many signalling pathways. Nature Reviews. Neuroscience. 2003;**4**:299-309. DOI: 10.1038/nrn1078

[13] Chen Z-Y, Chai Y-F, Cao L, Lu C-L, He C. Glial cell line-derived neurotrophic factor enhances axonal regeneration following sciatic nerve transection in adult rats. Brain Research. 2001;**902**:272-276. DOI: 10.1016/S0006-8993(01)02395-2

[14] Omura T, Sano M, Omura K, Hasegawa T, Doi M, Sawada T, et al. Different expressions of BDNF, NT3, and NT4 in muscle and nerve after

various types of peripheral nerve injuries. Journal of the Peripheral Nervous System. 2005;**10**:293-300. DOI: 10.1111/j.1085-9489.2005.10307.x

[15] Dieruf K, Poole JL, Gregory C, Rodriguez EJ, Spizman C. Comparative effectiveness of the GivMohr sling in subjects with flaccid upper limbs on subluxation through radiologic analysis. Archives of Physical Medicine and Rehabilitation. 2005;**86**:2324-2329. DOI: 10.1016/j.apmr.2005.07.291

[16] Cool JC. Biomechanics of orthoses for the subluxed shoulder. Prosthetics and Orthotics International. 1989;**13**:90-96. DOI: 10.3109/03093648909078219

[17] Meredith J, Taft G, Kaplan P. Diagnosis and treatment of the hemiplegic patient with brachial plexus injury. The American Journal of Occupational Therapy. 1981;**35**:656-660. DOI: 10.5014/ajot.35.10.656

[18] Kirjavainen M, Remes V, Peltonen J, Kinnunen P, Pöyhiä T, Telaranta T, et al. Long-term results of surgery for brachial plexus birth palsy. Journal of Bone and Joint Surgery. 2007;**89**:18-26. DOI: 10.2106/JBJS.E.00430

[19] Waters PM. Comparison of the natural history, the outcome of microsurgical repair, and the outcome of operative reconstruction in brachial plexus birth palsy. Journal of Bone and Joint Surgery. 1999;**81**:649-659. DOI: 10.2106/00004623-199905000-00006

[20] Hoeksma AF, ter Steeg AM, Nelissen RG, van Ouwerkerk WJ, Lankhorst GJ, de Jong BA. Neurological recovery in obstetric brachial plexus injuries: An historical cohort study. Developmental Medicine and Child Neurology. 2004;**46**:2. DOI: 10.1017/S0012162204000179

[21] Hale HB, Bae DS, Waters PM. Current concepts in the management of brachial plexus birth palsy. Journal of Hand Surgery. 2010;**35**:322-331. DOI: 10.1016/j.jhsa.2009.11.026

[22] Ögce F, Özyalçin H. Case study: A myoelectrically controlled shoulderelbow orthosis for unrecovered brachial plexus injury. Prosthetics and Orthotics International. 2000;**24**:252-255. DOI: 10.1080/03093640008726557

[23] Franzblau LE, Maynard M, Chung KC, Yang LJ-S. Medical treatment decision making after total avulsion brachial plexus injury: A qualitative study. Journal of Neurosurgery. 2015;**122**:1413-1420. DOI: 10.3171/2015.2.JNS132686

[24] Aszmann OC, Roche AD, Salminger S, Paternostro-Sluga T, Herceg M, Sturma A, et al. Bionic reconstruction to restore hand function after brachial plexus injury: A case series of three patients. The Lancet. 2015;**385**:2183-2189. DOI: 10.1016/S0140-6736(14)61776-1

[25] Hruby LA, Sturma A, Aszmann OC. Surface electromyographic biofeedback as a rehabilitation tool for patients with global brachial plexus injury receiving bionic reconstruction. Journal of Visualized Experiments. 2019;**151**. DOI: 10.3791/59839

[26] Justice D, Awori J, Carlson S, Chang KW-C, Yang LJ-S. Use of neuromuscular electrical stimulation in the treatment of neonatal brachial plexus palsy: A literature review. Open Journal of Occupational Therapy. 2018;**6**:10.15453/2168-6408.1431

[27] Gordon T, Sulaiman OAR, Ladak A. Chapter 24 electrical stimulation for improving nerve regeneration: Where do we stand? International Review of Neurobiology. 2009;**87**:433-444. DOI: 10.1016/S0074-7742(09)87024-4

[28] Knutson JS, Makowski NS, Kilgore KL, Chae J. Neuromuscular electrical stimulation applications. In: Atlas of Orthoses and Assistive Devices. US: Elsevier Health; 2019. pp. 432-439.e3. DOI: 10.1016/B978-0-323-48323-0.00043-3

[29] Wenjin W, Wenchao L, Hao Z, Feng L, Yan W, Wodong S, et al. Electrical stimulation promotes BDNF expression in spinal cord neurons through Ca^{2+}- and Erk-dependent signaling pathways. Cellular and Molecular Neurobiology. 2011;**31**:459-467. DOI: 10.1007/s10571-010-9639-0

[30] Urbanchek MG, Kung TA, Frost CM, Martin DC, Larkin LM, Wollstein A, et al. Development of a regenerative peripheral nerve interface for control of a neuroprosthetic limb. BioMed Research International. 2016;**2016**:1-8. DOI: 10.1155/2016/5726730

[31] Batty NJ, Fenrich KK, Fouad K. The role of cAMP and its downstream targets in neurite growth in the adult nervous system. Neuroscience Letters. 2017;**652**:56-63. DOI: 10.1016/j.neulet.2016.12.033

[32] Rosewilliam S, Malhotra S, Roffe C, Jones P, Pandyan AD. Can surface neuromuscular electrical stimulation of the wrist and hand combined with routine therapy facilitate recovery of arm function in patients with stroke? Archives of Physical Medicine and Rehabilitation. 2012;**93**:1715-1721.e1. DOI: 10.1016/j.apmr.2012.05.017

[33] Nascimento LR, Michaelsen SM, Ada L, Polese JC, Teixeira-Salmela LF. Cyclical electrical stimulation increases strength and improves activity after stroke: A systematic review. Journal of Physiotherapy. 2014;**60**:22-30. DOI: 10.1016/j.jphys.2013.12.002

[34] Knutson JS, Gunzler DD, Wilson RD, Chae J. Contralaterally controlled functional electrical stimulation improves hand dexterity in chronic hemiparesis: A randomized trial. Stroke. 2016;**47**:2596-2602. DOI: 10.1161/STROKEAHA.116.013791

[35] Meilink A, Hemmen B, Seelen H, Kwakkel G. Impact of EMG-triggered neuromuscular stimulation of the wrist and finger extensors of the paretic hand after stroke: A systematic review of the literature. Clinical Rehabilitation. 2008;**22**:291-305. DOI: 10.1177/0269215507083368

[36] Francisco G, Chae J, Chawla H, Kirshblum S, Zorowitz R, Lewis G, et al. Electromyogram-triggered neuromuscular stimulation for improving the arm function of acute stroke survivors: A randomized pilot study. Archives of Physical Medicine and Rehabilitation. 1998;**79**:570-575. DOI: 10.1016/S0003-9993(98)90074-0

[37] Howlett OA, Lannin NA, Ada L, McKinstry C. Functional electrical stimulation improves activity after stroke: A systematic review with meta-analysis. Archives of Physical Medicine and Rehabilitation. 2015;**96**:934-943. DOI: 10.1016/j.apmr.2015.01.013

[38] Mann G, Taylor P, Lane R. Accelerometer-triggered electrical stimulation for reach and grasp in chronic stroke patients: A pilot study. Neurorehabilitation and Neural Repair. 2011;**25**:774-780. DOI: 10.1177/1545968310397200

[39] Bioness H200 Functionele electrostimulatie voor handrevalidatie. n.d. Available from: https://www.ortho-kin.be/nieuws/nieuwsbericht/news/bioness-h200-functionele-electrostimulatie-voor-handrevalidatie/ [Accessed: November 20, 2022]

[40] Thrasher TA, Zivanovic V, McIlroy W, Popovic MR. Rehabilitation of reaching and grasping function in severe hemiplegic patients using functional electrical stimulation therapy. Neurorehabilitation and Neural Repair. 2008;**22**:706-714. DOI: 10.1177/1545968308317436

[41] Alon G, Levitt AF, McCarthy PA. Functional electrical stimulation enhancement of upper extremity functional recovery during stroke rehabilitation: A pilot study. Neurorehabilitation and Neural Repair. 2007;**21**:207-215. DOI: 10.1177/1545968306297871

[42] Knutson JS, Harley MY, Hisel TZ, Chae J. Improving hand function in stroke survivors: A pilot study of contralaterally controlled functional electric stimulation in chronic hemiplegia. Archives of Physical Medicine and Rehabilitation. 2007;**88**:513-520. DOI: 10.1016/j.apmr.2007.01.003

[43] Contralaterally controlled functional electrical stimulation (CCFES). ResearchGate. n.d. Available from: https://www.researchgate.net/figure/Contralaterally-controlled-functional-electrical-stimulation-CCFES-enables-stroke_fig 1_360552755 [Accessed: November 20, 2022]

[44] Rushton DN. Functional electrical stimulation and rehabilitation—An hypothesis. Medical Engineering & Physics. 2003;**25**:75-78. DOI: 10.1016/S1350-4533(02)00040-1

[45] De Marchis C, Santos Monteiro T, Simon-Martinez C, Conforto S, Gharabaghi A. Multi-contact functional electrical stimulation for hand opening: Electrophysiologically driven identification of the optimal stimulation site. Journal of NeuroEngineering and Rehabilitation. 2016;**13**:22. DOI: 10.1186/s12984-016-0129-6

[46] Fels M, Bauer R, Gharabaghi A. Predicting workload profiles of brain–robot interface and electromygraphic neurofeedback with cortical resting-state networks: Personal trait or task-specific challenge? Journal of Neural Engineering. 2015;**12**:046029. DOI: 10.1088/1741-2560/12/4/046029

[47] Kilgore KL, Bhadra N. Reversible nerve conduction block using kilohertz frequency alternating current. Neuromodulation: Technology at the Neural Interface. 2014;**17**:242-255. DOI: 10.1111/ner.12100

[48] Kilgore KL, Peckham PH, Keith MW, Montague FW, Hart RL, Gazdik MM, et al. Durability of implanted electrodes and leads in an upper-limb neuroprosthesis. Journal of Rehabilitation Research and Development. 2003;**40**:457. DOI: 10.1682/JRRD.2003.11.0457

[49] Grimm F, Walter A, Spüler M, Naros G, Rosenstiel W, Gharabaghi A. Hybrid neuroprosthesis for the upper limb: Combining brain-controlled neuromuscular stimulation with a multi-joint arm exoskeleton. Frontiers in Neuroscience. 2016;**10**:367. DOI: 10.3389/fnins.2016.00367

[50] Armeo®Spring. Hocoma. n.d. Available from: https://www.hocoma.com/solutions/armeo-spring/ [Accessed: November 20, 2022]

[51] Sterman MB, Macdonald LR, Stone RK. Biofeedback training of the sensorimotor electroencephalogram rhythm in man: Effects on epilepsy. Epilepsia. 1974;**15**:395-416. DOI: 10.1111/j.1528-1157.1974.tb04016.x

[52] Sanei S, Chambers JA. EEG Signal Processing. John Wiley & Sons Ltd.; 2007. pp. 35-125. DOI: 10.1002/9780470511923

[53] Pfurtscheller G, Flotzinger D, Neuper C. Differentiation between finger, toe and tongue movement in man based on 40 Hz EEG. Electroencephalography and Clinical Neurophysiology. 1994;**90**:456-460. DOI: 10.1016/0013-4694(94)90137-6

[54] Bauer R, Fels M, Vukelić M, Ziemann U, Gharabaghi A. Bridging the gap between motor imagery and motor execution with a brain–robot interface. NeuroImage. 2015;**108**:319-327. DOI: 10.1016/j.neuroimage.2014.12.026

[55] Vukelić M, Gharabaghi A. Oscillatory entrainment of the motor cortical network during motor imagery is modulated by the feedback modality. NeuroImage. 2015;**111**:1-11. DOI: 10.1016/j.neuroimage.2015.01.058

[56] Vukelić M, Gharabaghi A. Self-regulation of circumscribed brain activity modulates spatially selective and frequency specific connectivity of distributed resting state networks. Frontiers in Behavioral Neuroscience. 2015;**9**:181. DOI: 10.3389/fnbeh.2015.00181

[57] Vukelić M, Bauer R, Naros G, Naros I, Braun C, Gharabaghi A. Lateralized alpha-band cortical networks regulate volitional modulation of beta-band sensorimotor oscillations. NeuroImage. 2014;**87**:147-153. DOI: 10.1016/j.neuroimage.2013.10.003

[58] Gharabaghi A, Kraus D, Leão MT, Spüler M, Walter A, Bogdan M, et al. Coupling brain-machine interfaces with cortical stimulation for brain-state dependent stimulation: Enhancing motor cortex excitability for neurorehabilitation. Frontiers in Human Neuroscience. 2014;**8**:122. DOI: 10.3389/fnhum.2014.00122

[59] Naros G, Gharabaghi A. Reinforcement learning of self-regulated β-oscillations for motor restoration in chronic stroke. Frontiers in Human Neuroscience. 2015;**9**:391. DOI: 10.3389/fnhum.2015.00391

[60] Gharabaghi A, Naros G, Khademi F, Jesser J, Spüler M, Walter A, et al. Learned self-regulation of the lesioned brain with epidural electrocorticography. Frontiers in Behavioral Neuroscience. 2014;**8**:429. DOI: 10.3389/fnbeh.2014.00429

[61] Walter A, Murguialday AR, Rosenstiel W, Birbaumer N, Bogdan M. Coupling BCI and cortical stimulation for brain-state-dependent stimulation: Methods for spectral estimation in the presence of stimulation after-effects. Frontiers in Neural Circuits. 2012;**6**:87. DOI: 10.3389/fncir.2012.00087

[62] Leeb R, Sagha H, Chavarriaga R, Millán JdR. A hybrid brain–computer interface based on the fusion of electroencephalographic and electromyographic activities. Journal of Neural Engineering. 2011;**8**:025011, pp. 1-5. DOI: 10.1088/1741-2560/8/2/025011

[63] Sturma A, Hruby LA, Prahm C, Mayer JA, Aszmann OC. Rehabilitation of upper extremity nerve injuries using surface EMG biofeedback: Protocols for clinical application. Frontiers in Neuroscience. 2018;**12**:906. DOI: 10.3389/fnins.2018.00906

[64] Sturma A, Roche AD, Göbel P, Herceg M, Ge N, Fialka-Moser V, et al. A surface EMG test tool to measure proportional prosthetic control. Biomedical Engineering/Biomedizinische Technik. 2015;**60**(3):207-213. DOI: 10.1515/bmt-2014-0022

Chapter 12

Short-Segment Schanz Pedicle Screw Oblique Downward Fixation for Thoracolumbar Burst Fractures: A New Method for the Reduction of Intraspinal Bone Fragments

Sheng Yang and Chunyang Xia

Abstract

Short-segment pedicle screw internal fixation for thoracolumbar burst fracture has been widely used in clinic. When the fracture fragment enters the spinal canal seriously, it is often necessary to decompress. The authors pioneered the reduction of fracture fragments in the spinal canal by direct traction with pedicle screws implanted obliquely downward without lamina decompression. Compared with the previous pedicle screw parallel endplate fixation and lamina decompression, this new method has less trauma, better reduction and can remove the internal fixation after fracture healing. Compared with conventional pedicle screws, short-segment Schanz pedicle screws are more similar to normal posterior columns in structure and stress conduction and have better safety and stability, so the latter is more suitable for the treatment of severe burst fractures.

Keywords: thoracolumbar spine, burst fracture, short-segment pedicle screw, obliquely downward fixation, thoracolumbar burst fractures

1. Introduction

Thoracolumbar spinal fracture is the most common spinal fracture. When the fracture is serious, it often needs surgical treatment [1–5]. Previous studies have shown that it is difficult to reduce the intraspinal fracture fragments by direct distraction when the displacement distance is >0.85 cm, the turnover angle is >55° [6], the transverse diameter of fracture block/injured vertebral is >75%, and the height of displaced fracture block/injured vertebral height is >45% [7]. In this case, laminectomy combined with anterior surgery is usually required to directly reduce or treat intraspinal bone fragments. In 2018, the authors first reported a direct distraction and reduction of such intraspinal bone fragments by oblique downward insertion of Schanz pedicle screws in the adjacent upper and lower vertebrae without laminectomy and/or anterior surgery [8]. In this article, the authors will discuss the scoring criteria of thoracolumbar injuries, the advantages of Schanz screws, the mechanism of oblique downward screw distraction reduction, the indications and contraindications of the new method, and the role of thoracolumbar orthosis.

2. Thoracolumbar injury score criteria

Currently, commonly used scoring systems for thoracolumbar injury include Thoracolumbar Spine Injury Classification System (TL AOSIS) [3, 4], Thoracolumbar Injury Classification and Severity Score (TLICS) [2] and Load Sharing Classification (LSC) [5]. Both TLICS and TLAOSIS score thoracolumbar fractures from three aspects: fracture morphology, integrity of the posterior ligament complex (PLC), and nerve injury. Conservative treatment is recommended when the total score of TLICS is less than 4, and surgical treatment is recommended when the total score of TLICS is more than 4, and both are acceptable when the total score of TLICS is 4 [2]. TLAOSIS classifies neurological dysfunction on the basis of TLICS and adds clinical correction parameters. Conservative treatment is recommended when the total score of TLAOSIS is ≤3, surgery is recommended when it is >5, and surgery or conservative is recommended when it is 4–5 [3, 4].

Different from TLICS and TLAOSIS, LSC quantified and assigned values from three aspects, such as vertebral fracture degree, fracture block displacement range, and kyphosis correction angle. Each aspect was recorded as 1 point, 2 points, and 3 points, respectively, according to light, medium, and heavy, and the highest was 9 points [5]. Conservation is recommended when the total score of LSC is less than 4 points, and short-segment pedicle screw fixation is recommended when the total score of LSC is 4–6 points; posterior short segment fixation is not suitable when the total score is ≥7, and anterior fixation is recommended [5]. LSC only makes a detailed assessment of vertebral injury, but lacks the assessment of neurological function and posterior column (PLC), so it is not suitable to use LSC alone for assessment when combined with neurological and posterior column injuries. TLICS and TLAOSIS are more comprehensive in evaluating fractures than LSC, but their evaluation of fractured vertebral bodies is not detailed/lacks quantitative standards, so the authors use LSC + TLAOSIS to evaluate thoracolumbar fractures clinically.

LSC is an evaluation standard for judging the safety of short-segment pedicle screw fixation in the treatment of thoracolumbar fractures [5]. The higher the LSC score, the more unstable the injured vertebra and the worse the safety of short-segment pedicle screw fixation. Since this article mainly discusses the treatment of thoracolumbar burst fractures with pedicle screw fixation, the authors use LSC to evaluate the severity of fractures in this article. The accuracy of LSC has been questioned in recent years [9, 10]. Filgueira et al. reported in 2020 that LSC is safe and reliable when LSC is ≤6, and when LSC is ≥7, it is necessary to combine other evaluation criteria to select appropriate surgical methods [11]. Similarly, the author's finite element study on short-segment (T12 and L2) Schanz screw fixation for severe lumbar 1 fracture in 2021 also suggested that the scope/degree of posterior superior wall fracture of vertebral body is also one of the risk factors for fixation failure [12]. The authors believe that the evaluation of vertebral posterior superior wall injury should be increased when evaluating thoracolumbar fractures.

3. Advantages of Schanz Pedicle Screw

The purpose of surgical treatment is to rebuild the stability of thoracolumbar vertebrae, restore the height of injured vertebrae as much as possible, and reduce postoperative deformity and complications. At present, there are many surgical methods such as anterior approach, posterior approach, and anterior–posterior approach, but there is no best scheme due to the complexity of fracture [13]. Short-segment (adjacent to upper and lower vertebrae) conventional pedicle screw fixation for A3/A4 [2] thoracolumbar burst fracture has been applied clinically, but the complication of screw rod rupture in severe fracture (LSC $\geq$ 7) restricts its popularization [14–16]. Previous studies have shown that many factors, such as the degree of primary injury of fracture, pedicle screw diameter, screw depth, screw type, and bone abnormality (such as osteoporosis), are the risk factors for the failure of conventional pedicle screw fixation [17–20]. The successful treatment of thoracolumbar burst fractures with adjacent to upper and lower vertebrae Schanz screw fixation by the authors and Aono et al. shows that Schanz screws have better ability to maintain the stability of fixation segments [8, 17].

In 2018, the author put forward for the first time that Schanz screw is successful in treating severe fracture (LSC $\geq$ 7), mainly because Schanz screw is more similar to the posterior column structure of spine and its stress conduction than conventional nail [8]. The posterior column structure of normal lumbar spine (upper and lower articular processes, isthmus and lamina) is similar to "butterfly shape." The structure of Schanz screw rod is similar to "][" shape, while that of conventional pedicle screw rod is similar to "| |" shape [8]. The stress of normal posterior column of spine is transmitted through butterfly-like posterior column. The stress conduction of Schanz screw is from outside to inside, then down and finally to outside downward(like '][‘shape), and its connecting rod is located on both sides of spinous process and directly behind lamina [8, 19]. The stress of conventional pedicle screw is linear-like conduction, and its screw rods are located in the plane of upper and lower articular processes (see **Figure 1**) [8, 19].

Normal stress conduction between adjacent posterior columns (indirect conduction through intervertebral facet joint): from superior articular process along isthmus through lamina to inferior articular process and finally through intervertebral facet joint (indirect conduction) to superior articular process of the next vertebra. Stress conduction between Schanz screws and rods (indirect conduction through connecting clips): from upper screws to upper connecting clips (similar to isthmus), along connecting rods, through lower connecting clips (similar to intervertebral facet joints) and finally to lower screws. Direct conduction of stress between conventional screws and rods: from the upper screw to the lower screw directly through the connecting rod. Moderate fracture (LSC $<$ 7) had no significant effect on the stress of screw and rod because the injured vertebra could still bear part of the load. In severe burst fracture (LSC $\geq$ 7), when the loads of the anterior, middle, and posterior column are all (/most) transmitted across the injured vertebra through the posterior screw and moderate rod, this direct transmission may lead to excessive stress concentration in a certain part of the screw or rod (often at the root of the screw) and fatigue break. This view is first proposed by the author.

Because the connection clip has the adjustment function [8], there is no need to bend the connection rod to keep the Schanz screw-rod tightly combined. However, conventional screws often need to bend the connecting rod to ensure the tight combination of screw and rod [16]. The ability of conducting stress of straight rod is

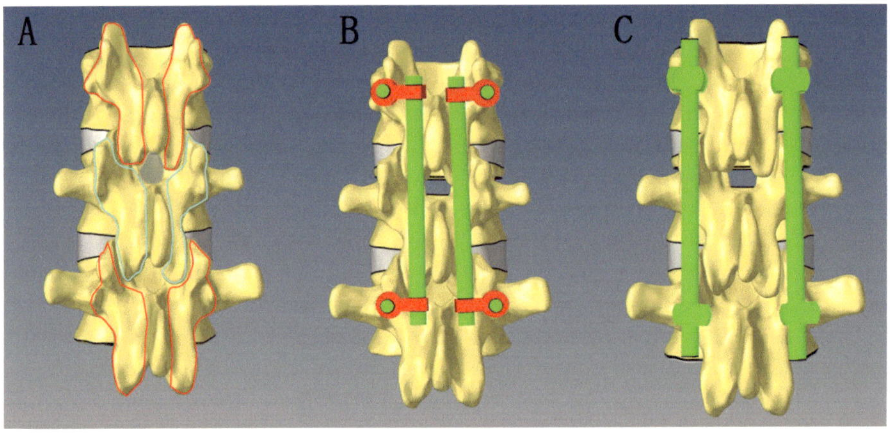

Figure 1.
Finite element simulation of posterior–anterior position of thoracic 12, lumbar 1, and lumbar 2 vertebrae. 1A. Normal T12, L1, and L2 butterfly-shaped rear column simulation diagram; 1B. T12 and lumbar 2Schanz pedicle screw fixation simulation diagram, Schanz screw rod is"][" shape, and its connecting rod is located on both sides of spinous process. 1C. Simulated images of routine pedicle screw fixation in T12 and L2. The structure of conventional pedicle screw rod is similar to "| |"shape, and its connecting rod is located in the plane of intervertebral facet joint outside the lamina.

better than that of bent rod. Compared with conventional screw, the straight rods of Schanz screw are located on both sides of spinous processes, while the curved rods of conventional screws are located on the planes of upper and lower articular processes, so the ability of Schanz screw to limit excessive flexion and extension of fixed segments is stronger than that of conventional screw. Namely, the straight rod of Schanz screw can also play a certain function similar to PLC [8]. The authors' previous finite element studies suggest that the anterior flexion of fixation segments is also one of the risk factors for the failure of pedicle screw fixation [12, 19]. Pedicle screws maintain the stability of fixed segments by bearing loads and conducting stresses. Compared with conventional screws, Schanz screws have better stress conduction and stronger unloading capacity, so that the screw can maintain the stability of the fixed segment without obvious stress increase (not exceeding the fatigue threshold of the screw) [8, 12, 19].

4. Mechanism and advantage of traction reduction of oblique downward screw

The typical imaging features of burst fracture are compression of anterior column, comminution of upper endplate, burst fracture fragments of middle column retropulsed into spinal canal [1]. When the burst vertebral body is compressed more than 30%, most of the burst bone fragments collapse and move backward and are mainly located in the middle and posterior part of the vertebral body and in the spinal canal (bone defects are often seen in the anterior part of the vertebral body). Only after the bone fragments located in the middle and posterior part of the vertebral body are reduced forward and upward can the intraspinal canal bone fragments have the space and possibility of reduction [8]. Unlike the backward and upward traction force of the screw parallel to the upper endplate, the traction force of the screw oblique downward is forward and upward (see **Figure 2**) [8].

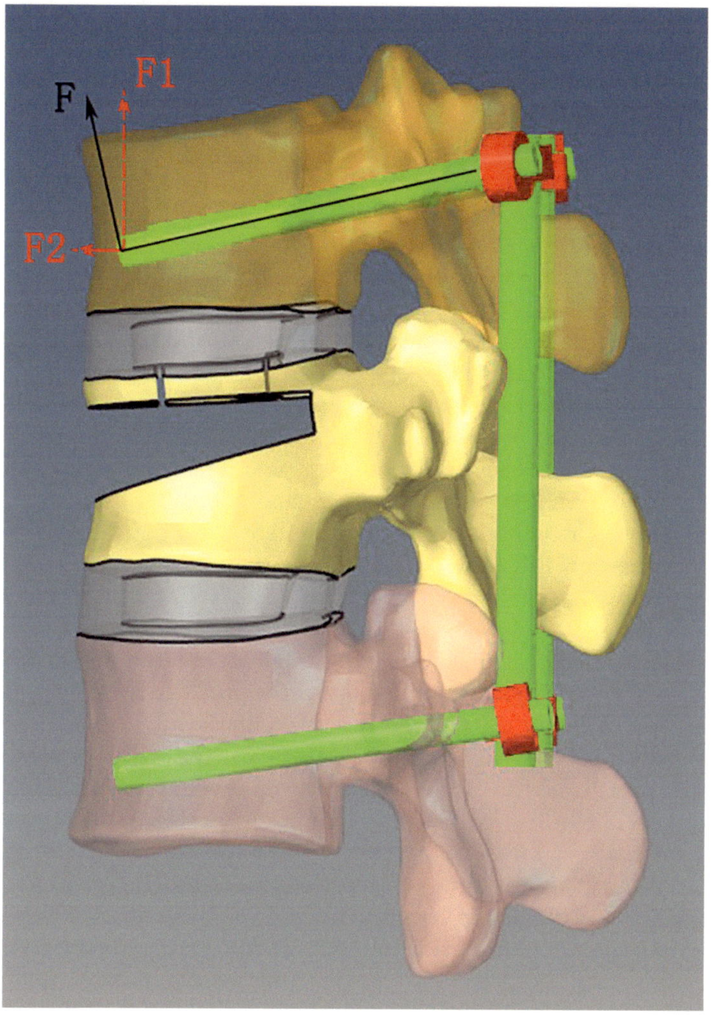

Figure 2.
Lateral finite element simulation of T12 and L2 Schanz pedicle screw oblique downward fixation of L1 severe burst fracture (LSC 9). The reduction traction F of the obliquely downward implanted screw in T12 includes an upward component F1 and a forward component F2.

In posterior column traction reduction, the forward and upward traction of the upper screw can not only elevate the height of vertebral body, but also move the bone fragments at the back of the vertebral body (in front of the spinal canal) forward and upward, providing enough reduction space for the bone fragments in the spinal canal to return [8]. Compared with the upward and backward traction of the conventional method, the forward and upward traction of the new method is more beneficial to the reduction of the intraspinal canal bone fragments and has less influence on the compressed dura sac and nerve [8]. In anterior column distraction reduction, the traction of upper screw is first forward and upward, then (beyond the level of upper endplate) backward and upward [8]. The forward and upward traction can make the collapsed and backward bones fragments move upward and forward. Upward and backward traction not only makes the bone fragments continue to be restored upward, but also makes the bone fragments displaced forward and downward return upward and backward [8]. The author's research based on his finite element model of burst fracture shows that it is safe to implant pedicle screw oblique downward within 15 degrees [19, 21].

5. Skills of oblique downward screw implantation and reduction

Due to limited space, the anesthesia, position and incision of this new method are detailed in the relevant paper published by the author in 2018 [8]. In this section, the authors focus only on the techniques of exposure of the operative area, oblique downward screw placement, and reduction (taking T12 and L2 Schanz pedicle screw fixation for lumbar 1 burst fracture as examples). Precautions for surgical site exposure: 1) subperiosteal dissection without transection of paravertebral muscles. The muscles at the attachment points of T12 transverse process and L2 superior articular process were turned upward and outward to expose intervertebral facet joints, so as to avoid damage to local intervertebral facet joints and joint capsule as much as possible; 2) avoid damage to supraspinous ligament and interspinous ligament; 3) only the paravertebral muscles of L1 need to be stripped to the extent that the connecting rod can be inserted; the lateral half of L1 lamina and T12L1 intervertebral facet joint need not be exposed.

Precautions for pedicle screw insertion: 1) Refer to the Roy-Camille method to select the nail entry point. 2) The parallel line of the upper endplate was the 0 degree reference line, and the pedicle screw was inserted into the middle and lower third of the vertebral body under the assistance of fluoroscopy (the angle between the long axis of the pedicle nail and the parallel line of the upper endplate was about 10°, not more than 15°). 3) According to the author's clinical experience, the sagittal position of the upper and lower screws should be as parallel as possible to achieve better reduction (based on the principle of force and reaction force). 4) The screw placement depth reaches 90% ~ 100% of the vertebral body. 5) Cyclic reduction was performed according to the sequence of posterior, anterior, and posterior column reduction: (1) during posterior column traction, the side with severe spinal stenosis was first reduced, and then the contralateral side was reduced. (2)Intraoperative lateral fluoroscopy is often difficult to directly observe the reduction of intraspinal fractures. The experience of the authors suggests that the angle change between the extension line of the upper endplate of the injured vertebral body and the extension line of the upper edge of the fracture fragment can indirectly judge whether the intraspinal canal fracture fragment is reduced or not. With the recovery of the height of the injured vertebral body, the angle between the two gradually decreased, indicating the reduction of the bone fragment, and the angle between the two was close to 0, indicating that the reduction was good. (3) The height of the anterior and posterior margins of the upper and lower intervertebral spaces of the injured vertebral body was similar to the height of the adjacent intervertebral discs, indicating that the anterior column was well reduced.

6. Indications and contraindications

The indications and contraindications of the new method are basically the same as those of the conventional screw. The author mainly discusses the characteristics of Schanz screw. Because the damage of Schanz pedicle screw to soft tissue is greater than that of percutaneous pedicle screw, the authors suggest using short-segment conventional percutaneous pedicle screw fixation for moderate fracture (LSC4–6) [5, 22, 23]. However, it is recommended to consider this new method when the fracture fragments retropulsed into the spinal canal seriously and requires lamina decompression. Indications of this new method are: (1) A3/A4 fracture [2, 3] with incomplete spinal cord/nerve injury with LSC ≥ 7 (fracture block protruding into spinal canal >40–50%); 2) fracture within 10 days; (3) MRI showed that the continuity of posterior longitudinal ligament (PLL) at the injured spinal canal level existed/did not break. Contraindications [2, 3]: 1) MRI showed that the PLL at the injured spinal canal level was broken, combined with cerebrospinal fluid leakage and/or complete paralysis (nerve injury); 2) unilateral pedicle fracture ≥90% or bilateral pedicle fracture ≥70%. 3) fracture with dislocation or C-type burst fracture [2, 3]; 4) congenital spinal malformation /severe degenerative scoliosis; 5) patients with severe osteoporosis (bone mineral density, BMD < −3.5); 5) Infectious/pathological fractures.

7. Thoracolumbosacral orthosis (TLSO)

The author's series of studies on the treatment of thoracolumbar fractures with short-segment pedicle screw fixation since 2018 showed that [8, 12, 18, 19, 21]: the maximum stress of pedicle screws increased with the aggravation of fracture degree, and the increase of screw stress in forward flexion was the most obvious. In moderate thoracolumbar fracture (LSC score 4–6), the risk of screw breakage is low with both types of screws, so brace assistance is not required. In severe fracture flexion, the fracture risk of conventional screws is increased while that of Schanz screws is low.

The maximum stress of these two screws in the upright position of severe fracture did not exceed the screw fatigue threshold, so the risk of fixation failure was low. In brief, maintaining an upright thoracolumbar position during early postoperative walking (within 3 months) reduces the risk of Schanz and conventional screw fixation failure. Although Schanz screws have a better ability to conduct stress compared with conventional screws, the authors' study [12, 19] showed that the bone defect area of the vertebral body after reduction of severe fractures has a slight movement during anterior flexion, and this micro movement is more severe in Schanz screws than in conventional screws. This slight movement may be one of the reasons for the re-collapse of the injured vertebra after Schanz screw fixation [8, 19, 24]. TLSO braces can keep the thoracolumbar and lumbar vertebrae upright, thereby reducing the micro movement of the injured vertebrae bone defect area and avoiding the re-injury of PLC and intervertebral disc caused by flexion and extension activities [24–26]. Early functional exercise (within 3 months) after short-segment pedicle screw fixation for severe thoracolumbar fractures requires TLSO assistance [8, 12, 19]. The time of wearing TLSO was adjusted according to the size of bone defect area and the growth of new bone during follow-up.

8. Typical case

A 45-year-old male patient. L2 burst fracture with incomplete nerve injury (Frankel C grade). Schanz pedicle screw was implanted obliquely downward in adjacent upper and lower vertebrae and then directly distracted reduction and fixation was performed. Lamina decompression and bone grafting were not performed.

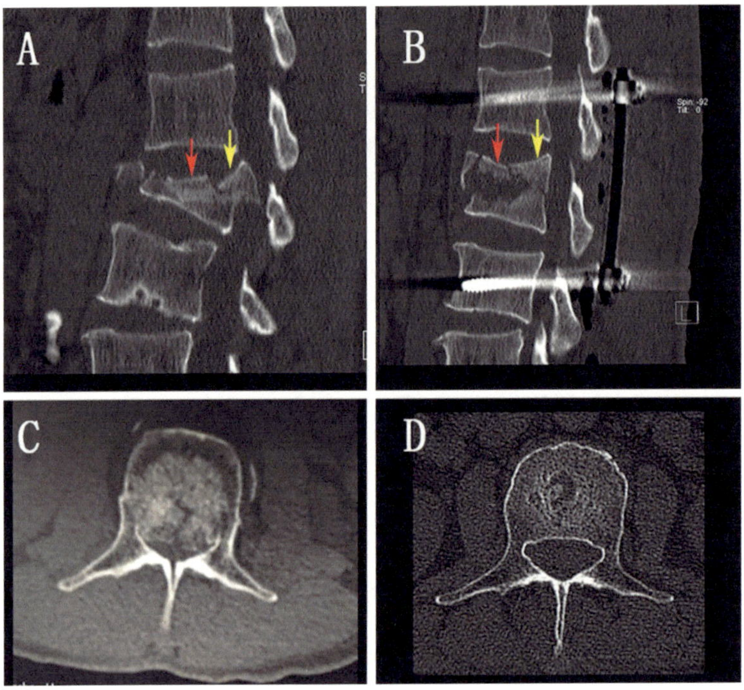

Figure 3.
3A preoperative sagittal CT image: Anterior column of L2 is compressed 80%, the middle column is comminuted, and the bone fragments enter the spinal canal ≥80%. The fracture fragment indicated by the red arrow shifts backward and downward, and the fracture fragment indicated by the yellow arrow obviously protrudes backward into the spinal canal; 3B. Sagittal CT image after L 1 and 3 Schanz pedicle screws oblique downward implantation and distraction reduction: Schanz pedicle screws were implanted obliquely downward in L1 and L3. The height of anterior and posterior edges of L2 vertebral body recovered to 90%, and the fracture fragments protruding into vertebral canal were basically reduced (the fracture blocks indicated by yellow and red arrows were reduced forward and upward), and there was a bone defect area in the anterior and middle part of the injured vertebral body. The kyphosis of injured vertebra was basically corrected, and the stenosis of spinal canal was obviously improved. 3C. Preoperative CT axial position showed that the vertebral body burst, the fracture fragments obviously protruded into the spinal canal, the spinal canal obviously narrowed, and the pedicle fracture. 3D. Axial CT images after fracture healing and internal fixation: The spinal canal is basically normal, and there is a small bone defect area in the middle of L2 vertebral body.

The neurological function was Frankel D 3 days after operation and Frankel E 1 month after operation (see **Figure 3**).

9. Conclusion

Compared with the previous pedicle screw fixation parallel to the end plate, the oblique downward Schanz pedicle screw can direct reduce the intraspinal fracture fragments without lamina decompression and does not increase the risk of nerve injury. This is a new safe and effective method for reduction of intraspinal fracture fragments. The treatment of severe thoracolumbar burst fracture with short-segment Schanz pedicle screw oblique downward fixation requires TLSO brace to help prevent the injured vertebra from re-collapse in the early stage after operation.

Author details

Sheng Yang* and Chunyang Xia
Department of Orthopedics, Affiliated Zhongshan Hospital of Dalian University, Dalian, Liaoning, China

*Address all correspondence to: yangsheng_88@163.com

References

[1] Magerl F, Aebi M, Gertzbein SD, et al. A comprehensive classification of thoracic and lumbar injuries. European Spine Journal: Official publication of the European Spine Society, the European Spinal Deformity Society, and the European Section of the Cervical Spine Research Society. 1994;**3**(4):184-201

[2] Vaccaro AR, Lehman RA Jr, Hurlbert RJ. A new classification of thoracolumbar injuries: The importance of injury morphology, the integrity of the posterior ligamentous complex, and neurologic status. Spine. 2005;**30**:2325-2333

[3] Vaccaro AR, Oner C, Kepler CK, et al. AOSpine thoracolumbar spine injury classification system: Fracture description, neurological status, and key modifiers. Spine. 2013;**38**(23):2028-2037

[4] Vaccaro AR, Schroeder GD, Kepler CK, et al. The surgical algorithm for the AOSpine thoracolumbar spine injury classification system. European Spine Journal: Official publication of the European Spine Society, the European Spinal Deformity Society, and the European Section of the Cervical Spine Research Society. 2016;**25**(4):1087-1094

[5] McCormack T, Karaikovic E, Gaines RW. The load sharing classification of spine fractures. Spine. 1994;**19**(15):1741-1744

[6] Peng Y, Zhang L, Shi T, et al. Relationship between fracture-relevant parameters of thoracolumbar burst fractures and the reduction of intracanal fracture fragment. Journal of Orthopaedic Surgery and Research. 2015;**27**(10):131. DOI: 10.1186/s13018-015-0260-2

[7] Wang XB, Lü GH, Li J, et al. Posterior distraction and instrumentation cannot always reduce displaced and rotated Posterosuperior fracture fragments in thoracolumbar burst fracture. Clinical Spine Surgery. 2017;**30**(3):E317-E322

[8] Yang S, Shang DP, Lu JM, et al. Modified posterior short-segment pedicle screw instrumentation for lumbar burst fractures with incomplete neurological deficit. World Neurosurgery. 2018;**119**:e977-e985

[9] Stam WT, Deunk J, Elzinga MJ, et al. The predictive value of the load sharing classification concerning sagittal collapse and posterior instrumentation failure: A systematic literature review. Global Spine Journal. 2020;**10**(4):486-492

[10] Wang K, Zhang ZJ, Wang JL, et al. Risk factor of failed reduction of posterior Ligamentatoxis reduction instrumentation in managing thoracolumbar burst fractures: A retrospective study. World Neurosurgery. 2018;**119**:e475-e481

[11] Filgueira ÉG, Imoto AM, Silva HECD, et al. Thoracolumbar Burst Fracture: McCormack Load-Sharing Classification - Systematic Review and Single Arm meta-Analysis. Spine (Phila Pa 1976). 2021 May 1;**46**(9):E542-E550. DOI: 10.1097/BRS.0000000000003826

[12] Xia C, Yang S, Liu J, et al. Finite element study on whether posterior upper wall fracture is a risk factor for the failure of short-segment pedicle screw fixation in the treatment of L1 burst fracture. Injury. 2021;**52**(11):3253-3260

[13] Anderson PA, Raksin PB, Arnold PM, et al. Congress of Neurological Surgeons systematic review and evidence-based

guidelines on the evaluation and treatment of patients with thoracolumbar spine trauma: Surgical approaches. Neurosurgery. 2019;**84**(1):E56-E58

[14] Liao JC, Chen WJ. Short-segment instrumentation with fractured vertebrae augmentation by screws and bone substitute for thoracolumbar unstable burst fractures. BioMed Research International. 2019;**26**(2019):4780426

[15] Kapoen C, Liu Y, Bloemers FW, Deunk J. Pedicle screw fixation of thoracolumbar fractures: Conventional short segment versus short segment with intermediate screws at the fracture level-a systematic review and meta-analysis. European Spine Journal. 2020;**29**(10):2491-2504

[16] Liao JC, Fan KF. Posterior short-segment fixation in thoracolumbar unstable burst fractures - Transpedicular grafting or six-screw construct? Clinical Neurology and Neurosurgery. 2017;**153**:56-63

[17] Aono H, Ishii K, Tobimatsu H, Nagamoto Y, Takenaka S, Furuya M, et al. Temporary short-segment pedicle screw fixation for thoracolumbar burst fractures: Comparative study with or without vertebroplasty. The Spine Journal. 2017;**17**(8):1113-1119

[18] Liu J, Yang S, Lu J, Fu D, Liu X, Shang D. Biomechanical effects of USS fixation with different screw insertion depths on the vertebrae stiffness and screw stress for the treatment of the L1 fracture. Journal of Back and Musculoskeletal Rehabilitation. 2018;**31**(2):285-297

[19] Zhou F, Yang S, Liu J, et al. Finite element analysis comparing short-segment instrumentation with conventional pedicle screws and the Schanz pedicle screw in lumbar 1 fractures. Neurosurgical Review. 2020;**43**(1):301-312

[20] Hishiya T, Ishikawa T, Ota M. Posterior spinal fixation using penetrating endplate screws in patients with diffuse idiopathic skeletal hyperostosis-related thoracolumbar fractures. Journal of Neurosurgery: Spine. 2021;**9**:1-6

[21] Liu J, Yang S, Zhou F, Lu J, Xia C, Wang H, et al. The feasibility of short-segment Schanz screw implanted in an oblique downward direction for the treatment of lumbar 1 burst fracture: A finite element analysis. Journal of Orthopaedic Surgery and Research. 2020;**15**(1):537

[22] Shao X, Peng P, Yang P, et al. A retrospective comparative study of clinical efficacy of percutaneous short segment pedicle screw fixation with or without screwing of the fractured vertebra with O-arm navigation. BMC Musculoskeletal Disorders. 2022;**23**(1):108

[23] Yang P, Chen K, Zhang K, et al. Percutaneous short-segment pedicle instrumentation assisted with O-arm navigation in the treatment of thoracolumbar burst fractures. The Journal of Orthopaedic Translation. 2019;**21**:1-7

[24] Lakshmanan P, Jones A, Mehta J, et al. Recurrence of kyphosis and its functional implications after surgical stabilization of dorsolumbar unstable burst fractures. The Spine Journal. 2009;**9**(12):1003-1009

[25] Hirota R, Teramoto A, Irifune H, et al. Risk factors for postoperative loss of correction in thoracolumbar injuries caused by high-energy trauma treated

via percutaneous posterior stabilization without bone fusion. Medicina (Kaunas, Lithuania). 2022;**58**(5):583

[26] Alan N, Donohue J, Ozpinar A, et al. Load-sharing classification score as supplemental grading system in the decision-making process for patients with thoracolumbar injury classification and severity 4. Neurosurgery. 2021;**89**(3):428-434

Section 4

Miscellaneous Spinal Procedures

Chapter 13

An Updated Review of the Surgical Techniques and Outcomes for Metastatic Spinal Cord Compression

Bhoresh Dhamija, Steven Tominey, Shabin Joshi, Rahim Hussain, Dheeraj Batheja and Birender Balain

Abstract

Metastatic spinal cord compression (MSCC) is a condition associated with high morbidity and mortality. It affects up to 5% of patients with cancer and continues to increase in prevalence with advances in cancer care. In certain cases, surgical management is required for management of pain, neurological decline, and mechanical instability. Various surgical approaches and techniques have been utilized with traditional open and minimally invasive surgery both shown to be effective in improving patients' function and quality of life. Predictors of survival and functional outcomes following surgery for MSCC include primary tumor type, performance status, and preoperative neurological status. Several prognostic models have been created and validated to assist clinicians in appropriate patient selection. Complications following surgery for MSCC are varied, with wound infection and dehiscence being the most frequently reported. There remains considerable variation in reported outcomes and the decision to pursue surgery should be carefully considered in the context of the individual patient's prognosis and goals of care.

Keywords: spinal metastases, spinal cord compression, surgical decompression, minimally invasive surgery, surgical techniques

1. Introduction

Metastatic spinal cord compression (MSCC) infers significant morbidity and mortality in patients with cancer and represents a significant clinical challenge. The incidence of spinal metastatic disease continues to increase due to an aging population and improved overall cancer survival [1]. It affects up to 5% of patients with cancer [2]. Primary tumors that more commonly spread to the spine include breast, lung, kidney, and prostate cancers [3]. The mean survival for patients with MSCC is dependent on a variety of factors including primary pathology, baseline performance status, and the number of extraspinal organs affected [4, 5].

Spinal metastases can cause a range of symptoms, including pain, weakness, paralysis, bowel and bladder dysfunction, and mechanical instability. A multidisciplinary collaborative approach involving radiologists, oncologists, and spinal surgeons has been shown to be effective in improving neurological function and reducing pain in patients with MSCC [6]. In around one-third of cases, patients experience symptoms refractory to medical management require timely surgical intervention. This is influenced by the primary pathological mechanism of MSCC causing damage to the spinal cord through direct tumor compression, resulting edema, venous congestion, and resultant demyelination and secondary vascular injury. These effects can eventually become irreversible if not timely acted on [6]. Surgical decompression has the potential to offer prompt resolution of this compression, while radiotherapy requires days and longer to take effect. Multiple studies including meta-analysis and a randomized-controlled trial have demonstrated a combined approach of surgery with radiotherapy, compared with radiotherapy alone results in better outcomes [6–8]. In addition, surgical management through instrumented fixation and stabilization of the spinal column can negate the effects following bony infiltration/destruction, causing instability, fracture, or collapse.

In this chapter, we provide a review of surgical techniques, predictors of patient outcomes, and the complications reported in the literature over the past two decades. This information is intended to support and inform clinicians and patients in making the most appropriate treatment decisions for spinal metastases.

2. Patient population, demographics, and surgical selection

The patient population affected by MSCC is diverse. Studies have shown that the incidence of MSCC is higher in males than females, with a male to female ratio ranging from 1.2:1 to 2:1 [6]. The age at diagnosis varies widely, with a mean age of around 60 years. However, MSCC can also occur in younger patients, particularly those with hematologic malignancies. The most common primary tumors leading to MSCC are lung, breast, prostate, and renal cell carcinomas [9]. The incidence also varies depending on the primary tumor, with lung cancer being the most common implicated association [9].

Generally, surgery is opted for in patients with severe or rapidly progressing neurological deficits, as well as those with a single level of compression or lesions causing spinal instability. In patients with a poor performance status or multiple levels of compression, surgery may not be beneficial, and palliative care or radiotherapy alone may be more appropriate [6]. The timing of surgery is also important, with emergent surgery indicated in cases of impending neurological compromise, and urgent or elective surgery recommended for stable patients with less severe symptoms. Patients with spinal metastases are often at increased risk of operative morbidity and mortality compared to the general population [10]. Therefore, informed consent and shared decision making between the patient and clinician are essential.

3. Surgical techniques

The choice of surgical technique used is dependent on several variables that comprise both clinician and patient factors. These include the tumor location, size, and degree of spinal cord compression, surgeon experience, and expertise with the options for approach. A significant factor is the patient's overall health status and expected survival.

Techniques can be categorized by approach (posterior, anterior, or combined) and exposure (open or minimally invasive surgery).

3.1 Posterior decompression

Posterior decompression techniques are the most common surgical approach used to treat MSCC. These techniques involve removal of the posterior elements of the vertebrae, to achieve decompression of the spinal cord and obtain a histological diagnosis. Simple decompression is a useful option for patients who require treatment to preserve neurology, while having significant frailty. However, additional instrumented fusion confers duration of benefit with mechanical stability.

Laminectomy involves removal of the laminae and spinous processes of the involved vertebrae; it provides direct access to the spinal cord and potentially allows for more extensive decompression but may result in spinal instability requiring additional fusion.

Laminoplasty involves making a hinge on one side of the laminae and opening it on the opposite side to create a channel facilitating decompression. Laminoplasty preserves the posterior spinal elements and can help maintain spinal stability, although it may not provide a sufficient channel for decompression in cases of extensive tumor involvement.

Surgical stabilization is achieved by use of rods fixed to pedicle screws commonly in unaffected vertebrae adjacent to the affected area of spine. This can involve use of inter-transverse grafts, metal cages, or bone grafts. Additional fusion in conjunction with decompression is preferred when there is significant anatomical instability, either due to the disease itself or created iatrogenically as a result of the necessary surgical decompression (**Figure 1**). Fusion allows reconstruction of the spinal column and mechanical stability, and confers longevity of surgical outcome. Surgical fusion is preferred in patients with good prognosis, and who are deemed medically fit for a more demanding surgical procedure.

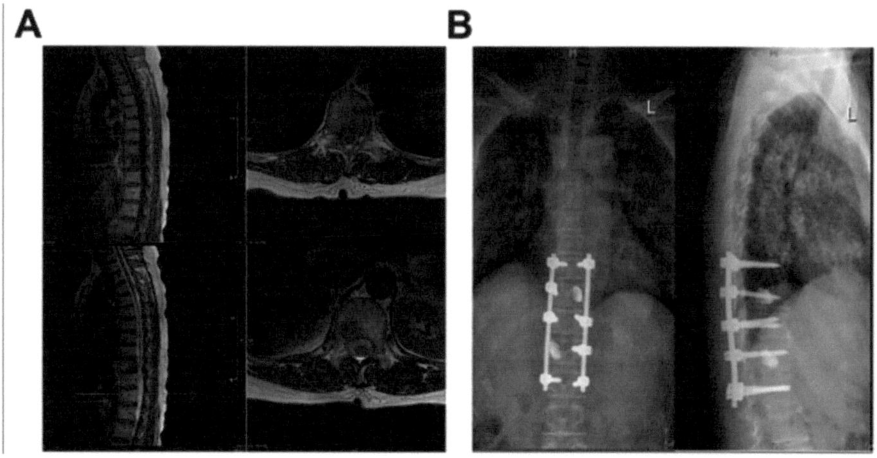

Figure 1.
65-year-old female with metastatic spinal lung cancer. Pre-operative MRI images with 4 week post-operative x-rays.

3.2 Anterior decompression

Anterior decompression techniques involve removal of the anterior elements of the vertebrae to achieve spinal cord decompression. These techniques are particularly useful for tumors that are located anteriorly or for tumors that cause instability of the vertebral body. Anterior corpectomy, or vertebrectomy, involves removal of the vertebral body and adjacent disc. It is often combined with fusion and instrumentation to stabilize the spine and is often used for patients with large tumors that involve multiple spinal levels (**Figure 2**). Anterior decompression is usually more invasive and may be associated with a longer recovery time than posterior decompression. A lack of surgeon familiarity with the techniques required and requirements for access surgeon participation can make this a less appealing option for many spinal surgeons. Additionally, depending on the level of the spine involved, anterior approaches can carry a higher risk of complications such as damage to the great vessels, esophagus, and nerves.

3.3 Traditional open surgery

The techniques described above represent in most cases a direct open approach, these being considered the recognized and more traditional methods to achieve MSCC decompression, with the posterior approach most used. The range of decompression can vary from a simple laminectomy to multi-level corpectomy depending on tumor involvement and desired operative outcome. Open surgery provides direct visualization of the tumor, allowing for improved and greater quantity of tumor resection, spinal reconstruction, and stabilization than minimally invasive techniques. Despite the advances in minimally invasive surgery,

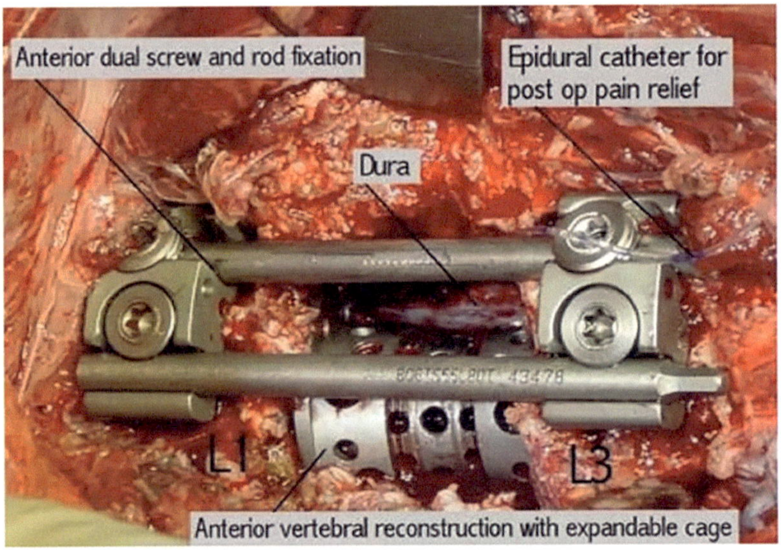

Figure 2.
Intra-operative image showing an anterior vertebral body reconstruction with metal cage, cement, ceramic spacer device with allograft. Fixation achieved with rods and screws.

open surgery remains a valuable option for selected patients with MSCC, especially those with large, complex, or unstable tumors that require extensive decompression and reconstruction.

3.4 Minimally invasive surgery

Minimally invasive surgery (MIS) has gained popularity for the treatment of MSCC due to its potential benefits over traditional open surgery, including reduced surgical trauma and blood loss, and faster recovery time with shorter hospital stay with good patient selection. Several MIS techniques have been used in the treatment of MSCC, including percutaneous vertebroplasty (**Figure 3**), percutaneous kyphoplasty, and minimally invasive decompression with or without spinal stabilization (**Figure 4**). However, MIS techniques may be associated with insufficient

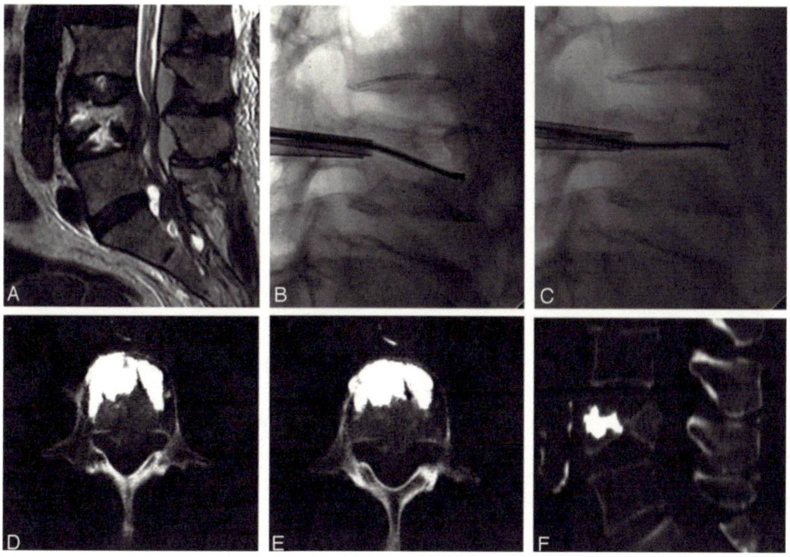

Figure 3.
A. MRI of 75-year-old female with an undifferentiated cancer associated with spinal metastasis and L4 vertebral compression. Fluoro images B and C, creation of a void in the vertebral body using a radiofrequency wand prior to vertebral body augmentation with bone cement. D–F, post-op CT images, axial (D and E), sagittal (F).

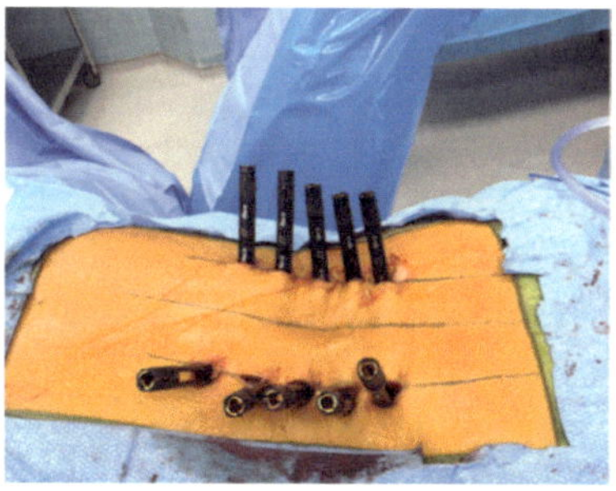

Figure 4.
Intra-operative image showing the construct for MIS thoracolumbar fixation in a MSCC patient.

	Description	Advantages	Disadvantages
Posterior	Removal, or opening of the posterior elements of the vertebrae. Commonly, laminectomy or laminoplasty.	Considered less technically challenging. Allows good exposure for spinal cord decompression. Less invasive.	Difficult access to anterior spine. Instability if not supplemented with fixation.
Anterior	Removal of the anterior elements of the vertebrae. Commonly, vertebrectomy or corpectomy.	Allows good exposure to anterior spine.	Often more technically challenging. Risk to anterior structures (aorta, esophagus, nerves). More invasive.
Open	Traditional open surgical access to the spine.	Better for extensive disease. Good visibility of affected areas. Allows for stabilization of the spine with direct open views of anatomical landmarks.	More invasive/traumatic.
Minimally invasive	Minimally invasive access to the spine.	Less invasive/traumatic. Potentially faster recovery time. Also allows for spinal stabilization using a percutaneous approach.	Reduced visibility of disease. Surgical skill set—additional training to perform.
Fixation	Additional intraoperative stabilization with a mechanical construct.	Provides added mechanical stability. Allows for prolonged duration of operative outcome.	Risk of construct failure. Risk to anterior structures (aorta, esophagus, nerves). More invasive.

Table 1.
Description of the surgical approaches used in MSCC along with advantages and disadvantages of each.

decompression of the spinal cord in cases of extensive tumor involvement or significant spinal cord compression. Additionally, the smaller exposure used in MIS may limit the surgeon's visualization and ability to fully resect tumor (**Table 1**).

4. Prognostic tools and predictors of survival

The prognosis for patients with MSCC can vary widely depending on several factors, including the patient's overall health, the extent and location of the metastases, and the effectiveness of the treatment approach (**Figure 5**). The one-year survival of patients with MSCC is poor at around 20%, and surgical treatment is targeted to preserve the remaining quality of life [9]. Prognostic tools and identified predictors of survival may help clinicians make informed decisions about the best treatment strategies for individual patients, avoiding inappropriate referrals and treatment.

4.1 Comprehensive scoring systems

The Tokuhashi scoring system is a widely used prognostic tool for predicting the survival time of patients with metastatic spinal *tumors* [11–13]. *It was developed by Tokuhashi and colleagues in 1990 and has since been modified* and validated by other researchers. The scoring system is based on six factors: primary tumor type, number

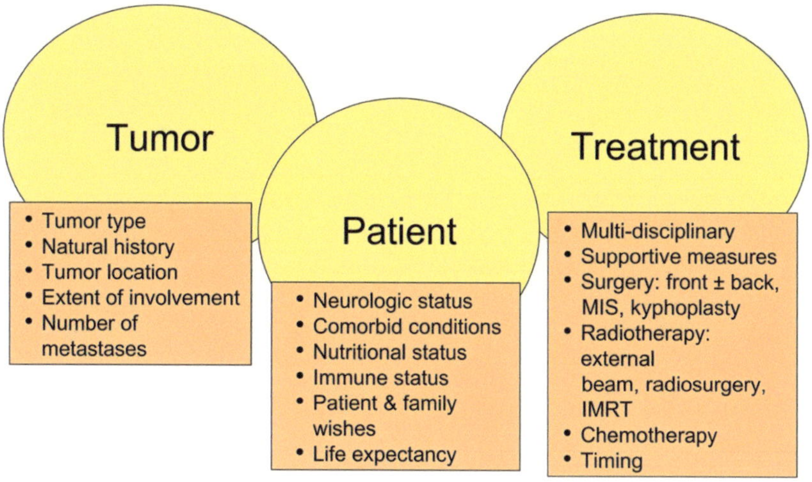

Figure 5.
Factors to consider when considering treatment options and outcomes for each MSCC patient.

of extraspinal bone metastases, number of spinal metastases, metastases to other organs, neurological deficit, and performance status. The system requires a bone scan to classify number of bony metastases and a CT/MRI to determine extraspinal metastases. The primary tumor type is scored based on its propensity to metastasize to bone, with lung and breast cancers receiving higher scores.

Each factor is assigned a point value ranging from 0 to 4, with a higher score indicating a more favorable prognosis. The total score ranges from 0 to 15. The scoring system is used to classify patients into one of three risk groups: A, B, and C. Group A patients have a poorer prognosis and are generally not considered candidates for aggressive surgical intervention. Group B patients have an intermediate prognosis and may benefit from surgery in some cases. Group C patients have the best prognosis and are generally considered candidates for surgical intervention.

Quraishi et al. conducted a semi-prospective study involving 201 patients to evaluate the usefulness of the Tokuhashi scoring system in predicting prognosis and decision making following surgery for MSCC [14]. The patients were divided into three groups based on their Tokuhashi score. Median survival was 93 days in Group A, 229 days in Group B, and 875 days in Group C. The predictive value of the Tokuhashi score using Cox regression for all groups was 66%. However, there was no significant difference in the neurological status between Group A and Group B or between Group B and Group C. However, Group C was found to have a significantly better neurological outcome than Group A patients.

The Katagiri scoring system was developed in 2005 and is based on the analysis of 1046 patients with spinal metastases [15]. The scoring system assigns points based on similar factors to the Tokuhashi system but utilizes degree of spinal cord compression in place of neurological status. Each factor is given a score ranging from 0 to 2, with a total possible score of 12.

Kobayashi et al. studied the merits of the Katagiri score in predicting survival outcomes in 201 patients with MSCC [16]. The authors concluded that faster rate of growth at the primary site, visceral metastases, and poorer performance status were the key significant independent prognostic factors showing correlation with decreased survival in patients.

4.2 Other scoring systems

The above scoring systems require comprehensive imaging and ideally multidisciplinary team discussion for proper functioning. Unfortunately, MSCC can present as a surgical emergency and require expedited decision-making in a patient's best interests. Additional scoring systems exist and may be of use in these circumstances.

The Oswestry Spinal Risk Index (OSRI) is a system that was developed by utilizing the two most predictive factors of some recognized studies: performance index (by Karnofsky score) /General Condition and the assumed Primary Tumor Type [17]. This allows for an estimation of prognosis without the need for additional imaging. The OSRI has been validated for use in several studies involving patients with MSCC. It was created as a means of comparison of three recognized scoring systems (Tokuhashi, Tomita, and modified Bauer). Here, a prospective cohort of 199 patients with spinal metastases was treated with either surgery and/or radiotherapy and used to compare these three systems. Each system was found to be equally as good as the others in terms of overall prognostic performance. By utilizing their most predictive items the OSRI was formulated. Namely the OSRI is a simple summation of two elements: primary tumor pathology (PTP) and general condition (GC): OSRI = PTP + (2-GC). OSRI was found to have similar concordance albeit with a larger coefficient of determination than the three scoring systems. This had been further validated in national cohort studies with similar excellent results [18, 19].

The American Society of Anesthesiologists (ASA) classification is a widely used system for assessing the risk of morbidity and mortality in patients undergoing surgery [20]. The ASA classification system is based on a patient's overall health status and helps guide the anesthetist and surgeon in making decisions about the type of anesthesia and surgical approach to use. The ASA classification system is divided into six categories depending on presence and generally perceived severity of disease.

The ASA classification system has been shown to be a useful tool in predicting surgical outcomes, as well as morbidity and mortality including in MSCC [21]. It is important to note, however, that the classification is based on a patient's overall health status and does not consider other factors that may impact surgical outcomes, such as the surgery itself or pathology treated. It is also largely based on operator/anesthetist subjective assessment of illness severity and does not control for severity of disease (e.g., uncontrolled vs. well-controlled hypertension) (**Table 2**) [22].

4.3 Other work examining survival

Out with these validation studies, one study found no significant difference in survival outcomes examining the surgical approaches (either anterior or posterior) in 282 patients who had surgery with overall survival rates of 63, 47, 30, and 16% at 3 months, 6 months, 1 year, and 2 years, respectively [23]. Neurological improvement in function was observed in most patients after surgery, but the complication rate was often high. Itshayek et al. identified a significant relation between duration of ambulation and both preoperative and post-operative ASIA grade, as well as a possible trend toward significance between preoperative ASIA grade and survival [24]. The importance of preoperative motor function was further highlighted by Lo et al. [25]. Patients who had an intact motor status preoperatively demonstrated improved survival compared to those with motor deficit. Survival was improved when surgery was performed within 7 days of the onset of motor deficit as opposed to when performed 7 days after onset.

Scoring system	Indicators associated with improved prognosis	Literature
Tokuhashi scoring system	Favorable primary tumor type.	[11–14]
	Lower number of extraspinal bone metastases.	
	Lower number of spinal metastases.	
	Lower number metastases to other organs.	
	Better baseline performance status.	
	Better baseline neurological function.	
Katagiri scoring system	Favorable primary tumor type.	[15, 16]
	Lower number of extraspinal bone metastases.	
	Lower number of spinal metastases.	
	Lower number metastases to other organs.	
	Better baseline performance status.	
	Lesser degree of cord compression.	
Oswestry spinal risk index (OSRI)	Favorable primary tumor type.	[17–19]
	Better baseline performance status.	
American Society of Anesthesiologists (ASA) classification	Healthier baseline (non-smoker, minimal alcohol).	[10, 20–22]
	Decreased number and severity comorbidities.	
	Decreased acute illness severity.	

Table 2.
Summary of prognostic indicators: An overview of the indicators used in discussed prognostic scoring systems and associated studies validating their use.

5. Predictors of function

5.1 Motor and ambulation

Several studies have investigated the association between surgical intervention and post-operative motor function and ambulation. Rades et al. reviewed patients who underwent spinal surgery with radiotherapy versus radiotherapy alone [26]. The surgical technique was operator dependent, but was described as simple laminectomy or decompression with fixation. An improved motor score was found in 22 and 16% of patients after surgery with radiotherapy and after radiotherapy alone, respectively. Post-treatment ambulatory rates were 67 and 61%, respectively. Of note, for patients who were non-ambulatory pre-intervention, 29 and 19% regained ambulatory status. Individuals who had MSCC from more unfavorable, radioresistant primary tumors had an improved functional outcome with decompressive surgery, stabilization, and radiotherapy compared to when only laminectomy and radiotherapy were performed.

A retrospective cohort study by Younsi et al. reviewed 101 patients undergoing decompressive laminectomy for spinal metastases [27]. At discharge, 83 patients (82%) stated an overall improvement in their symptoms. It was noted that 51% of all non-ambulatory patients had regained ambulation after surgery. Overall, 61 patients (60%) were ambulatory at discharge compared to 20 patients (20%) prior to surgery. Tateiwa et al. also showed the benefit of a posterior approach for direct decompression with or without subsequent stabilization [28]. In this study, 21 patients (68%) improved by at least one Frankel grade, and 17 patients (55%) became ambulatory post-operatively.

In summary, factors that affect post-operative motor and ambulatory function for patients with MSCC include the type of surgery performed, preoperative neurological function, pre-operative ambulatory status, and post-operative oncological treatment.

5.2 Neurological function

Several studies have examined the effect of surgical intervention on neurological outcomes. Cofano and colleagues conducted a retrospective study to investigate the impact of decompression type on neurological outcomes in patients with spinal metastases [29]. The study included 84 patients, and decompression types were divided into anterior/anterior-lateral (AD), posterior/posterior-lateral (PD/PDL), and circumferential (CD). The results indicated that patients who underwent AD/CD decompression had higher rates of improved neurology and lower rates of deterioration compared to those who underwent PD/PLD decompression. These findings suggest the importance of removing the source of epidural metastatic compression and targeting CD/AD decompression in cases of circumferential or anterior/anterolateral compression for good neurological outcome.

In a retrospective study by Lida et al., the neurological outcomes of radiotherapy and surgery were compared in patients with MSCC presenting with myelopathy [30]. The study found that radiotherapy alone was less effective compared to surgery in these patients. Of patients treated surgically, 30 (88%) showed neurological improvement compared to 1 patient (8%) in the radiotherapy group. In addition, ambulation and survival rates were significantly improved by surgery. Lak et al. also aimed to quantify the results of decompressive surgery on patients' quality of life in symptomatic metastatic spinal disease [21]. They reviewed 151 patients, where most patients had a posterior approach for their spinal metastases. The authors identified that surgical decompression provides considerable chances of neurological recovery and good functional performance in patients presenting with neurological deficits from MSCC. About 58.3% of patients improved, 31.5% had no improvement, and 10.0% had worsening of functional status. The findings also give support to surgical intervention in situations where life expectancy is less than 6 months, as significant QALY was gained at both 6 months and 1-year time points.

Walter et al. reported on the outcomes of patients with metastatic spinal disease treated with palliative considerations using the techniques of spinal decompression and posterior instrumentation [31]. In this study, 57 individuals underwent a posterolateral approach for decompression and posterior instrumentation, and the authors described excellent clinical outcomes with 13 (22.8%) patients demonstrating neurological improvement and 43 (75.5%) remaining stable at follow-up. In another study, nerve root palsies showed good recovery following decompressive laminectomy, and pain relief was provided in most cases [27]. Pre-operatively impaired neurological function had improved by at least one grade in 61% of patients at discharge. However, sensory deficits and bladder/bowel dysfunction were often persistent.

A subgroup analysis by the global spine tumor study group suggested that post-operative improvement in neurological function may not always be sustained, and long-term follow-up is required [32]. This review of 914 patients undergoing decompressive debulking surgery with fixation demonstrated an initial improvement in post-operative Frankel scores in 25% of patients; however, it was found that approximately 20% of patients had deteriorated between 6 and 12 months post-op.

6. Complications

Complications following surgical treatment of MSCC have been reported in the literature and can be defined broadly as surgical and non-surgical (**Table 3**).

6.1 Surgical complications

Across the literature, multiple surgical complications have been reported including worsening pain or neurology, wound infection, dural tears/CSF leak, significant operative hemorrhage, and construct failure. Wrong level surgery has also been recognized in this setting. Wound infection or wound dehiscence were the most frequently reported complication in the studies reviewed. In one study, rates of wound infection were found to be significantly higher in open compared with MIS surgery [41].

The loosening rate of implants was also studied with an overall loosening rate of 44% [46]. Luque rods and sublaminar wire system were the most affected systems (70%). Despite this, no cases needed revisional surgery or implant removal at 1 year post-operatively. The authors postulated that the loosening rate of implants was high

Type	Complication	Rates Reported
Surgical	*Worsening neurology*	1 (1.9%) Iida [30], 17 (1.9%) Depreitere [32], 4 (2%) Quraishi [14], 4 (2.4%) Vanek [33]
	Wound problem (infection/ dehiscence)	2 (3.5%) Lak [21], 2 (3.6%) Uei [34], 1 (2.9%) Li [35], 5 (5.2%) Pessina [36], 3 (5.5%) Iida [30], 2 (6.7%) Gallazzi [37], 42 (4.6%) Depreitere [32], 3 (5%) Chen [38], 2 (3.5%) Xiaozhou [39], 2 (3.8%) Colangeli [40], 7 (4.5%) Zhu [41], 15 (8%) Quraishi [14], 13 (7.8%) Vanek [33], 3 (2.1%) Hohenberger [42], 1 (3.3%) Gao [43]
	CSF leak	1 (2.9%) Li [35], 1 (1.9%) Xiaozhou [39], 2 (3.8%) Colangeli [40], 3 (1.9%) Zhu [41], 34 (12.1%) Jansson [23], 4 (4.3%) Hohenberger [42], 6 (6.3%) Rustagi [44]
	"Significant" hemorrhage	5 (9%) Uei [34], 1 (2.0%) Hamad [45]
	Epidural hematoma	2 (3.6%) Uei [34], 1 (2.9%) Li [35], 2 (3.7%) Iida [30], 1 (1.9%) Colangeli [40], 6 (3.6%) Vanek [33]
	Gastric perforation	1 (1.9%) Iida [30]
	Construct failure	2 (2.1%) Pessina [36], 1 (3.3%) Gallazzi [37], 7 (0.8%) Depreitere [32], 3 (5.9%) Hamad [45], 4 (2%) Quraishi [14], 4 (2.4%) Vanek [33]
	Wrong level surgery	2 (0.7%) Jansson [23]
Medical	*Pulmonary embolism*	1 (3.3%) Gallazzi [37], 3 (1.5%) Quraishi [14], 2 (4.3%) Hohenberger [42]
	Deep vein thrombosis	3 (3.1%) Rustagi [44]
	Post-operative pneumonia	(3.7%) Iida [30], 8 (4%) Quraishi [14]
	Medical unspecified	1 (2.9%) Li [35], 7 (7.6%) Pessina [36], 32 (3.5%) Depreitere [32], 7 (4.2%) Vanek [33]

Table 3.
Summary of reported complications: An overview of surgical and medical complications following operative treatment of MSCC as reported in the literature. Total number reported (percentage of cohort) [study]: N (%) [Author Year].

and would be expected to grow even higher as oncological patients continue to show improved level of survivorship with medical advances, for example, target therapy. However, there remain no definitive studies on how the loosening of implants would impact patients' quality of life and clinical performance.

6.2 Medical complications

Where documented in these studies, systemic/medical complications tended to concentrate on cardiorespiratory events particularly venous thromboembolism and post-operative pneumonia.

7. Conclusion

Surgical treatment for MSCC typically involves decompression with or without spinal stabilization with various approaches used to address this condition. Minimally invasive surgery has been shown to be non-inferior to open surgery in improving patients' motor and neurological function. Multiple validated prognostic scoring systems exist to assist surgical decision making and patient selection. Wound infection and dehiscence are the most common complications of surgical management. However, there is a notable incidence of construct/implant failure, epidural hematoma, incidental durotomy, and venous thromboembolism. Further research is required directly comparing surgical approaches and techniques for MSCC along with the adjunctive treatment measures used. This needs to be tailored to the tumor type, extent, and levels of spinal involvement and consideration given to the goals for patient care.

Conflict of interest

The authors declare no conflict of interest.

Author details

Bhoresh Dhamija[1*], Steven Tominey[1], Shabin Joshi[2], Rahim Hussain[2], Dheeraj Batheja[3] and Birender Balain[3]

1 Charing Cross Hospital, Imperial College Healthcare NHS Trust, London, UK

2 University Hospital of Coventry and Warwickshire NHS Trust, Coventry, UK

3 Center for Spinal Studies, Robert Jones and Agnes Hunt Orthopaedic Hospital, Shropshire, UK

*Address all correspondence to: bhoresh.dhamija1@nhs.net

References

[1] Boussios S, Cooke D, Hayward C, Kanellos FS, Tsiouris AK, Chatziantoniou AA, et al. Metastatic spinal cord compression: Unraveling the diagnostic and therapeutic challenges. Anticancer Research. 2018;**38**(9):4987-4997

[2] Robson P. Metastatic spinal cord compression: A rare but important complication of cancer. Clinical Medicine (London, England). 2014;**14**(5):542-545

[3] Loblaw DA, Laperriere NJ, Mackillop WJ. A population-based study of malignant spinal cord compression in Ontario. Clinical oncology (Royal College of Radiologists (Great Britain)). 2003;**15**(4):211-217

[4] Lei M, Liu Y, Tang C, Yang S, Liu S, Zhou S. Prediction of survival prognosis after surgery in patients with symptomatic metastatic spinal cord compression from non-small cell lung cancer. BMC Cancer. 2015;**15**(1):853

[5] Weber A, Bartscht T, Karstens JH, Schild SE, Rades D. Survival in patients with metastatic spinal cord compression from prostate cancer is associated with the number of extra-spinal organs involved. Anticancer Research. 2013;**33**(10):4505-4507

[6] Patchell RA, Tibbs PA, Regine WF, Payne R, Saris S, Kryscio RJ, et al. Direct decompressive surgical resection in the treatment of spinal cord compression caused by metastatic cancer: A randomised trial. Lancet (London, England). 2005;**366**(9486):643-648

[7] Sarri G, Patorno E, Yuan H, Guo JJ, Bennett D, Wen X, et al. Framework for the synthesis of non-randomised studies and randomised controlled trials: A guidance on conducting a systematic review and meta-analysis for healthcare decision making. BMJ Evidence-based Medicine. 2022;**27**(2):109-119

[8] Klimo P, Thompson CJ, Kestle JRW, Schmidt MH. A meta-analysis of surgery versus conventional radiotherapy for the treatment of metastatic spinal epidural disease. Neuro-Oncology. 2005;**7**(1):64-76

[9] Cardiff (UK): National Collaborating Centre for cancer (UK). NICE clinical guidelines 75: Metastatic spinal cord compression: Diagnosis and management of patients at risk of or with metastatic spinal cord compression. [Internet]. NICE Clinical Guidelines; 2008. Available from: https://www.ncbi.nlm.nih.gov/books/NBK55011/

[10] de Araujo BLC, Theobald D. Letter to the editor: ASA physical status classification in surgical oncology and the importance of improving inter-rater reliability. Journal of Korean Medical Science. 2017;**32**(7):1211

[11] Tokuhashi Y, Kawano H, Ohsaka S, Matsuzaki H, Toriyama S. A scoring system for preoperative evaluation of the prognosis of metastatic spine tumor (a preliminary report). Nihon Seikeigeka Gakkai Zasshi. 1989;**63**(5):482-489

[12] Tokuhashi Y, Matsuzaki H, Toriyama S, Kawano H, Ohsaka S. Scoring system for the preoperative evaluation of metastatic spine tumor prognosis. Spine. 1990;**15**(11):1110-1113

[13] Tokuhashi Y, Matsuzaki H, Kawano H, Sano S. The indication of operative procedure for a metastatic spine tumor: A scoring system for the preoperative evaluation of the prognosis.

Nihon Seikeigeka Gakkai Zasshi. 1994;**68**(5):379-389

[14] Quraishi NA, Manoharan SR, Arealis G, Khurana A, Elsayed S, Edwards KL, et al. Accuracy of the revised Tokuhashi score in predicting survival in patients with metastatic spinal cord compression (MSCC). European Spine Journal: Official Publication of the European Spine Society, the European Spinal Deformity Society, and the European Section of the Cervical Spine Research Society. 2013;**22**(Suppl. 1):S21-S26

[15] Katagiri H, Okada R, Takagi T, Takahashi M, Murata H, Harada H, et al. New prognostic factors and scoring system for patients with skeletal metastasis. Cancer Medicine. 2014;**3**(5):1359-1367

[16] Kobayashi K, Ando K, Nakashima H, Sato K, Kanemura T, Yoshihara H, et al. Prognostic factors in the new Katagiri scoring system after palliative surgery for spinal metastasis. Spine. 2020;**45**(13):E813-E819

[17] Balain B, Jaiswal A, Trivedi JM, Eisenstein SM, Kuiper JH, Jaffray DC. The Oswestry risk index: An aid in the treatment of metastatic disease of the spine. The Bone & Joint Journal. 2013;**95-B**(2):210-216

[18] Fleming C, Baker JF, O'Neill SC, Rowan FE, Byrne DP, Synnott K. The Oswestry spinal risk index (OSRI): An external validation study. European Spine Journal. 2016;**25**(1):252-256

[19] Kramer A, Coßmann T, Jägersberg M, Preuß A, Meyer B, Ringel F. The Oswestry spinal risk index (OSRI) in assessing prognosis of patients with spinal metastases. Brain Spine. 2022;**2**:100875

[20] Hurwitz EE, Simon M, Vinta SR, Zehm CF, Shabot SM, Minhajuddin A, et al. Adding examples to the ASA-physical status classification improves correct assignment to patients. Anesthesiology. 2017;**126**(4):614-622

[21] Lak AM, Rahimi A, Abunimer AM, Tafel I, Devi S, Premkumar A, et al. Quantifying the impact of surgical decompression on quality of life and identification of factors associated with outcomes in patients with symptomatic metastatic spinal cord compression. Journal of Neurosurgery. Spine. 2020;**33**(2):237-244

[22] Mayhew D, Mendonca V, Murthy BVS. A review of ASA physical status - historical perspectives and modern developments. Anaesthesia. 2019;**74**(3):373-379

[23] Jansson KÅ, Bauer HCF. Survival, complications and outcome in 282 patients operated for neurological deficit due to thoracic or lumbar spinal metastases. European Spine Journal. 2006;**15**(2):196-202

[24] Itshayek E, Candanedo C, Fraifeld S, Hasharoni A, Kaplan L, Schroeder JE, et al. Ambulation and survival following surgery in elderly patients with metastatic epidural spinal cord compression. The Spine Journal. 2018;**18**(7):1211-1221

[25] Lo WY, Yang SH. Metastatic spinal cord compression (MSCC) treated with palliative decompression: Surgical timing and survival rate. PLoS One. 2017;**12**(12):e0190342

[26] Rades D, Huttenlocher S, Bajrovic A, Karstens JH, Adamietz IA, Kazic N, et al. Surgery followed by radiotherapy versus radiotherapy alone for metastatic spinal cord compression from unfavorable tumors. International Journal of Radiation Oncology, Biology, Physics. 2011;**81**(5):e861-e868

[27] Younsi A, Riemann L, Scherer M, Unterberg A, Zweckberger K. Impact of decompressive laminectomy on the functional outcome of patients with metastatic spinal cord compression and neurological impairment. Clinical & Experimental Metastasis. 2020;**37**(2):377-390

[28] Tateiwa D, Oshima K, Nakai T, Imura Y, Tanaka T, Outani H, et al. Clinical outcomes and significant factors in the survival rate after decompression surgery for patients who were non-ambulatory due to spinal metastases. Journal of Orthopaedic Science. 2019;**24**(2):347-352

[29] Cofano F, Di Perna G, Alberti A, Baldassarre BM, Ajello M, Marengo N, et al. Neurological outcomes after surgery for spinal metastases in symptomatic patients: Does the type of decompression play a role? A comparison between different strategies in a 10-year experience. Journal of Bone Oncology. 2021;**26**:100340

[30] Iida K, Matsumoto Y, Setsu N, Harimaya K, Kawaguchi K, Hayashida M, et al. The neurological outcome of radiotherapy versus surgery in patients with metastatic spinal cord compression presenting with myelopathy. Archives of Orthopaedic and Trauma Surgery. 2018;**138**(1):7-12

[31] Walter J, Reichart R, Waschke A, Kalff R, Ewald C. Palliative considerations in the surgical treatment of spinal metastases: Evaluation of posterolateral decompression combined with posterior instrumentation. Journal of Cancer Research and Clinical Oncology. 2012;**138**(2):301-310

[32] Depreitere B, Ricciardi F, Arts M, Balabaud L, Bunger C, Buchowski JM, et al. How good are the outcomes of instrumented debulking operations for symptomatic spinal metastases and how long do they stand? A subgroup analysis in the global spine tumor study group database. Acta Neurochirurgica. 2020;**162**(4):943-950

[33] Vanek P, Bradac O, Trebicky F, Saur K, de Lacy P, Benes V. Influence of the preoperative neurological status on survival after the surgical treatment of symptomatic spinal metastases with spinal cord compression. Spine. 2015;**40**(23):1824-1830

[34] Uei H, Tokuhashi Y, Maseda M, Nakahashi M, Sawada H, Nakayama E, et al. Clinical results of multidisciplinary therapy including palliative posterior spinal stabilization surgery and postoperative adjuvant therapy for metastatic spinal tumor. Journal of Orthopaedic Surgery. 2018;**13**(1):30

[35] Li Z, Long H, Guo R, Xu J, Wang X, Cheng X, et al. Surgical treatment indications and outcomes in patients with spinal metastases in the cervicothoracic junction (CTJ). Journal of Orthopaedic Surgery. 2018;**13**(1):20

[36] Pessina F, Navarria P, Carta GA, D'Agostino GR, Clerici E, Nibali MC, et al. Long-term follow-up of patients with metastatic epidural spinal cord compression from solid tumors submitted for surgery followed by radiation therapy. World Neurosurgery. 2018;**115**:e681-e687

[37] Gallazzi E, Cannavò L, Perrucchini GG, Morelli I, Luzzati AD, Zoccali C, et al. Is the posterior-only approach sufficient for treating cervical spine metastases? The evidence from a case series. World Neurosurgery. 2019;**122**:e783-e789

[38] Chen LH, Chen WJ, Niu CC, Shih CH. Anterior reconstructive spinal surgery with Zielke instrumentation for

metastatic malignancies of the spine. Archives of Orthopaedic and Trauma Surgery. 2000;**120**(1-2):27-31

[39] Xiaozhou L, Xing Z, Xin S, Chengjun L, Lei Z, Guangxin Z, et al. Efficacy analysis of separation surgery combined with SBRT for spinal metastases—A long-term follow-up study based on patients with spinal metastatic tumor in a single-center. Orthopaedic Surgery. 2020;**12**(2):404-420

[40] Colangeli S, Capanna R, Bandiera S, Ghermandi R, Girolami M, Parchi PD, et al. Is minimally-invasive spinal surgery a reliable treatment option in symptomatic spinal metastasis? European Review for Medical and Pharmacological Sciences. 2020;**24**(12):6526-6532

[41] Zhu X, Lu J, Xu H, Tang Q, Song G, Deng C, et al. A comparative study between minimally invasive spine surgery and traditional open surgery for patients with spinal metastasis. Spine. 2021;**46**(1):62-68

[42] Hohenberger C, Schmidt C, Höhne J, Brawanski A, Zeman F, Schebesch KM. Effect of surgical decompression of spinal metastases in acute treatment – Predictors of neurological outcome. Journal of Clinical Neuroscience. 2018;**52**:74-79

[43] Gao X, Zhang K, Cao S, Hou S, Wang T, Guo W, et al. Surgical treatment of spinal cord compression caused by metastatic small cell lung cancer: Ten years of experience in a single center. Cancer Management and Research. 2020;**12**:3571-3578

[44] Rustagi T, Mashaly H, Ganguly R, Akhter A, Mendel E. Transpedicular Vertebrectomy with circumferential spinal cord decompression and reconstruction for thoracic spine metastasis: A consecutive case series. Spine. 2020;**45**(14):E820-E828

[45] Hamad A, Vachtsevanos L, Cattell A, Ockendon M, Balain B. Minimally invasive spinal surgery for the management of symptomatic spinal metastasis. British Journal of Neurosurgery. 2017;**31**(5):526-530

[46] Chong-chung C, Martin WC t, Eleanor W, Wing-ngai Y, Hung-on C, Ka-kin C. Decompression and instrumentation without fusion for spinal metastases: Loosening rate and consequences. Journal of Orthopaedics, Trauma and Rehabilitation. 2018;**25**(1):82-86

Chapter 14

Lumbar Interspinous Devices: Indications, Surgical Aspects, Clinical Considerations

Claudio Irace

Abstract

Interspinous devices (or spacers) are currently used in lumbar spine surgery, but their use is still controversial, mainly due to confusion between so-called first and second-generation spacers, and unrespect of formal indications to implant. Our first aim is trying to offer an interpretation for a correct indication of surgical implantation, paying additional attention to those pathological conditions in which these devices must not be used; second, to identify the right clinico-surgical method to avoid potential errors in this surgery; third, to stress those surgical tricks directed to perform a successful implant of these spacers.

Keywords: interspinous device, interspinous spacer, lumbar spine stenosis, lumbar spine surgery, neurogenic intermittent claudication

1. Introduction

Nowadays, surgical implantation of lumbar interspinous devices (ISDs) has a widely accepted role in the management of spinal degenerative disorders, and this is confirmed by the current high number of scientific papers dealing with their use. Nevertheless, the issue of ISDs still remains quite controversial, and this is mainly due to two reasons: first, experimental data are often misinterpreted and therefore not considered strong enough to justify a clinical application; second, sometimes, indication to an ISD implant isn't done in a correct way and the subsequent potential poor surgical outcome being then attributed to the ISD itself (and not to the surgeon!); third, the technique of implantation of an ISD is too often deemed 'easy' and, hence, those basic surgical steps not respected, so opening the way to poor postoperative results.

2. Historical remarks

We are indebted to Prof. Jacques Sénégas, who first elaborated the concept of 'lumbar dynamic fixation' about forty years ago and developed the ISD named Wallis [1]. Since then, a deluge of ISDs, often having different experimental and clinical

 IntechOpen

supports, have been marketed and scientific papers concerning their use go on to be published; this context led to an unfavourable confusion about their correct use and, of course, careful and free from prejudices evaluation of clinical application and outcome.

3. Experimental data

Biomechanical studies have shown that all of ISDs act grossly in the same way: they enlarge spinal canal dimensions, increase neuro-foramina height, reduce intradiscal pressure in neutral and extended position [2]; moreover, they have a 'primary stabilizing effect' [3]. The ISDs designed 'for fusion' additionally show to promote bone fusion at the instrumented level.

4. Interspinous devices

ISDs may be grouped into two categories: the first group includes the so-called 'simple' spacers (first-generation), and the second one is constituted by the spacers 'for fusion' (second-generation); 'simple' spacers maybe static or dynamic (the term 'elastic' is sometimes used to indicate some dynamic devices). We'll here take in consideration some of the most frequently implanted (and studied) devices, remembering that some of them are no more marketed.

4.1 Spacers 'simple'

Wallis (Abbott, USA). It's made of polyetheretherketone (PEEK) and two flat woven Dacron bands; experimentally these latter resist traction of 200 decaNewton (daN) and stretch approximately 20% before failure by overloading; biomechanical studies demonstrated that, after a surgical decompression, the Wallis implant produces a significant restriction of segmental range of motion (ROM), limiting the flexion–extension plane, having no effect on lateral bending and minimal impact on axial rotation [4]; moreover it's able to markedly release the intradiscal pressure in extension (**Figure 1**).

DIAM (Medtronic, USA). It's a dynamic stabilizer, made of a silicone core with polyester sleeve, providing segmental stability and restoring foraminal height, particularly in those disorders accompanied by hyperlordosis [5].

4.2 X-STOP (taken off the market)

SUPERION (Vertiflex, USA). This device may be a valid alternative to laminectomy in a well-restricted population of patients affected by one- or two-level lumbar spinal stenosis (LSS); however, patients should be informed of the high rate of possible reintervention [6].

COFLEX (Paradigm Spine, USA). It was the first of the so-called titanium 'U-devices', also due to its appearance as a 'U-shape' on lateral radiographs; it received FDA approval for implant in one- or two-level lumbar stenosis; later there were some observations concerning its use at the superior stenotic level of a decompression/fusion operation, to reduce the incidence of adjacent segment disease (ASD) (the 'topping-off' technique) [7].

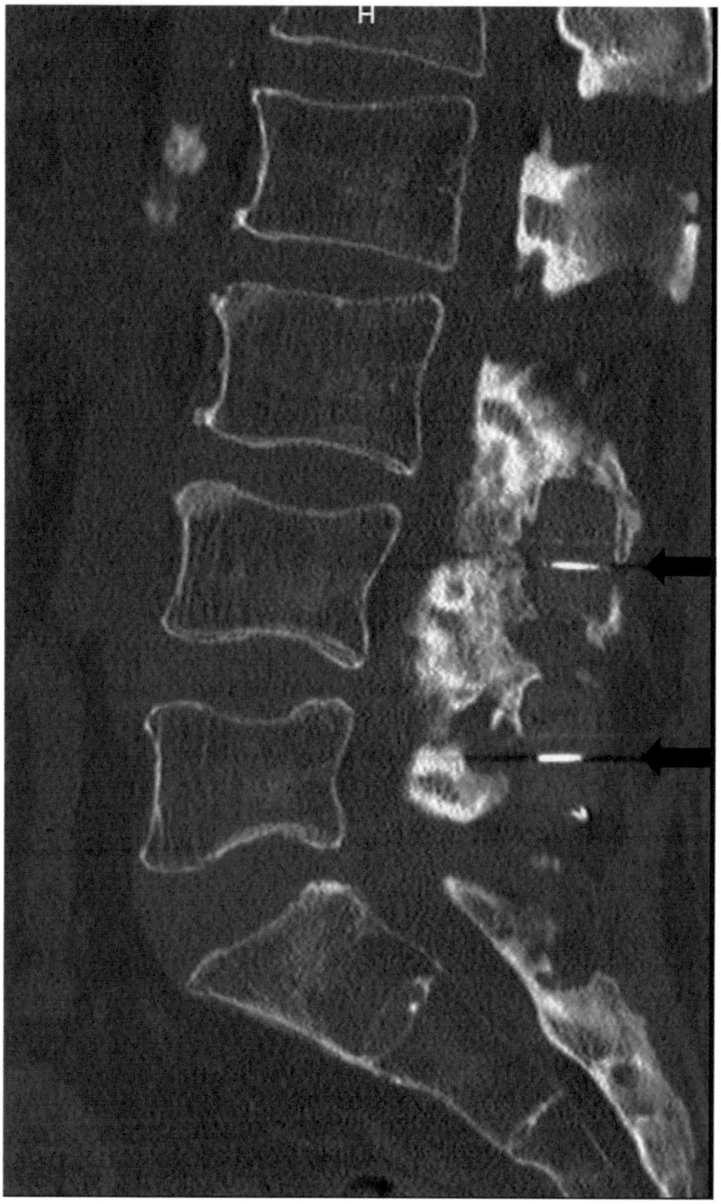

Figure 1.
*Lumbar stenosis. Sagittal CT scan at 15-year follow-up: the Wallis spacers, correctly placed, are visualized at L3-L4 and L4-L5 (*black arrows*).*

BACJAC (Surgalign, USA). It's made of PEEK, a bioplastic which has an elastic modulus close to that of bone [e.g., human femur has a flexural modulus of about 20 gigaPascal (GPa), and PEEK Optima has about the same value]; its advantages are a self-deploying way of insertion, tissue-sparing technique, minimal (or absent) risk of subsidence, no MR/CT artefacts [8]. Stand-alone implant or following uni- or bilateral decompression provides mid-term relief of low-back and radicular pain, and improvement of neurogenic intermittent claudication (NIC), in the following lumbar spine disorders: central and foraminal stenosis, recurrent disc protrusion associated with foraminal stenosis, mild antero- or retrolisthesis, degenerative disc disease (DDD), synovial cysts associated with pseudospondylolisthesis. When considering these disorders, this device seems to provide a 'primary stabilizing effect'; a 2-year follow-up confirms that this effect is still active, with no need for subsequent more invasive fixation surgical procedures [3].

APERIUS (Medtronic, USA). It was the first percutaneous titanium ISD available on the market; it was designed to be used as a stand-alone implant [9]; a good outcome at six months follow-up in LSS patients, with no migration of the device has been reported [10].

4.3 Spacers 'for fusion'

ASPEN, ALPINE (Zimmer, USA). The ASPEN was the first device projected to achieve bone fusion, so revolutioning the market of existing spacers, which were simple distances. Experimentally it showed a reduced range of motion (ROM) in flexion/extension about equal to anterior lumbar interbody fusion (ALIF) [11]. Moreover, it remains one of the few devices which may also be implanted at the thoracic segment (**Figure 2**), and it's worth that a 'flared' model is available to be best adapted to the L5-S1 level. The ALPINE differs from the ASPEN device because it's adaptable in length and may be inserted in compression or extension.

ROMEO 2 PAD (Spineart, CH). It's composed of two plates, one polyaxial, and a central core, made in PEEK or titanium; compared to the other devices, it has the advantage of being applied in a pre-assembled format, so making the surgical procedure faster and easier.

MINUTEMAN G3 (Spinal Simplicity, USA). This device for fusion is probably one of the fewest to be implanted percutaneously.

PITBULL (BMK, Korea). This device probably has one of the largest central cores to be filled with bone (to promote fusion).

SEASPINE (SeaSpine Orthopedics Corporation, USA). This spacer may also be applied at the thoracic segment (**Figure 3**), and a dedicated model for L5-S1 is available.

BACFUSE (taken off the market). It derived from the BacJac spacer (see above) and was designed to act as a device for fusion; despite its somewhat bulky design, which probably contributed to its scarce diffusion, our long-term follow-up showed optimal bone incorporation without loss of regional lordosis (**Figure 4**).

5. Indications

Main indications for an ISD implant are grouped under the wide term of lumbar spine degenerative disorder; although this comprehensive definition may represent a protective shield for the surgeon, we strongly recommend trying to obtain an exact preoperative diagnosis, not only because 'the more correct the indication, the higher the rate of success of the intervention', but also because, concerning the term of lumbar degenerative conditions, instructions for use (IFUs) of different ISDs may vary. Therefore, we'll here describe different degenerative lumbar disorders amenable to ISD implants.

5.1 Central stenosis

Central lumbar canal stenosis probably represents the most important indication of an ISD implant, and this has been extensively confirmed. Having this said, the main

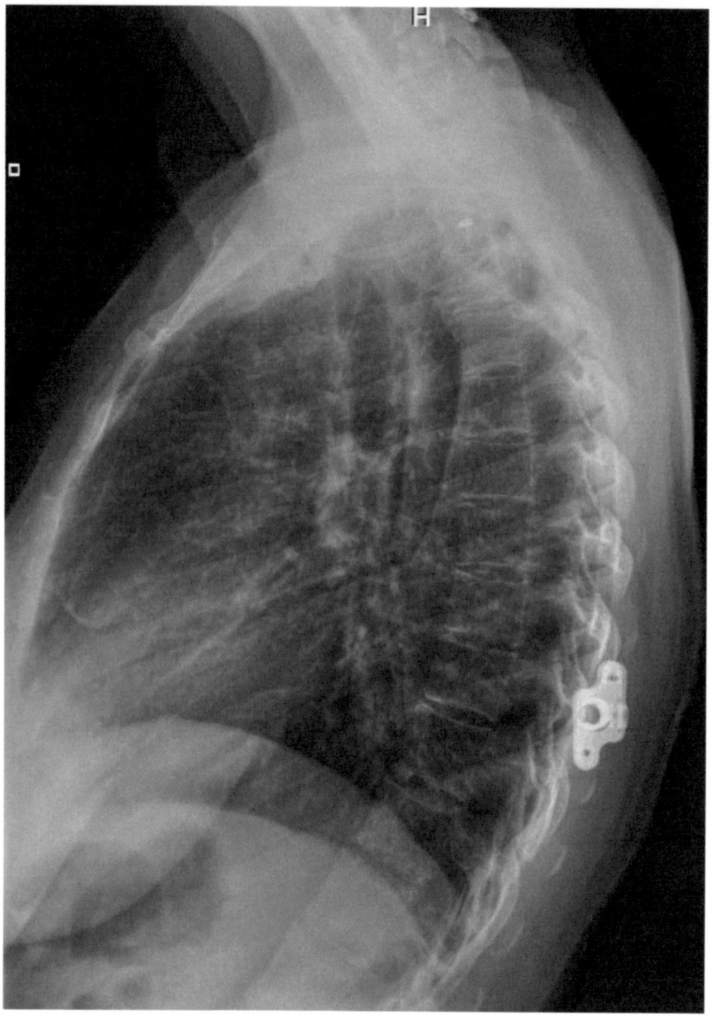

Figure 2.
Thoracic degenerative disc disease. Lateral x-ray film: the ASPEN device is correctly inserted at the mid-thoracic indexed level.

relevant aspects are two: performing or not decompression of neural structures before ISD implant, and coexistence of a listhesis which could be not adequately treated by ISD. About the first point, the decision to perform a decompressive step may be taken simply based on preoperative magnetic resonance (MR) or computed tomography (CT) scans and this is unequivocally true for severe stenosis causing bilateral NIC (**Figure 5**). Milder degrees of central stenosis could not necessarily require pre-ISD neural decompression; in such an occurrence, intraoperatively we behave as follows: after having skeletonized the indexed level, the application of traction on spinous processes (using two Backhaus forceps) is made; if frank hypermobility is appreciated, the ISD is inserted without delivering a flavo-laminotomy, because we know that it will realize an enlargement of the central canal and restore the bi-foraminal height, such to obtain a sufficient neural decompression (as we say, '*we let the ISD make its dirty job*'). It goes without saying that paracentral canal stenosis causing 'intractable' ipsilateral symptoms always needs a unilateral decompression before ISD insertion.

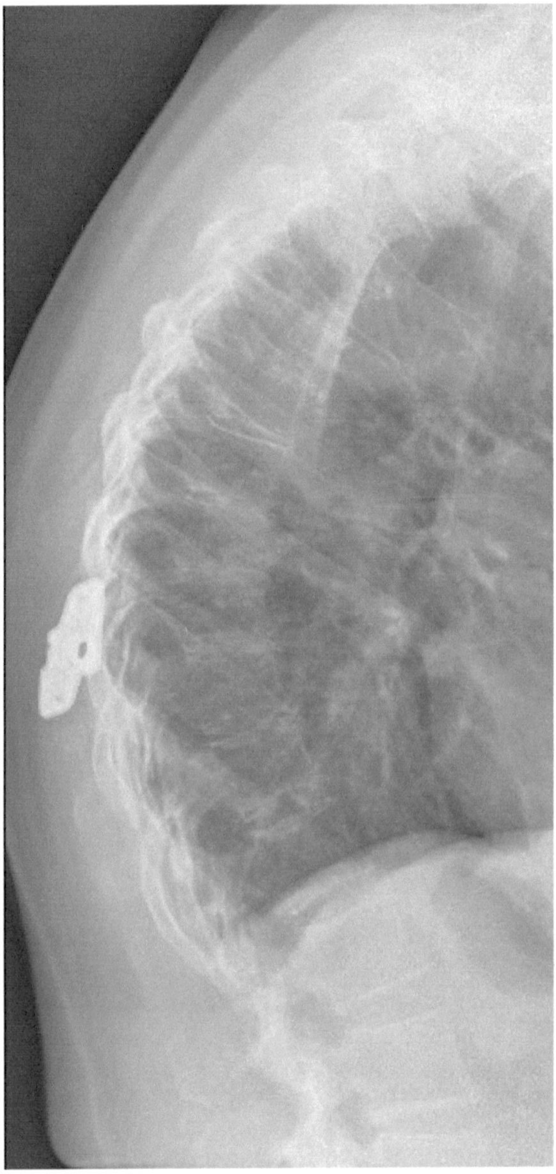

Figure 3.
Thoracic degenerative disc disease. Lateral x-ray film: the SEASPINE device is well visualized at the mid-thoracic indexed level.

5.2 Foraminal stenosis

This is probably one of the most correct and valuable indications (**Figure 6**). Intraoperatively, after having performed a plain microsurgical foraminotomy on the affected side, only minimal contralateral skeletonization will be necessary before applying the ISD. We here must remember that in these cases, the choice of the ISD could favour those spacers, which can be inserted by sparing the supraspinous ligament.

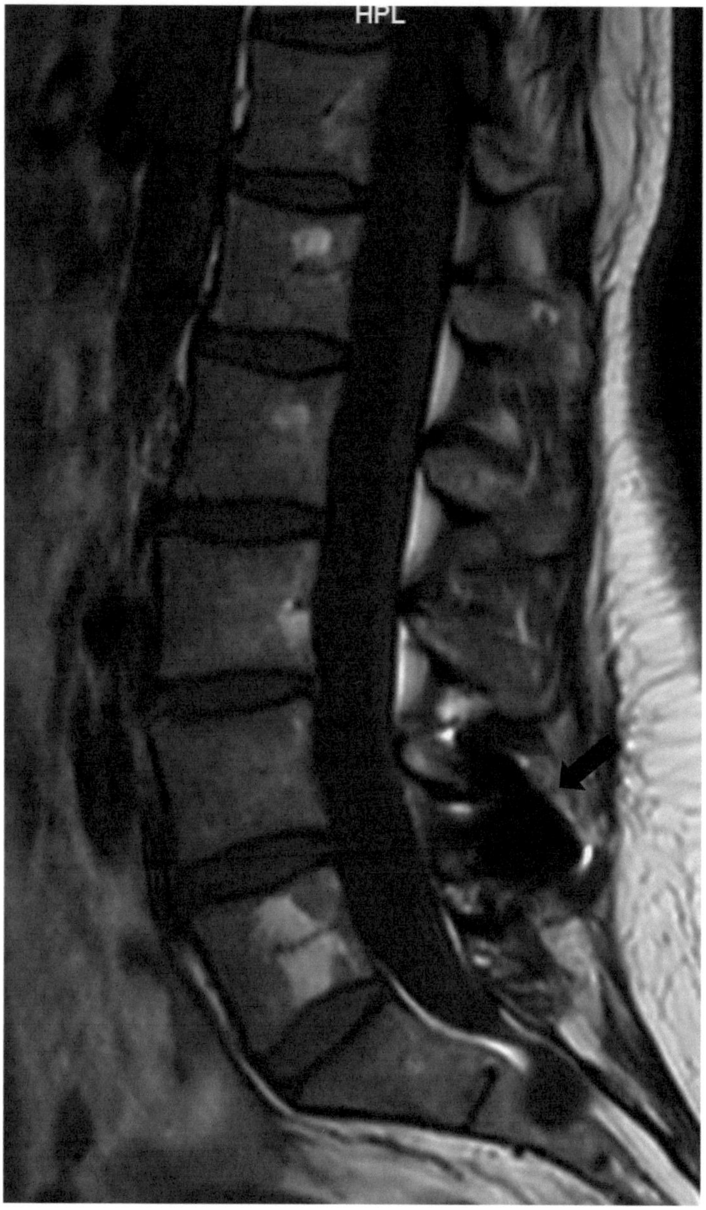

Figure 4.
Spacers 'for fusion'. Sagittal MR T1-weighted image at 2-year follow-up: the BACFUSE spacer is seen at L4-L5 (black arrow)*; the regional lordosis is unchanged.*

5.3 Recurrent disc herniation

Operated lumbar disc herniations may recur in different ways; clinical presentation is often persistent back pain, exacerbated by movements, associated with radicular irradiation, and the MR scan may show a small extruded disc fragment, surrounded by scar tissue, just at the entry of the neuroforamen; such condition,

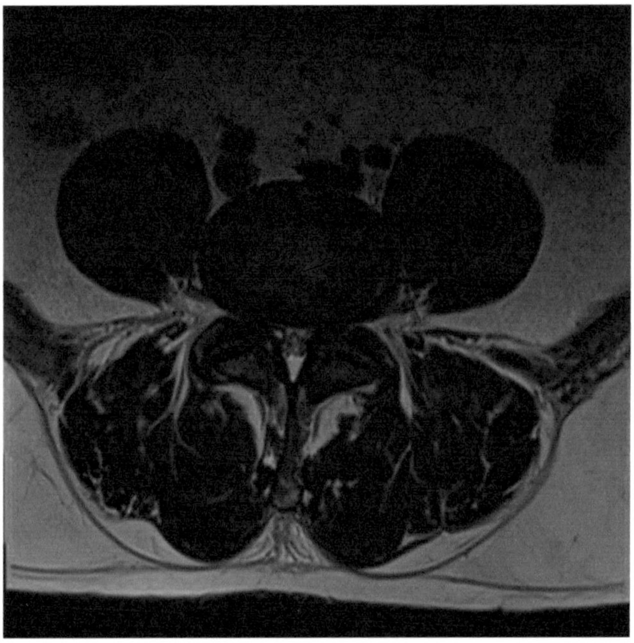

Figure 5.
Severe lumbar central stenosis. Axial MR T2-weighted image: preoperative study.

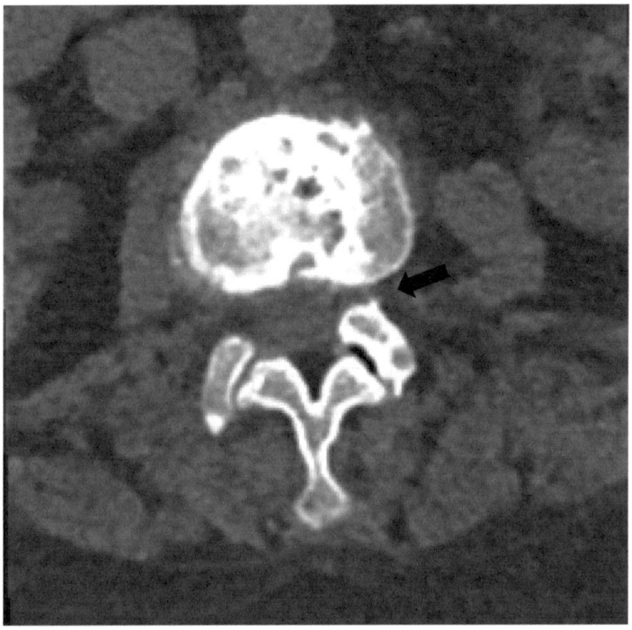

Figure 6.
*Lumbar foraminal stenosis. A preoperative axial CT scan shows the marked narrowing of the left neuroforamen (*black arrow*).*

usually refractory to medical and physical therapy, is the ideal target for a micro-surgical decompression of the involved nerve root(s), associated with a selective discectomy, followed by ISD implant.

5.4 Isolated disc herniation

Implantation of an ISD has no role in treating an isolated primary lumbar disc herniation; however, some empirical evidence delineates a long-term reduced rate of recurrent disc herniation when a spacer is applied at the end of the removal of the extruded disc. In those selected cases in which the herniated fragment is associated with a frank degenerated disc, causing intense low-back pain, the option of the additional insertion of an ISD may be considered [12].

5.5 DDD

As already stated in Section 3, ISDs reduce intradiscal pressure and have a stabilizing effect [which is quantitatively comparable to ALIF, meaning about 50% reduction of range of motion (ROM)]; basing upon these experimental data, we implanted ISD in several cases of single DDD, obtaining good results in terms of long-lasting back pain relief (**Figure 7**). We wish to stress the occurrence of a hyperintense signal of interspinous ligament in MR T2-weighted images, which must be considered an additional element of disc disease, hence supporting the indication of an ISD implant (**Figure 8**).

5.6 Post-surgical instability

This is a well-known condition, which may follow one or more lumbar surgical procedures: refractory pain is mainly located at the low-back and flexion–extension x-ray films usually show minimal or no listhesis; these patients may be adequately treated by an ISD implant, which is safer than other invasive fixation procedures.

5.7 Spondylolisthesis

During a procedure aiming to stabilize a lumbar anterolisthesis, the matter of reducing the slipped vertebrae occurs, considering that reduction may potentially result in permanent nerve root damage; our experience led us to the conclusion that spinous fixation by means of a second-generation ISD plus additional bone fusion provides a valid result when used in those cases of spondylolisthesis up to grade-1 (**Figure 9**).

5.8 Synovial cyst

Lumbar synovial cysts are frequently diagnosed as the cause of lumbar and sciatic pain; except for rare instances of spontaneous resorption, most of these cysts require surgical removal; because of the association of satellite spondylolisthesis, which in our experience occurs in almost all cases, it may be advisable to correct the vertebral slippage contextually to the excision of the cyst. Associated anterolisthesis is never grade-2, so we routinely insert an ISD once the cyst is removed; our long-term follow-up x-ray controls demonstrate no need for additional stabilization procedures.

5.9 Transitional vertebra

Vertebral anomalies at the lumbosacral junction, named as sacralization of L5 or lumbarization of S1, are frequent and may give rise to refractory, mechanical back

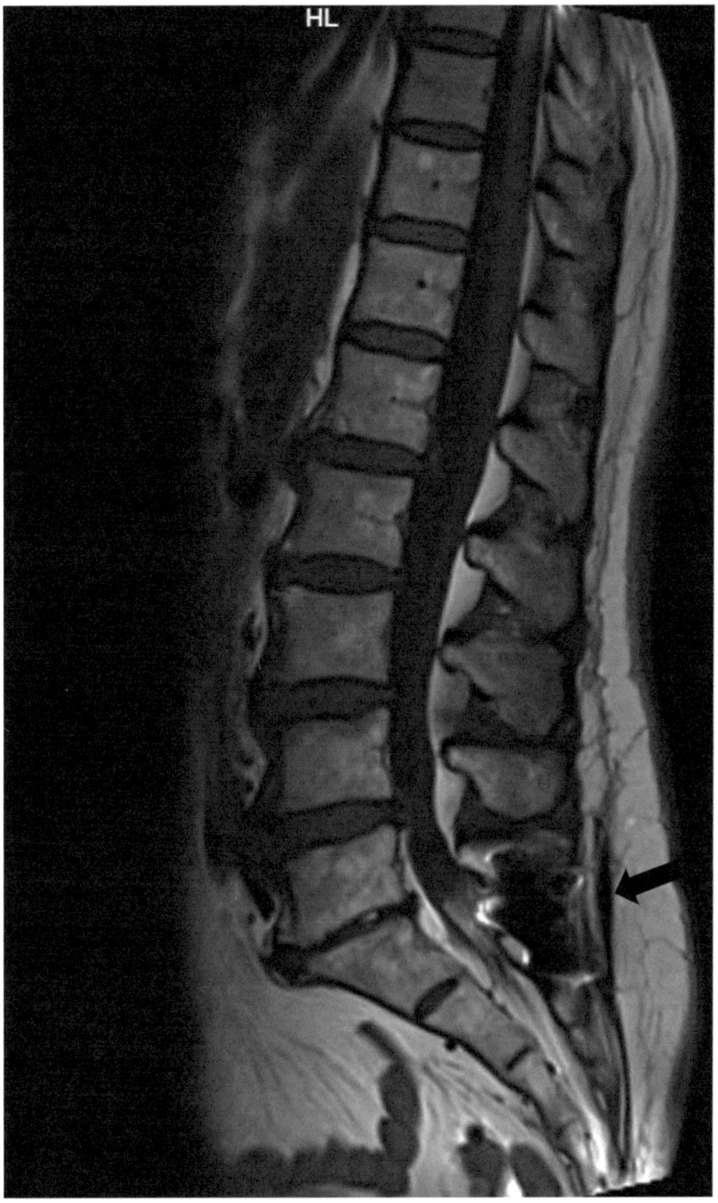

Figure 7.
*Lumbar DDD. Sagittal MR T1-weighted scan at 6-year follow-up: the L5-S1 degenerated disc is well seen, and the spacer is correctly inserted between the two spinous processes (*black arrow*).*

pain; in these cases, x-ray films usually show mild instability, which may appear as L5-S1 retrolisthesis. ISD implants proved to be effective in providing long-lasting, excellent back pain relief (**Figure 10**).

5.10 Adjacent segment disease

As already stated before (see Section 4), the implant of an ISD at the rostral level of a multilevel fixation may be useful to reduce the future risk of ASD. We never

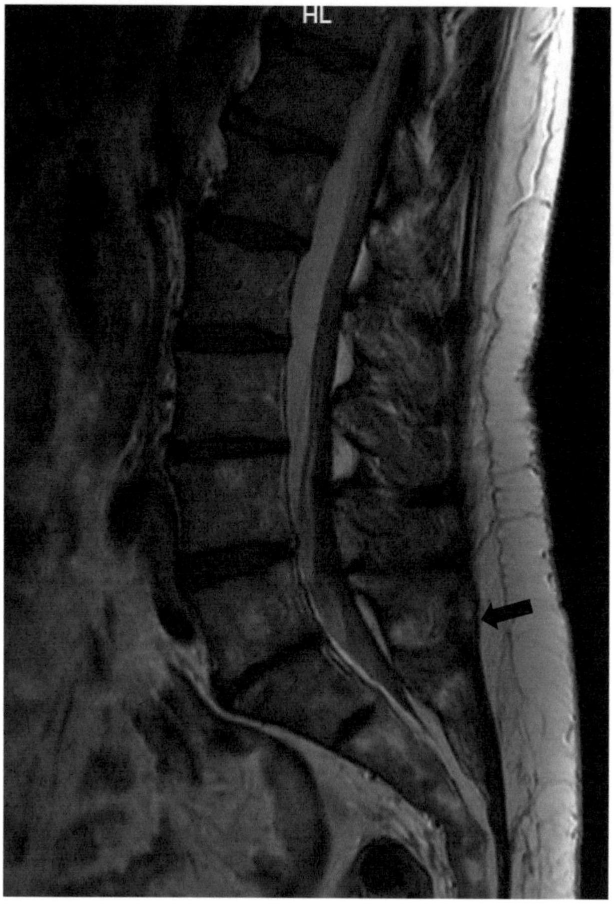

Figure 8.
*Lumbar degenerative disc disease (DDD). Preoperative sagittal MR T2-weighted image: the L5-S1 degenerative disc is shown, as well the hyperintense signal of the interspinous ligament (*black arrow*), which may be considered an additional element of the degenerative process.*

adopted this technique in a prophylactic way; however, we implant a second-generation ISD to treat those cases of ASD, in which a lumbar stenosis w/wo associated listhesis occurs rostrally or caudally to a previous posterior pedicular fixation (**Figure 11**). Of course, a careful evaluation of preoperative neuroradiological examination is mandatory to check the shape and volume of the spinous process to be included in the ISD anchor; intraoperatively, the terminal part of rods and the surgical scar may hinder skeletonization of the indexed spinous processes, but we never had to temporarily remove one of them to insert the ISD.

6. Contraindications

ISDs may differ from each other in several aspects; however, all of them share two important features: first, they cannot be implanted at the level of a pars defect; second, they cannot be used in case of a spondylolisthesis >grade-1.

Concerning the first occurrence, it must be stressed that sometimes preoperative neuroradiological exams may scotomize an isthmic defect and the related mild

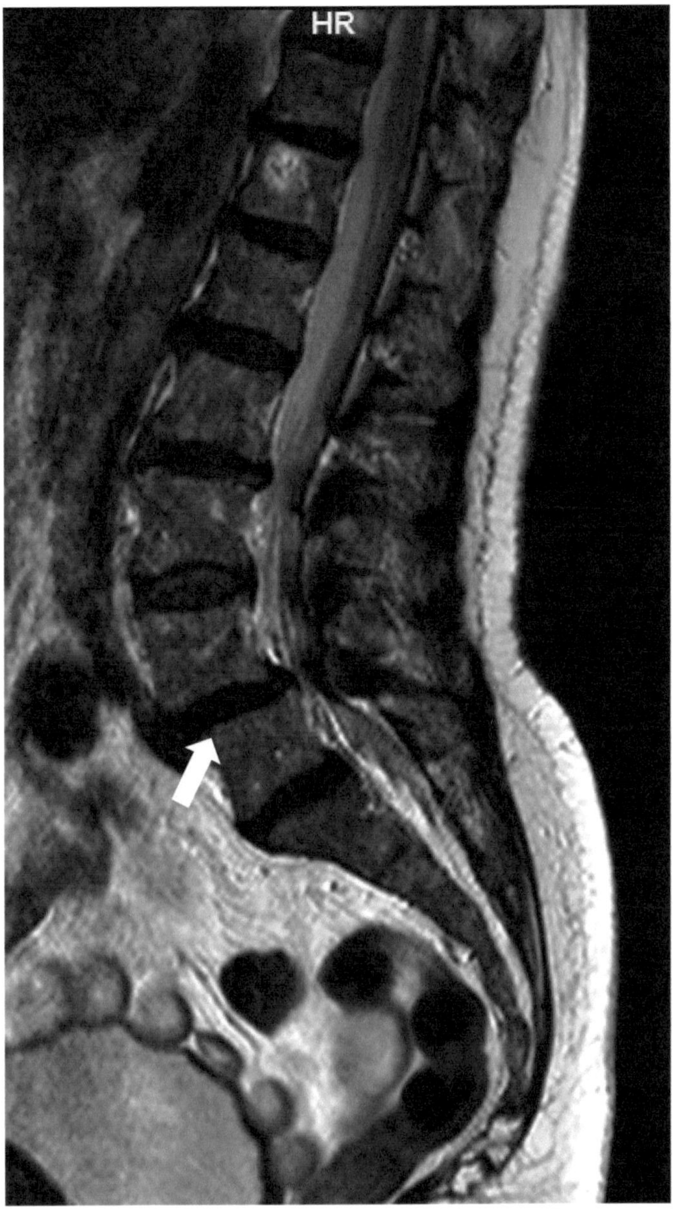

Figure 9.
Lumbar spondylolisthesis. Preoperative sagittal MR T2-weighted scan: the L4–L5 stenosis and listhesis grade-1 (white arrow) *is well seen.*

listhesis be wrongly attributed to a degenerative disorder; if so, intraoperatively, the surgeon will have to face an unexpected pathoanatomical finding and be obviously addressed to change surgical strategy timely.

Anterolisthesis grade-2 may involve different scenarios. A surgeon may incorrectly interpret preoperative images and judge a borderline slippage as grade I instead of grade II, often due to a misleading neuroradiological report; this is why a flexion–extension x-ray film is mandatory in the preoperative setup of a lumbar instability.

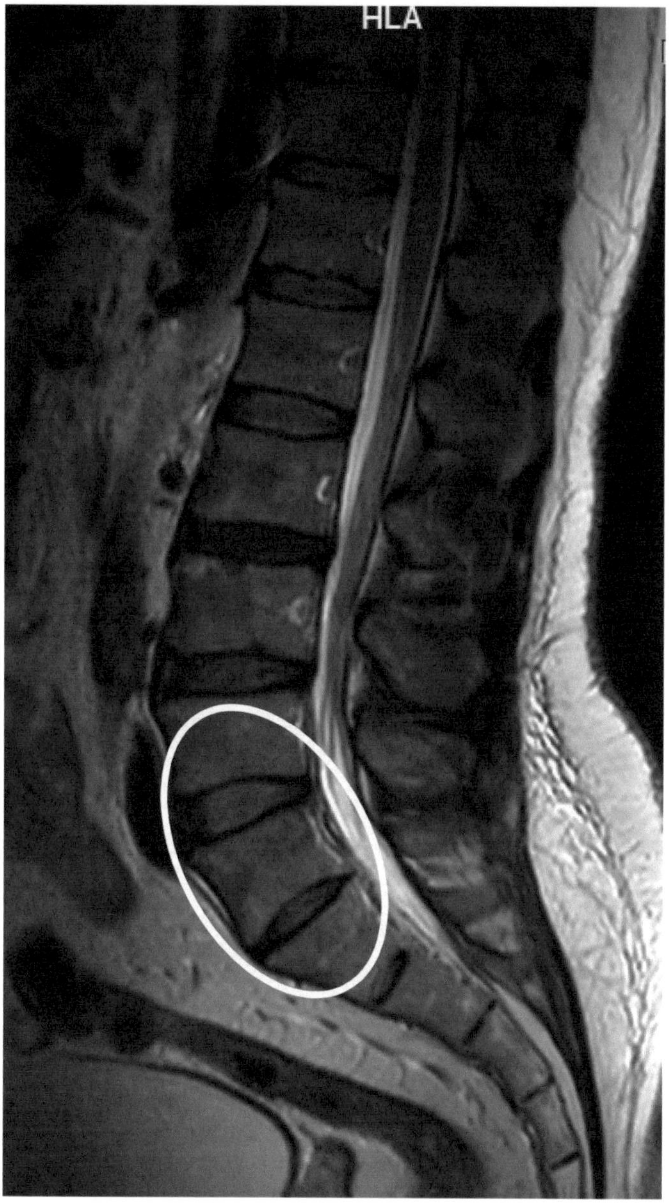

Figure 10.
Transitional vertebra. Preoperative sagittal MR T2-weighted scan: typical appearance of vertebral bodies and discs at the lumbosacral passage (white oval)*; L5-(lumbarized)S1 retrolisthesis may be appreciated too.*

Or, a frank listhesis, deemed by the experienced surgeon when unexpectedly found out at surgery, will discourage him from implanting the scheduled ISD and possibly shift to a pedicle fixation.

Of course, several additional disorders (such as osteoporosis, coexisting infective states, bone anomalies of the posterior vertebral arch, etc.) constitute a contraindication to the implant of an ISD, but they are easily ascertained at the time of preoperative consultation.

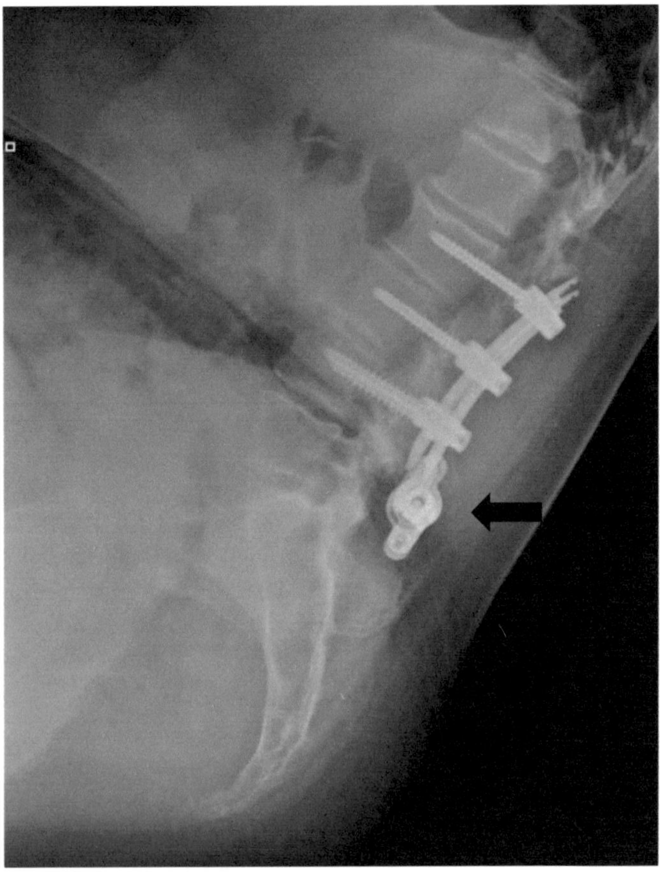

Figure 11.
*Adjacent segment disease (ASD). Lateral x-ray film at 2-year post-ISD implant: pedicular fixation L2-L3-L4 is seen; the spacer at the caudal ASD level is well inserted between the spinous processes (*black arrow*).*

7. Surgical tricks

The interspinous space may present multiple anatomic variations, and this must be kept in mind by the surgeon, particularly the shape of the space and its matching with the shape of the spacer [13].

The L5-S1 level. Anatomy of the passage L5-S1 may be quite variable, and this is mainly due to the shape and height of sacrum protuberance; when an ISD implant at L5-S1 is planned, great attention must be paid to the preoperative study, and if the MR scan is not clear about bone aspects of sacrum, a CT examination must be done before surgery.

Regardless of the type of ISD, the basic rule to implant it successfully is to insert it as deep as possible, and the right placement is at the line of articular processes (**Figure 12**); suboptimal insertion of the spacer does not necessarily involve a poor clinical outcome, but x-ray follow-up controls, at least over the first postoperative year, are strongly recommended.

The surgical technique to implant an ISD may differ, and it's also due to the type of spacer and the strumentarium to implant. Some spacers are to be applied through the

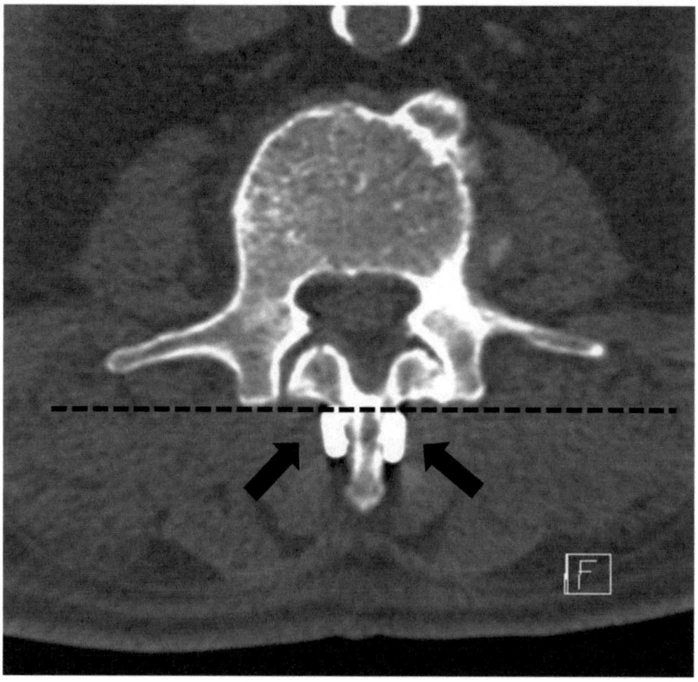

Figure 12.
*Depth of ISD implant. Postoperative axial CT scan: the base of lateral plates of the spacer (*black arrows*) are correctly placed at the level of articular processes (*black dotted line*).*

interspinous ligament, assembling the two parts once they are *in situ*; this implies that the supraspinous ligament has not to be sacrificed (sparing technique) offering an additional barrier to potential superficial dislocation of the device. Alternatively, if you use a 'U'-spacer or opt for a not-sparing technique, attention must be paid not to over-decorticate the facing surfaces of spinous processes because this manoeuvre does not enhance bone incorporation and may result in the spinous process weakening.

The last step of implantation is clamping the lateral plates of the spacer against spinous processes; this is probably the most hazardous manoeuvre in terms of risk of rupture of spinous process and must be done cautiously, squeezing the dedicated compressors in a step-by-step alternate way. Once you have compressed the device in situ, we suggest checking its final mechanical seal: the spacer is grabbed by a needle-holder and pulled superficially and horizontally, so observing that the lumbar segments move as a unique block.

Multilevel stenosis of the lumbar canal, though usually symptomatic at just one level, may be encountered in the daily practice and the matter of operate upon two or three levels is not trivial; are ISDs insertable at multiple levels? Yes, they are. However, much attention must be paid to the preoperative CT scan: the decisive factor is represented by the height of the middle of the three indexed spinous processes, which must be high enough to receive plates of both spacers (**Figure 13**). Based on our experience, the implant of two spacers having a metal-to-metal final construct at one or both sides of the middle spinous process may result in a poor clinical outcome in terms of back and/or radicular pain.

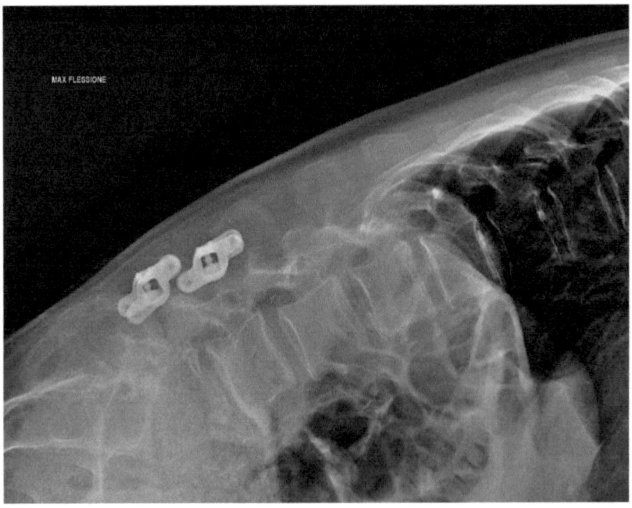

Figure 13.
Two-level lumbar spinal stenosis. Flexion x-ray film at 2-year follow-up: the spacers are correctly placed, and the construct is no metal-to-metal.

8. Complications

Wrong level. Although bizarre to comprehend, an ISD may be implanted at the wrong level (**Figure 14**); this may occur when 'kissing' spinous processes are found at surgery, often in an obese patient, so making intraoperative fluoroscopic controls incorrectly interpreted.

Spinous process rupture. In most of cases in which this complication happens, this occurs intraoperatively; factors leading to such a complication are incorrectly sized device selection and poor surgical technique; we never encountered early or late postoperative rupture of a spinous process in an ISD-implanted patient, and in those rare cases in which we found out this complication, retrospective review of postoperative x-ray and/or CT exams indeed revealed that the rupture had occurred at surgery.

Regardless of the type of ISD used, most of the fractures involve the junction of the inner and middle thirds of the cranial spinous process. When we started inserting a PEEK ISD, the first bone fracture case was discovered only through CT scan, which we routinely performed on postoperative day 1, and it passed clinically unnoticed (*e.g.*, postoperative pain was the same that uncomplicated patients referred). How to manage this complication? It must be remembered that the lateral plates of the ISD (especially those of second-generation) act as fixators of the ruptured spinous process, usually making revision surgery unnecessary; the use of a lumbar corset for two months (instead of one) is advisable.

Dislocation of ISD. When a spacer migrates into the spinal canal, urgent revision surgery, aimed to remove it and repair the dural sac, if lacerated, is mandatory. Migration of ISD in the paravertebral soft tissues is far more frequent and may be accompanied by recurring pain or claudication; in such cases, an election revision operation is planned, and two options are available: once the displaced spacer has been removed, a new, different-type ISD is inserted; alternatively, transpedicular fixation is performed.

Miscellaneous. Scientific literature reports different complications: dural tear, nerve root injury, late lumbar/radicular recurrent pain, neurological impairment, and chronic lumbar pain.

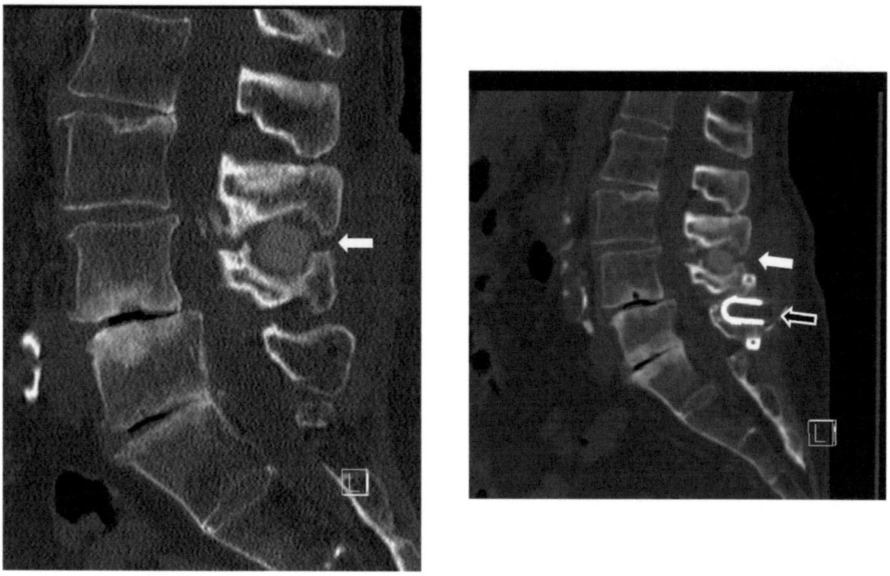

Figure 14.
'Wrong level'. Sagittal reformatted CT scans: this patient came to our attention after having performed an "interspinous stabilization L4-L5" elsewhere (as reported in medical discharging chart); soon after surgery her bilateral claudicatio radicolaris *started to worsen;* on the left, *the DIAM device applied at the L3-L4 (wrong level), and,* on the right, *the COFLEX device correctly inserted at L4-L5; the DIAM at L3-L4 was intentionally left in place to avoid late compromise of segmental stability.*

9. Personal considerations

Dutch school of neurosurgery goes on to keep a leading role in the management of spinal stenosis; over 70 years ago, in a tribute to another giant of spinal surgery (Clovis Vincent), Prof Verbiest first described the pathophysiological correlation between symptoms of cauda equina compression and spinal stenosis, which, curiously and interestingly, he defined as 'rare' [14]. Nowadays, the group of Moojen goes on sharing elegant works concerning the outcome of patients receiving an ISD implant: in their very recent randomized control trial paper, a 5-year follow-up good outcome in ISD implant, if compared to conventional lumbar decompression was reported [15]. Moreover, it's worth that they also state that the ISD group seems to have less back pain during long-term follow-up; this constitutes a very important issue: our experience, using different types of ISD, supports the same conclusion: ISD patients, implanted for treating lumbar stenosis (and, above all, for a DDD), early in the postoperative course refer that back pain is of different quality and far milder than preoperatively, and this substantial pain relief maintains over time.

We started to implant ISDs in 2005, and since then, we have used different types of spacers; on time, we realized that each of them has its own pros and cons, which must be well-known by the surgeon to best adapt to any patient elected for this kind of surgery.

In my daily activity, patients affected by spondylolisthesis grade 2, in which implanting an ISD represents a formal contraindication, are very few; on the contrary, the number of cases harbouring a listhesis up to grade- 1 is far larger, and almost all of them are ideal candidates to ISD implant; this means that at least as first surgical management step, more invasive procedures (such as transpedicular fixation, anterior lumbar interbody fusion, XLIF, etc.) are not necessary.

Lumbar spinal stenosis affects about one-third of people aged 70, and those of them requiring a surgical treatment are offered different options, the first of whom being a decompressive one- or more-level laminectomy. Based upon our 30-year experience, we think that: a] standard one- or multilevel laminectomy [*e.g.*, with the removal of spinous process(es)] for the management of lumbar stenosis has to be abandoned; b] of course, minimally invasive decompressive procedures [with sparing of spinous process(es)] are still highly valid and have to be correctly proposed to the 'stenotic' patients as a first surgical option; c] ISD implant, coupled or not with a decompressive step, actually represents the ideal treatment for one-level lumbar stenosis w/wo listhesis up to grade1; d] empirically, if compared, the group of decompressed-only and that of ISD-implanted patients share about the same high rate of improvement of NIC, but the latter seems to fare largely better in terms of relief of lumbar pain.

Most of the scientific papers dealing with the outcome of different surgical operations, performed to achieve lumbar stabilization take bone fusion rate into account as the main indicator of success. This methodological approach was developed and consolidated more than 50 years ago when global aspects concerning this kind of surgery were different: hardware, age of patients (usually less than 80 years), and

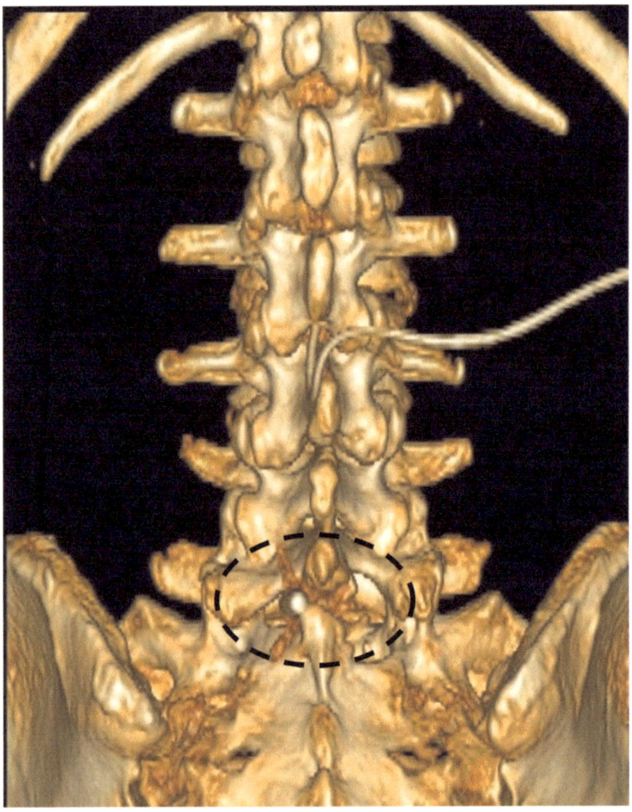

Figure 15.
Lumbar DDD. Three-dimensional reformatted coronal CT scan at 13-year follow-up: the BACJAC spacer is well inserted between the spinous processes of L5 and S1 (dotted black oval)*; a spinal cord stimulation electro-catheter is also seen at L2-L3.*

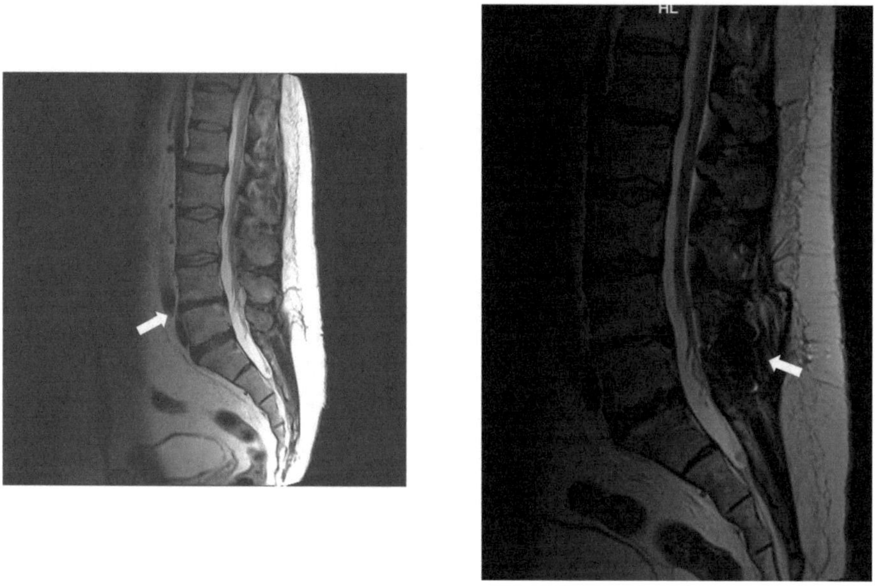

Figure 16.
*Lumbar DDD. Preoperative (*left*) and 10-year follow-up (*right*) sagittal MR T2-weighted scans: the L4-L5 degenerated disc (*left, white arrow*) and the long-term correctly placed ROMEO 2 PAD spacer (*right, white arrow*) are well seen.*

diagnostic tools (grossly limited to x-ray films). Nowadays, we feel that the concept of bone fusion, adopted to evaluate the outcome of surgical options for DDD and lumbar stenosis, should be replaced by that of 'bone synthesis', which is more helpful and adherent to global (functional, clinical, and radiological) analysis of operated patients.

One of most frequent criticisms made to ISDs is the absence of long-term follow-up studies; this may be partially true and it's also due to the replacement of the first-generation spacers with the newest ones, probably making ongoing studies obsolete and, therefore, abandoned. Moreover, recent covid-19 epidemics determined a tremendous gap in the follow-up studies, especially concerning many aged patients operated upon for lumbar stenosis, who deceased or were lost over last three years. Currently, our documented experience with hundreds of implanted ISDs allows us to affirm that: (a) a first-generation PEEK spacer demonstrates no neuroradiological migration or bone spinous process rupture at a 13-year follow-up (**Figure 15**); (b) a second-generation device shows the same good result at a 10-year follow-up (**Figure 16**).

10. Final reflections

Of course, most of the spinal disorders described in Section 5 may be treated by means of other surgical techniques; concerning this statement, some observations help both the surgeon and the patient. First, a '(at least) second opinion' will help the patient to take the right decision to manage his/her problem; second, ISD implant may be considered as an 'intermediate step in the continuum of care for patients with NIC associated with lumbar spinal stenosis' [16].

In some western countries ISDs are widely implanted by physiatrists and interventional pain specialists; recently, a small series of complications related to ISD implants, in particular, the migration of the spacer in the spinal canal, performed by pain specialists, was reported [17]. Over the last two decades, the industry has promoted the ISD surgical implant and, based upon its presumed 'easiness of technique', it forced its use by 'non-spine surgeons'; the matters of incorrect surgical indication, poor knowledge of the biomechanics of the spinal column, inability to manage potential complications, have rocketed. It has been strongly recommended that 'spinal instrumentation, however minimally invasive, should be performed by fellowship-trained spine surgeons' and, in the same way, a consultation with an experienced spine surgeon before an ISD implantation should be performed [17].

As for most lumbar spine surgical procedures, the problem of costs exists for ISD implant too; this directly leads to our (as surgeons) formidable task to conciliate budget-based medicine and the goal of 'best treatment for the ideal patient'; therefore, settings of clinical assessment, surgical experience, profound knowledge of available spacers, must be managed with skill and simultaneously by the experienced surgeon. This goal will revitalize the somewhat abandoned 'ancient doctor-patient relationship' and decrease the high rate of litigation in spinal surgery [18].

Very recently, the experience of ISD implantation was reported as being very satisfying in terms of minimal surgical invasiveness and good clinical outcome [19]; based upon our 20-year ISD-dedicated surgery, we truly share these observations: early in the postoperative course, most of our ISD-implanted patients refer to stand and walk with a straight back after a long time of pain and claudication, and this excellent result usually maintains over time.

Acknowledgements

Our huge thanks run to Dr Susanna USAI (Acting Director, Neurologia 3, Istituto Neurologico 'Carlo Besta', Milan, Italy): her acute and stimulating observations are always precious to us.

Conflict of interest

The Author declares no conflict of interest.

Author details

Claudio Irace
Department of Orthopedics, 'Piccole Figlie' Hospital, Parma, Italy

*Address all correspondence to: clauirax@gmail.com

References

[1] Sénégas J. Lumbar dynamic stabilization with the Wallis implant. Argospine News & Journal. 2009;**21**(2): 48-55

[2] Kabir SMR, Gupta SR, Casey ATH. Lumbar interspinous spacers; a systematic review of clinical and biomechanical evidence. Spine. 2010;**35**: E1499-E1506

[3] Irace C, Giannachi L, Amato V, Corona C. The BacJac interspinous device in the treatment of lumbar spine degenerative disorders: A prospective study and 2-year follow-up results. Journal of Spine. 2014; **3**:163-168

[4] Schulte TL, Hurschler C, Haversath M, Liljenqvist U, Bullmann V, Filler TJ, et al. The effect of dynamic, semi-rigid implants on the range of motion of lumbar motion segments after decompression. European Spine Journal. 2008;**17**:1057-1065

[5] Kim KA, McDonald M, Pik JHT, Khoueir P, Wang MY. Dynamic intraspinous spacer technology for posterior stabilization: case-control study on the safety, sagittal angulation, and pain outcome al 1-year follow-up evaluation. Neurosurgery Focus. 2007; **22**(1):E7

[6] Caporlingua F. (Editorial on): Superion® InterSpinous Spacer treatment of moderate spinal stenosis: 4-year results. Journal of Spine Surgery. 2018;**4**(3):666-667. DOI: 10.21037/jss.2018.08.01

[7] Gala RJ, Russo GS, Whang PG. Interspinous implants to treat spinal stenosis. Current Review Musculoskeletal Medicine. 2017;**10**: 182-188

[8] Giltaij L, Timothy J, Derks M. BacJac interspinous decompression system: another me-too or an improvement? Spinal Surgery News. 2008;**2008**:29-34

[9] Pintauro M, Duffy A, Vahedi P, Rymarczuk G, Heller J. Interspinous implants: are the new implants better than the last generation? A review. Current Review in Musculoskeletal Medicine. 2017;**10**:189-198

[10] Assietti R, De Falco R. The first multicenter, prospective 6 month follow-up study of 21 patients treated with the Aperius Perclid system. In: 13th European Congress of Neurosurgery – EANS. Glasgow, United Kingdom; 2007. pp. 607-613

[11] Karahalios DG, Kaibara T, Porter RW, Kakarla UK, Reyes PM, Baaj AA, et al. Biomechanics of a lumbar interspinous anchor with anterior lumbar interbody fusion. Journal of Neurosurgery Spine. 2010;**12**(4):372-380

[12] Plasencia Arriba MA, Maestre C, Martin-Gorrono F, Plasencia P. Analysis of long-term results of lumbar discectomy with and without an interspinous device. International Journal of Spine Surgery. 2022;**16**(4): 681-689

[13] Barbagallo GM, Olindo G, Corbino L, Albanese V. Analysis of complications in patients treated with the X-Stop Interspinous Process Decompression System: proposal for a novel anatomic scoring system for patient selection and review of the literature. Neurosurgery. 2009;**65**:111-120

[14] Verbiest H. Sur certaines forms rares de compression de la queue de cheval. Hommage à Clovis Vincent. Paris: Maloine; 1949. pp. 161-174

[15] Schenck CD, Terpstra SES, Moojen WA, van Zwet E, Peul W, Arts MP, et al. Interspinous process device versus conventional decompression for lumbar spinal stenosis: 5-year results of a randomized controlled trial. Journal of Neurosurgery Spine. 2022;**36**:909-917

[16] Carl L. Appropriate selection of patients with lumbar spine stenosis for interspinous process decompression with the X STOP device. Neurosurgery Focus. 2007;**22**(1):E5

[17] Florence TJ, Say I, Patel KS, Unterberger A, Laiwalla A, Vivas AC, et al. Neurosurgical management of interspinous device complications: a case series. Frontiers in Surgery. 2022;**9**:1-9

[18] Irace C. Wrong level (reply to letter). Journal of Neurosurgery Spine. 2011;**12**:689-690

[19] Gilbert JW, Christensen B, Matheny S. Interspinous process device clinical practice experience. Journal of Neurosurgery Spine. 2022;**25**:1-2. DOI: 10.3171/2022.7.SPINE22831

Chapter 15

The Application of Multi-Modal Image Fusion Combined with Navigation Technology to Precisely Localize Spinal Cord Lesions

Peihai Zhang and Xuejun Yang

Abstract

Objective: To study the application value of multi-modal image fusion combined with navigation for precise localization of spinal cord lesions. Methods: From November 2015 to January 2022, a total of 28 patients with spinal cord lesions were enrolled in the study, and intraoperative CT images were obtained by O-arm, and preoperative MRI and intraoperative CT were fused by the navigation system to reconstruct 3D models of the spine and lesion. Complete the localization and resection of spinal cord lesions during navigation, and record basic patient information, image fusion time, and navigation accuracy. Results: All 28 patients successfully localized spinal cord lesions with multi-modal image fusion combined with navigation. The time of image processing was between 7 min and 19 min, and the mean value was 15.3 ± 2.2 min. The navigation error was between 0.9 mm and 5.3 mm, and the mean value was 1.8 ± 0.9 mm. Conclusion: The multi-modal image fusion combined with navigation can be used to precisely localize spinal lesions, providing a more objective basis and a new approach for individualized and precise surgical planning.

Keywords: O-arm, navigation, multi-modal, image fusion, spinal cord lesions

1. Introduction

Spinal cord lesions, also known as spinal canal lesions, account for about 4.3% ~ 10.4% of all central nervous system lesions and an annual incidence of about 0.97/100,000 people. Lesions can occur in the spinal cord, nerve roots, and meninges [1, 2], and surgical resection is the preferred treatment. The intraoperative precise localization of spinal cord lesions is one of the crucial factors affecting the quality of surgery. Determining the lesion location mainly relies on the vertebral body being inferred indirectly, while the localization of spinal segments lacks consistent standards. It has been reported that the risk of surgical exposure or exploration in the wrong segment is between 0.032 and 15% [3–7]. This is likely to cause unnecessary spinal cord injuries, especially for lesions that extend into the foramen area. Due to the difficulty of exposure and the complex spatial structure of lesions, a large amount of lamina milling is required to remove part of the small joints, which may lead to accelerated spinal degeneration and instability in the long term. Glioma and intramedullary tiny lesions of the spinal cord can be difficult to locate and require the surgeon's experience to determine the extent of resection. However, the spinal cord lacks a functional dummy area, and blind exploration is bound to cause nerve function injury, which is far from the standard of accurate neurosurgery.

In 2015, the study team started using multi-modal image fusion techniques to identify intraoperative spinal cord lesions. The O-arm was used to capture intraoperative CT images of the patients, which were then uploaded to the navigation system and combined with other images for intraoperative localization of spinal cord lesions. Previous investigations [8–10] have confirmed the technique's viability and accuracy. The intangible surgical experience can be made concrete through preoperative MRI images that clearly show the lesions. The use of multi-modal image fusion technology in treating spinal cord lesions can be encouraged by summarizing and updating existing data.

2. Methods

28 patients with spinal cord lesions who underwent surgical treatment in our hospital's neurosurgery department between November 2015 and January 2022 were selected, including 13 men and 15 women, with cases affecting the cervical segment 6, thoracic segment 10, and lumbar segment 12. Patients' ages ranged from 14 to 78, with an average age of 41. During postoperative pathology, 8 cases of neurofibroma, 3 cases of schwannoma, 2 cases of meningioma, 3 cases of capillary hemangioma, 6 cases of spinal cuff cyst of nerve roots, 1 case of intramedullary vascular malformation of the spinal cord, 3 cases of cavernous hemangioma, and the remaining 4 cases of ependymoma were identified.

Prior to surgery, patients underwent regular CT (64-slice spiral CT, GE, USA) and MRI (3.0 T, GE, USA) scans. After scanning, axial, sagittal, and crown pictures were captured, recorded in DICOM format, and stored at the Stealth station 7 navigation workstation. The enhanced inspection is selected based on the relationship between the lesions and significant blood vessels.

Before surgery at Synergy Cranial, the intraoperative O-arm was used to take CT images of the patient's spinal segments, which were then registered and merged with CT and MRI images sent to the navigation workstation. Operate in the Stealth Merge module, select the O-arm CT images as the reference, verify the fusion image's accuracy by combining or separating Windows, choose the appropriate transparency, and ensure that the bone cortex is consistently aligned on both pictures. Additionally, the key to a successful fusion was to maintain the continuous union of vertebrae and facet joints in the diseased segment due to intraoperative spinal flexion and rotation, which could not align with preoperative imaging. Two senior neurosurgeons collaborated to achieve image fusion.

In the Synergy Cranial software's building 3D model module, the target structure's 3D model is reconstructed. Blood vessels and the spine can be reconstructed using modules including bone and vessel using preoperative CT and O-arm scans as data sources. and enhanced by tools such as Push, Threshold, and others. Based on preoperative MRI data that can be reconstructed using programs like Lasso, the 3D model of spinal cord occupation was created. Once the 3D model reconstruction is complete, it is possible to display the integrated model of the spine, blood vessel, and lesion in the same spatial coordinate system by varying the model's size and transparency. At this stage, the operation path can be virtually created and planned at any level.

With reference to multi-modal 3D fusion images, surgical incisions, laminae milling, facet joint grinding, and other precise locations were designed. Prior to the surgical exploration of the spinal cord using anatomical markers on the bones, such as the spinous process and facet joints, the precision of navigation was examined. The degree of lesion excision was determined, the lesion location was found, navigation accuracy was validated, and CT or MRI images were switched to display in accordance with the operation's goals.

The time for image processing included the time for acquiring the image using O-arm and the time for image fusion. Navigation errors were evaluated by measuring the maximum distance between the end of the lesion in MRI images and its real position. Descriptive statistics were used to calculate the mean and standard deviation. SPSS (version 13.0 SPSS Inc) was used for the analysis.

3. Results

The findings showed that only a small portion (2.29%–15.66%) of the entire operation time (83–400 min) was accounted for by the operating time for O-arm scanning and image fusion (7–19 min). For the high cervical-level spinal cord lesion, O-arm scanning was not necessary. The posterior fossa bone can usually be used for automatic fusion, and the procedure is quick overall. Patients with lumbar lesions undergo O-arm scanning and image fusion in a shorter time (10–17 minutes) than those with cervical and thoracic lesions (15–19 minutes).

MRI and CT image fusion for patients with spinal cord lesions in the high cervical segment was successful (**Figure 1**). O-arm scanning was omitted, and intraoperative

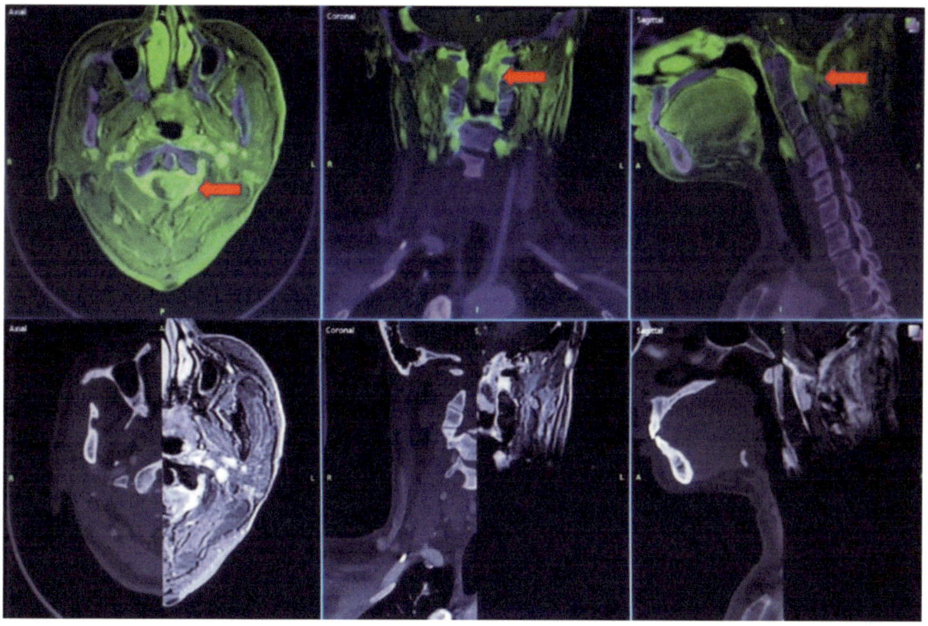

Figure 1.
Shows the image fusion of patients with meningioma from the foramen magnum to C2. The MRI T1WI axial image was combined with the CT image and the red arrow shows the location of C1–2. The accuracy of the fusion was verified by adjusting transparency and separate windows.

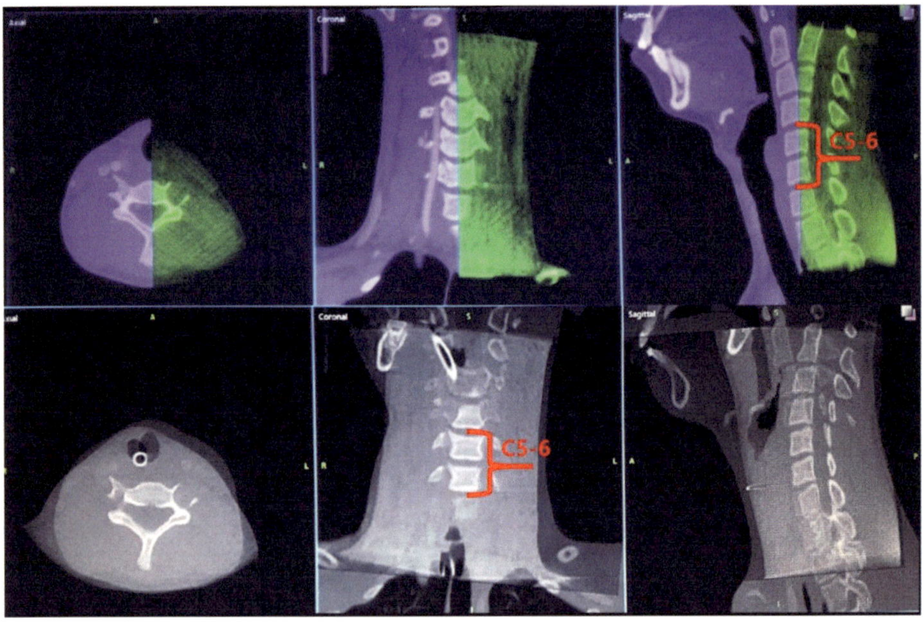

Figure 2.
Image fusion of patients with C5–6 ganglion lesion: Preoperative enhanced CT was combined with intraoperative O-arm images. The red figure indicated the C5–6 vertebral body where the lesion was located. The registration time maximized the C5–6 fusion.

contour registration was performed using MRI data. The intraoperative O-arm scanning was performed according to the schedule of all the other patients. During the procedure, one patient with a cervical 5–6 ganglion lesion was lying on their side with their neck partially extended to the healthy side. The preoperative CT and MRI images and the intraoperative O-arm image did not integrate well, and the image fusion was finished using the principle of maintaining continuous fusion of vertebral body and joint bone in lesion segments (**Figure 2**). A patient with a thoracic spinal cord intramedullary vascular malformation paraplegic had an acute intramedullary hemorrhage and only an emergency thoracic MRI scan was performed before surgery. Sagittal T2-weighted sequences were used to fuse the MRI with intraoperative O-arm images (**Figure 3**).

After the image fusion was completed, Synergy Cranial software was used to reconstruct the patient's 3D model and plan the surgical path. To completely remove the lesion and minimize spinal and paravertebral muscle damage, minimally invasive surgical incisions were made in 2 cases of lumbar schwannoma and 1 case of thoracic nerve root rotator cuff cyst. **Figure 4** depicts a case of minimally invasive image-assisted navigation for lumbar 3–4 schwannoma resection. Under the microscope, the lesion was completely removed while only a part of the patient's lamina was ground. The minimally invasive incision is based on the body surface projection of the lesion recorded by navigation, and the accurate finding of the lesion through minimally invasive channels is defined by letters A, B, and C. A is the navigational interface of CT images during O-arm surgery; B is the navigational interface of synchronous T2WI imaging on MRI.

An example of lumbar schwannoma with L3–5 posterior pedicle screw placement due to injury to the L4 vertebrae. The O-arm scan immediately confirmed that all screws were in their proper places (**Figure 5**). During intraoperative 3D model reconstruction, a patient with ganglioblastoma at the C5–6 level (**Figure 6**)

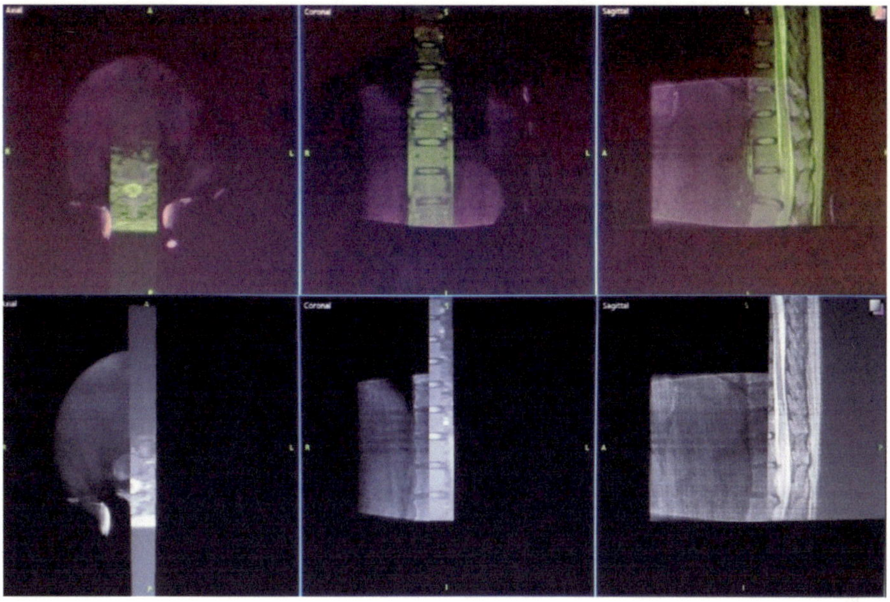

Figure 3.
Image registration of patients with intramedullary vascular malformation of the thoracic spinal cord. Sagittal images of patients with MRI T2WI were fused with intraoperative 3D images of an O-arm, and the accuracy of fusion was verified by adjusting transparency and separate windows, respectively.

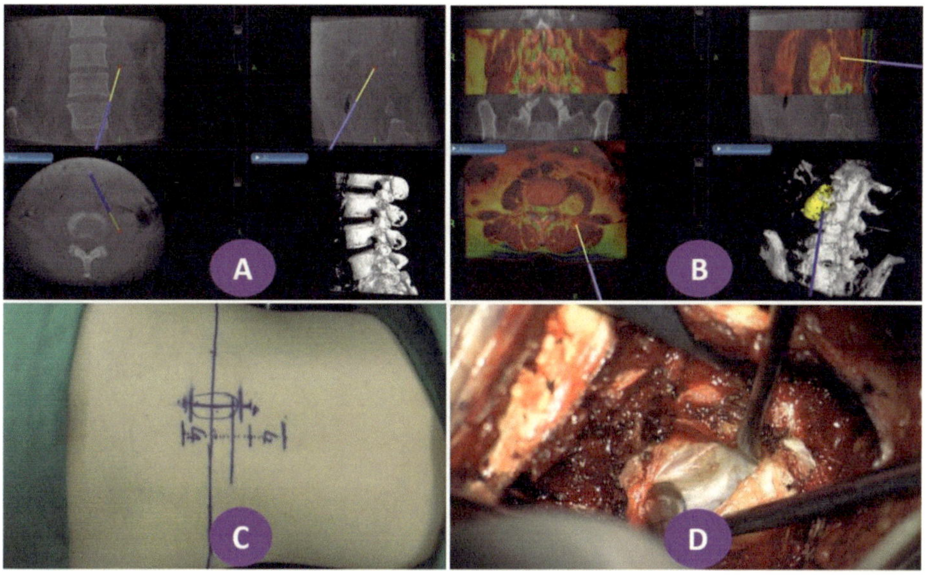

Figure 4.
Navigation and operation of lumbar 3–4 schwannoma using rainbow mode for MRI images, greyscale mode for O-arm images, yellow for lesion models, and white for lumbar models.

had a satisfactory union of the C5–6 vertebrae and tiny joints, while the remaining vertebrae showed significant deviation due to changes in body position. A and B used data from intraoperative O-arm scanning to create a 3D reconstruction of the cervical spine, while C and D used preoperative CT data to create a reconstruction

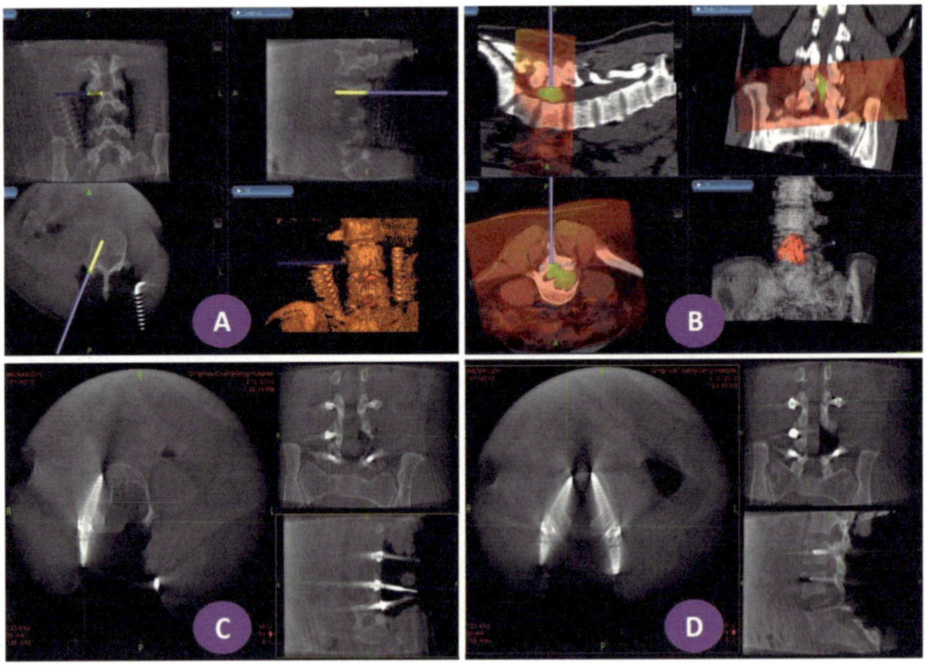

Figure 5.
O-arm scanning of patients with lumbar 4–5 schwannoma after navigation and screw placement. The lesion model was red, the orange spinal model was reconstructed from intraoperative O-arm 3D CT data, and the white spinal model was reconstructed from preoperative CT images.

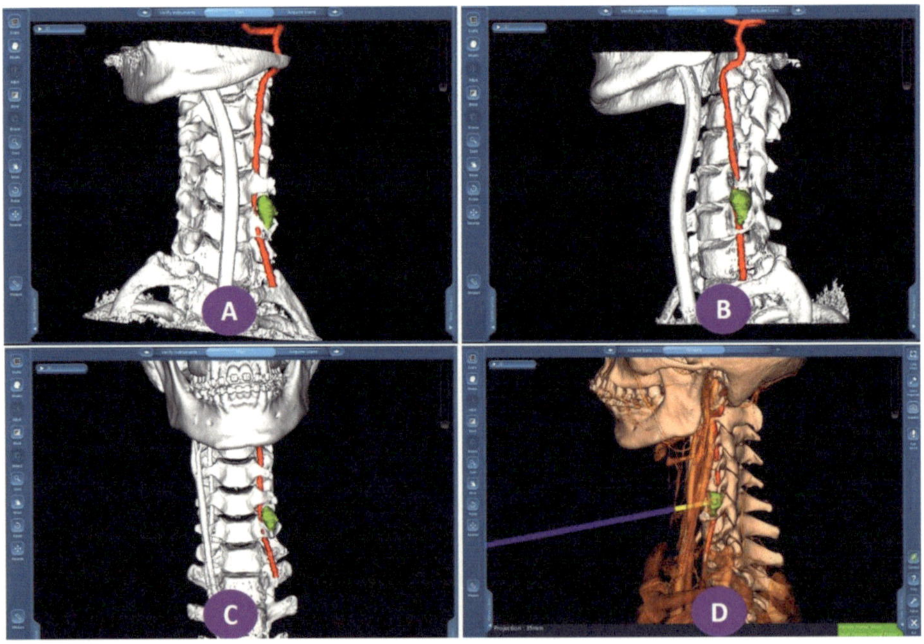

Figure 6.
3D model reconstruction and navigation of patients with C5–6 ganglioblastoma: The spine and other bony models were set in white, the left vertebral artery was set in red, and the lesion was set in green.

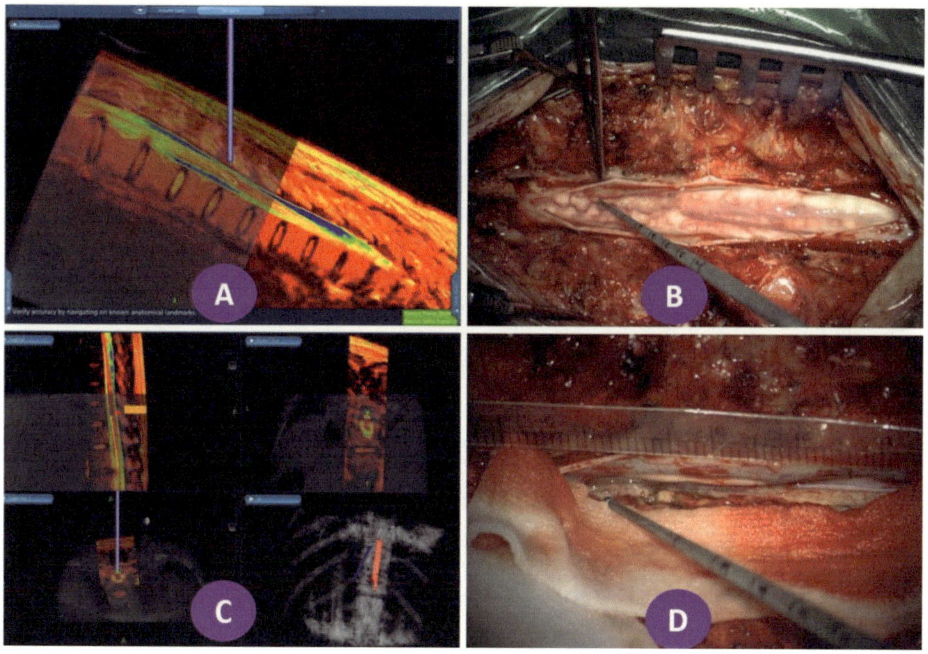

Figure 7.
Navigation and operation of patients with 10–12 intramedullary vascular malformations of the spinal cord in the chest. A and B show the location of intramedullary lesions under navigation; C and D show the extent of lesions during surgery to verify the accuracy of navigation. The spine and lesion are reconstructed in white and red, respectively.

of the cervical spine. To reach the base of the skull, the left vertebral artery may be seen passing through the neck's transverse foramen 1–6. According to figures A and B, the vertebral artery outside of the C5–6 vertebrae was shifted significantly from the cervical vertebrae. Surgical navigation requirements can be met due to intraoperative navigation, which also confirmed the high accuracy of navigation within the neck's fifth and sixth vertebrae. A navigation stick was used to assess the extent of the lesion in a patient with intramedullary spinal vascular malformations at the T10–12 level before exploring the spinal cord, and the position of the upper and lower poles of the lesion was consistent with the position shown by the navigation stick (**Figure 7**).

4. Discussion

Intraoperative localization of spinal segments is a unique problem in spinal surgery. Jillian E [11] et al., in a survey of 2338 members of the North American Spinal Association, which included 173 physicians, showed that fluoroscopy was the most commonly used method for thoracic and lumbar spine localization (89% and 86%, respectively). This was followed by intraoperative plain radiographs (54% vs. 58%, respectively), and fluoroscopy plus plain radiographs were used by 43.9% of physicians, even though 68% of the physicians reported having misidentified the segment. Currently, the chance of incorrect exposure and milling of incorrect segments is estimated to be between 0.032 and 15% [3–7]. Although the probability is low, incorrect localization can not only increase the trauma and cost of patients, but also prolong their hospital stay, and sometimes even lead to legal disputes for doctors.

The O-arm can collect intraoperative 3D CT images of the spine and then transfers them to the neural navigation system to complete real-time spine navigation. It changes the traditional localization based on intraoperative plain X-rays and fluoroscopy, with extremely high localization accuracy. In recent years, reports on its clinical application in spinal cord surgery have been increasing year after year [12–16]. Jang, Sang Hoon et al. [12] reported in 2015 that 31 patients undergoing anterior cervical surgery used an O-arm image navigation system during surgery. The statistical navigation errors showed that the horizontal deviation was 0.49+/–0.71 mm, and the vertical deviation was 0.88+/– 0.93 mm. The sagittal plane deviation Angle is 0.59+/–0.55°. Silbermann, J et al. [13] conducted a study of 187 screws inserted under an O-arm image-guided navigation in 37 patients, with an accuracy of 99%. Hand insertion was performed in 30 patients in the control group, with an accuracy of 94.1%, while 187 screws were inserted by hand in 37 patients, with an accuracy of 94.1%. In conclusion, the O-arm image navigation system is fully qualified for its requirements and provides accurate localization of spinal segments, eliminating the risk of radiation [14], and reducing the long-term cost of patients [15, 16]. However, it is challenging to display spinal cord lesions using O-arm scanning.

The multi-modal image fusion technology is based on the information fusion of images from two or more sources, which is helpful in obtaining a more accurate, comprehensive, and reliable image description of the same scene [17–19]. With the advancements in medical imaging and computer technology, neural navigation systems have evolved from simple anatomical navigation to functional navigation. Through multi-modal image fusion technology, functional brain images are combined with anatomical images such as CT and MRI, 3D reconstruction is performed, and space occupation, functional cortex, white matter conduction tract, and blood vessels are visually recorded. Assisted in creating virtual surgical plans before surgery and continued with localization and navigation during surgery. In the past 20 years, studies on multi-modal image fusion technology and neural navigation systems have mainly been seen in cases of craniocerebral lesions [20–27], with glioma being the most common. Glioma is an invasive growth that lacks a clear boundary, especially in middle and low-grade lesions. It is often difficult to distinguish the boundary between glioma and normal brain tissue during surgery. Studies [25, 27–28] have shown that this technique can significantly improve the lesion resection rate and reduce postoperative complications in patients.

In this study, the innovative Synergy Cranial software was used to integrate intraoperative O-arm 3D CT images with patients' preoperative high-definition CT and MRI for image fusion and navigation surgery, reducing navigation errors caused by spinal flexion and rotation and ensuring accurate localization of spinal segments while completing spinal lesions development. All 28 patients successfully underwent image fusion and underwent guided lesion resection. The intraoperative findings were completely in line with those indicated by navigation. Navigation localization was accurate, giving objective reliance on the operation, reducing unnecessary spinal cord exploration, and improving the surgeon's confidence. In the study, no patient opened the lamina by mistake and no patient damaged important blood vessels. It is worth mentioning that the results of the study on intramedullary spinal cord lesions showed that the sagittal and navigational boundaries under the microscope were completely consistent, which is of great significance for the accurate localization of intramedullary spinal cord lesions, the improvement of resection rate, and the reduction of reducing nerve injury.

The 3D lesion model, which is based on multi-modal image fusion reconstruction, can adjust transparency to meet the needs of the operation, perform free cutting, measure the distance between the lesion and any location, observe the direction and branch of blood vessels throughout the entire process, and assist the surgeon in creating a surgical plan and evaluating the degree of lesion resection. The digital model can help junior doctors understand the 3D anatomy of lesions, overcome the limitations of traditional anatomy teaching, and provide a good learning platform for young doctors to grow.

In conclusion, this study conducted multi-modal image fusion and precision navigation surgery on spinal cord lesions, which established the clinical operation process of multi-modal image fusion technology in precision surgical treatment and the modern surgical treatment concept of minimally invasive, individualized treatment [29, 30].

Acknowledgements

This work was supported by Tsinghua Precision Medicine Foundation (20219990008), Tsinghua University, Beijing, China.

Author details

Peihai Zhang and Xuejun Yang*
Beijing Tsinghua Changgung Hospital, Tsinghua University, Beijing, China

*Address all correspondence to: zpha00855@btch.edu.cn

References

[1] Duong LM, McCarthy BJ, McLendon RE, et al. Descriptive epidemiology of malignant and nonmalignant and primary spinal cord, spinal meninges, and cauda equina tumors, United States, 2004-2007. Cancer. 2012;**118**:4220-4227

[2] Dolecek TA, Propp JM, Stroup NE, et al. CBTRUS statistical report: Primary brain and central nervous system tumors diagnosed in the United States in 2005-2009. Neuro Oncology. 2012;**14** (Suppl. 5):v1-v49

[3] Siminski CP, Carr CM, et al. Fluoroscopy- and CT-guided gold fiducial marker placement for intraoperative localization during spinal surgery: Review of 179 cases at a single institution-technique and safety profile. AJNR. American Journal of Neuroradiology. 2023;**44**(5):618-622

[4] Hsu W, Kretzer RM, Dorsi MJ, et al. Strategies to avoid wrong-site surgery during spinal procedures. Neurosurgical Focus. 2011;**31**:E5

[5] Hsu W, Sciubba DM, Sasson AD, et al. Intraoperative localization of thoracic spine level with preoperative percutaneous placement of intravertebral polymethylmethacrylate. Journal of Spinal Disorders & Techniques. 2008;**21**:72-75

[6] Paolini S, Ciappetta P, Missori P, et al. Spinous process marking: A reliable method for preoperative surface localization of intradural lesion of the high thoracic spine. British Journal of Neurosurgery. 2005;**19**:74-76

[7] Mayer JE, Dang RP, Duarte Prieto GF, Cho SK, Qureshi SA, Hecht AC. Analysis of the techniques for thoracic- and lumbar-level localization during posterior spine surgery and the occurrence of wrong-level surgery: Results from a national survey. Spine J. 1 May 2014;**14**(5):741-748

[8] Zhang P, Sun Z, et al. Preliminary application of multimodal image fusion technique to treatment of lesions within the spinal canal. Chinese Journal of Neurosurgery. 2016;**32**(12):1239-1243

[9] Zhang P, Wang G, Sun Z, Lv X, Guo Y, Wang J, et al. Application of multimodal image fusion to precisely localize small intramedullary spinal cord Tumors. World Neurosurgery. 2018;**118**:246-249

[10] Zhang P, Liu H, Sun Z, Wang J, Wang G. The application of O-arm and navigation system in precise localization of spinal cord lesions: A case series study. Clinical Neurology and Neurosurgery. 2020;**196**:105922

[11] Jillian E, Mayer BA, et al. Analysis of the techniques for thoracic- and lumbar-level localization during posterior spine surgery and the occurrence of wrong-level surgery: Results from a national survey. The Spine Journal. 2014;**14**:741-748

[12] Jang SH, Cho JY, et al. Novel method for setting up 3D navigation system with skin-fixed dynamic reference frame in anterior cervical surgery. Computer Aided Surgery. 2015;**20**(1):24-28

[13] Silbermann, J Riese, F, et al. Computer tomography assessment of pedicle screw placement in lumbar and sacral spine: Comparison between free-hand and O-arm based navigation techniques. European Spine Journal. 2011;**20**(6):875-881

[14] Grelat, M. Zairi, F, et al. Assessment of the surgeon radiation exposure during

a minimally invasive TLIF: Comparison between fluoroscopy and O-arm system. Neurochirurgie. 2015;**61**(4):255-259

[15] Dea N, Fisher CG, et al. Economic evaluation comparing intraoperative cone beam CT-based navigation and conventional fluoroscopy for the placement of spinal pedicle screws: A patient-level data cost-effectiveness analysis. The Spine Journal. 2016;**16**(1):23-31

[16] Sclafani JA, Regev GJ, et al. Use of a quantitative pedicle screw accuracy system to assess new technology: Initial studies on O-arm navigation and its effect on the learning curve of percutaneous pedicle screw insertion. SAS Journal. 2011;**5**(3):57-62

[17] Maintz JBA, Viergever MA. A survey of medical image registration. Medical Image Analysis. 1998;**1**:1-36

[18] Moche M, Busse H, Dannenberg C, et al. Fusion of MRI, fMRI and intraoperative MRI data: Methods and clinical signance examplified by neurosugical interventions. Radiologe. 2001;**41**:993-1000

[19] Nimsky C, Kuhnt D, Ganslandt O, et al. Multimodal navigation integrated with imaging. Acta Neurochirurgica. Supplement. 2011;**109**:207-214

[20] Baum KG et al. Fusion viewer: A new tool for fusion and visualization of multimodal medical data sets. Journal of Digital Imaging. 2008;**21**(Suppl. 1): S59-S68

[21] Inoue A et al. Usefulness of an image fusion model using three-dimensional CT and MRI with Indocyanine green fluorescence endoscopy as a multimodal assistant system in endoscopic Transsphenoidal surgery. International Journal of Endocrinology. 2015;**2015**:694273

[22] Kin T et al. A new strategic neurosurgical planning tool for brainstem cavernous malformations using interactive computer graphics with multimodal fusion images. Journal of Neurosurgery. 2012;**117**(1):78-88

[23] Mirzadeh Z et al. Validation of CT-MRI fusion for intraoperative assessment of stereotactic accuracy in DBS surgery. Movement Disorders. 2014;**29**(14):1788-1795

[24] Pichler BJ et al. Multimodal imaging approaches: PET/CT and PET/MRI. Handbook of Experimental Pharmacology. 2008;**185 Pt 1**:109-132

[25] Rajasekar D et al. Multimodality image fusion in dose escalation studies of brain tumors. Journal of Applied Clinical Medical Physics. 2003;**4**(1):8-16

[26] Wakabayashi T et al. Advanced new neurosurgical procedure using integrated system of intraoperative MRI and neuronavigation with multimodal neuroradiological images. Nagoya Journal of Medical Science. 2009;**71**(3-4):101-107

[27] Xiao BX, Xu BN, Chen XI, et al. Assessment of complete resection of gliomas by intraprative high-field magnetic resonance imaging. Zhonghua Yi Xue Za Zhi. 2010;**26**:320-322

[28] Zhang JS, Chen XL, Li FY, et al. Influences of high-field intraoperative magnetic resonance imaging on the extent of resection in low-grade gliomas. Zhonghua Yi Xue Za Zhi. 2012;**92**:1738-1741

[29] Stellato TA. Humanism and the art of surgery. Surgery. 2007;**142**(4):433-438

[30] Brooke B, Nathan H, Pawlik TM. Trends in the quality of highly cited surgical research over the past 20 years. Annals of Surgery. 2009;**249**(1):162-167

Chapter 16

The Multiple Trajectory Anchoring Technique for Lumbar Sacral Fusion: An Alternative Solution for Spinal Fixation

Yuzeng Liu, Yong Hai, Hongtao Ding and Mingzheng Zhao

Abstract

Cortical bone trajectory (CBT) screw was firstly utilized by Santoni in 2009, which had been proved to have stronger hold force, especially in the osteoporosis vertebrae compared with the pedicle screw (PS). In this study, we developed a technique combining pedicle screw, cortical bone trajectory screw, and sacral alar screw, which was named as multiple trajectory anchoring (MTA) technique for patients who underwent lumbar-sacral fusion. The technique comes with the following improvements and advantages. First, the satellite rods are fixed with the additional screws which makes the tension more dispersed and avoids stress concentration. Second, the interaction between the multi-trajectory screws anchoring on one vertebra makes the screws stronger and reduce the risk of screw loosening. Third, the MTA screw can provide better stability for the anterior column. Forth, the MTA fixation can not only strengthen the construct, but also provide additional correction force. In this chapter, we aimed to introduce an original lumbar-sacral strengthening technique, multiple trajectory anchoring(MTA), for lumbar-sacral fusion. It is a safe and effective means to strengthen lumbar-sacral internal fixation as well as provide additional correction force for patients with lumbar-sacral degeneration, deformity and tumor. More importantly, it provides an alternative solution for pelvic fixation.

Keywords: cortical bone trajectory, pedicle fixation, lumbar fusion, multiple trajectory anchoring fixation, spinal fixation

1. Introduction

Pedicle screws (PS) are the most common method of sacral fixation. Spinal fusion with traditional bilateral PS fixation has been described for a variety of surgical indications, such as spinal canal stenosis, spinal degenerative disc disease, spinal slip, spinal tumor, spinal trauma, and malformations [1–5]. However, the main defects of the sacral PS fixation are screw loosening and pseudarthrosis, especially in the long-segment surgery and in fixation for osteoporotic patients. While a percutaneous pedicle screw (PPS) technique is an alternative, it requires an additional method of decompression and bone

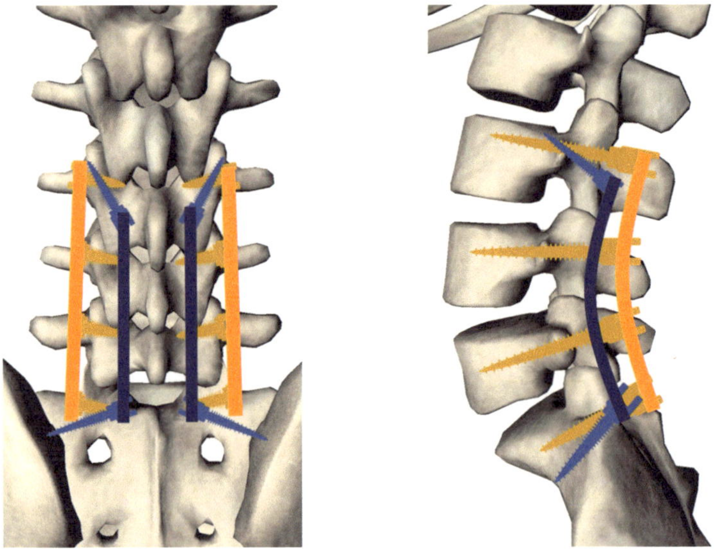

Figure 1.
The schematic diagram of the multiple trajectory anchoring (MTA) technique. Pedicle screws are in yellow. CBT and sacral alar screws are in blue.

grafting. In addition, the PPS technique relies on intraoperative multiplanar fluoroscopy, which leads to high radiation exposure risk for surgeons and patients. In addition, screw loosening is known to be a complication of PS fixation, especially in osteoporotic patients. There are several methods to enhance the purchase of screws, such as modifying screw design and strengthening the vertebrae with augmentation materials or the combination of cortical pedicle screw techniques. However, they remain unavailable for severe osteoporosis. Weaknesses of bone cement include its high exothermic polymerizing temperature, high monomer toxicity, and high risk of cement leakage into vertebrae. Cortical bone trajectory (CBT) screw was first utilized by Santoni [6] in 2009, which had been proved to have stronger hold force, especially in the osteoporosis vertebrae, compared with the pedicle screw. In 2013, Masaki [7] put forward the double-trajectory technique, cortical bone trajectory combined with traditional pedicle trajectory, in a patient with degenerative lumbar scoliosis and osteoporosis. We developed a technique combining pedicle screw, cortical bone trajectory screw, and sacral alar screw, which was named as the multiple trajectory anchoring (MTA) technique, for patients who underwent lumbar-sacral fusion (**Figure 1**). It provided an alternative solution for pelvic fixation and kept the motion of sacroiliac joint in the lumbar-sacral fusion surgery. With the MTA technique, CBT screws were selectively implanted in the lumbar spine and sacral alar screws were inserted on the same side of the sacrum, after completing the pedicle screw fixation and interbody fusion. And the screws were then connected with titanium or cobalt rod(s), which increased the strength of the internal fixation and provided additional strength for compression or distraction.

2. Anatomy and biomechanics of the MTA technique

As described by Masaki [7], the combined application of the CBT and PS in the same vertebrae was safe and feasible. The entry point of CBT screw was the intersection point of the vertical line at the midpoint of the superior articular process and a line 1 mm below the inferior edge of the transverse process. CBT screws rely on 4-point purchase between the dorsal cortex at the site of insertion, the medial and lateral cortex of the pedicle wall, and the curvature of the vertebral body wall, to maximize the cortical bone contact to improve purchase strength. The CBT screw followed a caudal-to-cephalad path in the sagittal plane and a medial-to-lateral path in the transverse plane through the pedicle, which maximized the thread contact of the screws with the vertebral cortical bone and offered stronger fixation strength. In the MTA technique, the sacral alar screw is inserted additionally based on the PS fixation and connected with the cranial CBT screw to enhance the fixation and reduce the incidence of pseudarthrosis. The entry point of the sacral alar screw is in the lower edge of the L5-S1 articular process, which is medial to the pedicle screw and can be well aligned with CBT screws. The outreach angle is 35 to 45 degrees and the sagittal inclination angle is 30 to 35 degrees. The length of the sacral alar screw can range from 35 to 45 mm. Breaking through the ventral cortical bone can maximize the anti-pullout strength. With the MTA technique, CBT screws were selectively implanted in the lumbar spine and sacral alar screws were inserted on the same side of the sacrum, after completing the pedicle screw fixation and interbody fusion. And the screws were then connected with titanium or cobalt rod(s), which increased the strength of the internal fixation and provided additional strength for compression or distraction.

Santoni found that CBT screws and PS have comparable pullout strengths and switching characteristics. Compared to PS, CBT screws showed a 30% increase in uniaxial pullout strength. However, the traditional pedicle trajectory screws are different from CBT. It is unclear whether screws and trajectory affect the uniaxial pullout strength of a single axis. Ueno studied the relationship between thread screw entry trajectory or thread characteristics and pullout strength in pig cadaver experiments. The results showed that the cortical screw was able to improve fixation strength but not significantly improve pullout strength. This specific trajectory appeared to have a major impact on pullout force. The biomechanical properties of PS and CBT screws were investigated by Calvert in which each screw was used to rescue the other in the setting of revision in 10 fresh-frozen human lumbar spines. The results of this study showed that CBT rescue screws retained 60% of the original pullout strength of PS, while traditional salvage screws retained 65% of the original CBT screw pullout strength. Either CBT or PS use as a rescue choice in the setting of a failed or compromised pedicle screw construct in the lumbar spine is supported by it. Baluch found that the CBT screw had greater loosening resistance in the fatigue tests when compared to the PS. According to Perez-Orribo, there was no significant difference in the mean range of motion or area of laxity of the CBT screw and PS during any mode of loading. Matsukawa [8] reported that CBT screws have 2.01 Ncm (Newton centimeter units) higher insertion torque than PS in vivo. CBT screw's fixation strength is superior to those of the traditional pedicle screws, as loading the flexing and stretching load resistance is higher, but its ability to fight the lateral bending and axial rotation is poorer. The mechanical performance of the CBT screw is attributed to such factors as the position of the screw specifications, placement, and patient's bone. One of the most critical factors is the size and length of the screw, the factors in the subsequent have also been confirmed in the experiments of other relevant bodies [9]. Compared with the traditional technique of pedicle screws, the use of CBT of bigger size and length can enhance biomechanical properties of the screw. Xiao-yu wu et al. [10] established a finite element model through a case of osteoporosis, simulated traditional pedicle screw and CBT screw in a two-way fixed effect. The results suggested that the stability of CBT group under flexion extension and rotation was greater than that of conventional pedicle screw group; extension and rotation was greater than that of conventional pedicle screw group; The CT values of the CBT group nail way around the bone are greater than conventional pedicle screws. The CBT screw technology is one of the preferred methods for lumbar internal fixation in patients with osteoporosis. CBTS internal fixation technology provides biomechanically stronger pullout forces and yield loads, and has similar flexion and extension resistance to PS. The screwing torque is about 1.7 times that of traditional PS internal fixation technology, but it has poor effect on lateral bending and axial rotation resistance. The results of biomechanical experiments and finite element analysis showed that the biomechanical properties of multi-trajectory screw internal fixation were significantly better than those of traditional PS internal fixation. Under the condition of simulating real human movement, multi-trajectory screw internal fixation technique can increase the strength of internal fixation, thereby improving the stability of lumbar fusion segment, reducing the risk of loosening of internal fixation and the incidence of pseudarthrosis, and improving the success rate and satisfaction of surgery. CBTS internal fixation technique can fully protect the posterior paravertebral muscles and facet joints of the spine to avoid postoperative paravertebral atrophy and facet joint degeneration. In addition, the combined application of CBTS internal fixation technique, SAS internal fixation technique, and PS internal fixation technique in lumbar fusion surgery can further increase the mechanical strength of the surgical segment, while obtaining a similar intervertebral stress environment, and effectively increase the mechanical stability of the surgical segment.

The MTA technique we are reporting on has the following biomechanical characteristics. First, compared with the existing multi-rod construct technique, the satellite rods in MTA are fixed on the additional screws that make the stress to be more dispersed and avoid stress concentration. Second, the interaction between the multi-trajectory screws anchoring on one vertebra makes the screws stronger and reduces the risk of screw loosening. Third, the MTA screw can provide more stability to the anterior column and help in interbody bone healing. Fourth, in the lumbar sacral deformity cases, MTA fixation could not only strengthen the construct, but also provide additional correction force to restore both coronal and sagittal balance. Fifth, the MTA technique is based on the usage of CBT screws and sacral alar screws, which provides an alternative for pelvic fixation and preserves the movement of sacroiliac joints. As we know, pelvic fixation may cause dysfunction and even seriously affect the patients' quality of life. With the application of the MTA technique, pelvic fixation can be reduced and the sacroiliac joint can be preserved. The MTA technique provides additional orthopedic strength and makes the lumbosacral internal fixation more solid. Meanwhile, CBT screw and sacral wing screw insertion through a medial entry point demands no additional exposure of the wound. When inserting the CBT screw, it may cross with pedicle screw, so there are three points to be noted. First, the insertion point of the pedicle screw should be lateral and close to the lower part of the pedicle, so as to leave enough space for the CBT screw. Second, CBT screws should be thinner and shorter than pedicle screws, generally 4.5 mm in diameter and 3.0 mm in length. Before CBT screws are inserted, probe detection can be applied to ensure that the inner wall of the vertebral pedicle is not breached. Third, if the pedicle is too thin to hold two screws, do not proceed with the insertion by force, and the alternative vertebrae can be selected as the upper hook point.

3. Clinical application of the MTA technique

Recent years have seen an increase in the incidence of lumbar degenerative disc disease (DDD) in older adults. There are significant changes in spinal anatomy and curvature with age. Hegazy [11] confirmed changes in the shape and size of lumbar kyphosis in older adults and recommended that more attention be paid to anatomy and curvature during surgery. Furthermore, osteoporosis is fairly common in older people. For this reason, another key treatment strategy for lumbar DDD in older adults is osteoporosis management. In the elderly, osteoporosis may cause loosening of internal fixation. One study reported a pedicle screw loosening rate of 12.8–25% in osteoporotic patients. Furthermore, the risks of both proximal and distal junctional kyphosis also rise as a result. Thus, internal fixation stability in patients with osteoporosis should be improved intraoperatively by employing expansive pedicle screws, bone cement screws, or cortical bone path screws. Expansive pedicle screws can increase the intensity of internal fixation, but there are obvious shortcomings such as complicated placement, high rate of screw breakage, and limited clinical applicability. Compared to the traditional technique, CBT increases the area of contact between the screws and the cortical bone, and all of the screws used in the CBT technique are encircled by cortical bone. Thus, this technique is best suited to the treatment of lumbar DDD patients with osteoporosis. In addition, in 2014, Mizuno proposed the combination of this technique with posterior lumbar midline fixation and fusion in lumbar midline fusion surgery (MIDLF). The CBT technique in MIDLF surgery has been used extensively in cases of lumbar DDD, adjacent spinal disease, and postoperative revision because of its poor invasiveness and high-safety advantages. Recently, with the widespread application of internal fixation of the spine, the incidence of failed back surgery syndrome and autism spectrum disorder (ASD) has increased, resulting in a high proportion of lumbar revision surgeries [12]. The risk of nerve structure and blood vessel exposure is significantly increased in revision surgery due to hypertrophic scar tissue and imprecise spinal anatomy. Minimizing exposure risk in revision surgery is another benefit of the MTA technique. During revision surgery, when the adjacent segment is decompressed and fixed, the internal fixation of the original operation usually needs to be replaced. However, internal fixation replacement may not only increase operative time and surgical risk, but also lead to more blood loss. As a result, decompression, fixation, and fusion on adjacent segments without removal of internal fixation from the original surgical procedure has become a key technique in the treatment of ASD. The CBT technique, which has a single-entry site and trajectory, allows for decompression, complete screw placement, and fusion of adjacent segments through a small incision while preserving the original internal fixation, thus avoiding significant dissection and reducing operative time and surgical risk. For example, the MTA technique can be used to place two groups of screws within the same vertebral body [13]. In a study by Takata et al. [14], it was shown that the CBT technique combined with MIDLF in lumbar revision surgery has the benefits of less soft tissue damage, less postoperative complications, and improved internal fixation stability compared to traditional revision surgery. Lumbosacral spinal fusion is a common surgical procedure for the treatment of spinal pathologies including degenerative disc disease, lumbar spinal stenosis, malformations, trauma, and neoplasms. Fixation in lumbar fusion requires screws to be inserted into the vertebrae. Traditionally, these procedures have been performed via pedicle screw augmentation of the posterior lumbosacral spine in the manner first described by Boucher in 1959. However, advances in spine surgery and a broader trend toward less invasive procedures have resulted in the development of novel and innovative techniques, which are intended to achieve spinal fixation while causing less damage to the surrounding tissues. The traditional PS approach to lumbosacral spine surgery, which is the current standard of care, requires extensive lateral vertebral dissection for screw placement. In contrast, the CBT procedure requires less soft tissue exposure as screws are placed medially to laterally with a starting point at the junction between the lateral pars interarticularis and superior articular process (1 mm inferior to the inferior border of the transverse process, which was projected at the 5 o'clock orientation in the left pedicle and at the 7 o'clock orientation in the right pedicle). Recent trends have demonstrated a shift toward minimally invasive surgical approaches as opposed to traditional invasive approaches. Since CBT involves less spinal dissection and smaller incisions than PS, of the two approaches, it is considered to be the least invasive. Multi-rod technique has been tried in many centers so as to achieve a more rigid construct [15–18]. Robert [17] performed a retrospective review for consecutive adult spinal deformity patients who underwent long fusion to the pelvis. He concluded that patients treated with multi-rod constructs had a statistically lower incidence of lumbosacral pseudarthrosis and implant failure than those treated with dual-rod constructs. Seung-Jae et al. [16] compared the radiographic outcomes after the use of a standard 2-rod construct versus similar outcomes after the use of a multiple-rod construct, and they thought that using a multiple-rod construct is an effective method to enhance the stability across 3-column osteotomy site, and further to significantly prevent implant failure and symptomatic pseudarthrosis. Yu et al. [18] retrospectively analyzed a consecutive case of patients with adult spinal deformity who underwent 3-column osteotomy with pelvic fixation. He concluded that additional rods covering the osteotomy site and lumbosacral junction can reduce the incidence of rod fracture following 3-column surgery with pelvic fixation. Meanwhile, biomechanical studies have also proved that accessory rods improved the stability and reduced the motion and rod strain at the osteotomy site [19–21]. However, according to a systematic review of treatment strategies for the prevention of junctional complications after long-segment fusions in the osteoporotic spine conducted by Murray [22], there is less or insufficient evidence to recommend the use of multi-rod constructs. Moreover, there were also some shortcomings in the multi-rod constructs that need to be modified. First, the accessory rods were linked by side-by-side connectors with the primary rods, which might concentrate more stress on the junction of screws and rods. Furthermore, the application of the connector would increase the possibility of mechanical failure, such as the disengagement of the rod from the connector [23, 24]. Second, the multi-rod constructs mainly increased the rigidness of the posterior column, but the reinforcement for anterior column was not achieved. Andrea [25] considered that the high loads acting on the rods with respect to the physiologic condition could slow down the bone healing at the osteotomy site. Furthermore, according to the study of Tomohiro, the use of multi-rod constructs led to a higher incidence of junctional iliac screw loosening than the use of conventional a two-rod construct, especially for patients with osteoporosis, following the adult spinal deformity surgery.

Degenerative diseases of the spine are a common condition affecting the quality of life of middle-aged and elderly people, affecting about 32–68% of people over 65 years of age [26]. Degenerative scoliosis is among the more complex issues, often with vertebral canal and nerve root canal stenosis, vertebral rotation, intervertebral joint subluxation, and sagittal balance loss due to pathological changes. Among them, the incidence of female is higher than that of male. Due to the degeneration of thoracolumbar segment, it can lead to asymmetric joint space stenosis, small joint hyperplasia, osteophyte formation, yellow ligament hypertrophy and spinal canal stenosis, and even vertebral rotation and intervertebral joint subluxation. The clinical and imaging manifestations are often complicated. The treatment is mainly intended to alleviate symptoms, to improve the function of the spine status, to bring about reconstruction of spinal stability, to restore the spinal sagittal balance, and to handle the individual situation of treatment according to different choices of different surgical strategies. Currently, pedicle screw internal fixation is the preferred surgical method to reconstruct spinal stability and restore spinal sequence, but the patients on the receding side are often complicated with osteoporosis. Simple pedicle screw fixation often results in internal fixation loosening and pseudarthrosis formation. The long-term complication rate of 5-year follow-up has been reported to be about 59%. Adult patients with degenerative scoliosis tend to be aging, more often combined with osteoporosis, at the time of long-segment fixation fusion, there is the possibility of internal fixation loosening, pseudojoint, and other complications. A study by Stanley et al. [27] reviewed internal fixation-related complications in patients over 65 years of age who underwent multi-level spinal fusion surgery for bone weakness. A total of 38 patients were included in the study, all of whom underwent more than five levels of surgery. Follow-up time was greater than 5 years, and the incidence of short-term postoperative complications (less than 3 months, vertebral fracture, pedicle fracture) was about 13%, and the incidence of long-term complications (longer than 3 months) was about 59%, including the failure of pseudarthrosis combined with internal fixation 11%, internal fixation loosening 7%, and pelvic internal fixation prolapse 11%. In a large sample of more than 140,000 people, Lee et al. [28] found that osteoporosis significantly lengthens hospital stay for spinal surgery, increases readmission rates, and increases healthcare costs. Therefore, how to reduce the complications related to internal fixation after spinal surgery in the elderly and improve the intensity of fixation should be paid clinical attention and solved. The common ways to improve the strength of the internal fixation in clinic include increasing screw size, using specially designed expansion screws, and vertebral body bone cement reinforcement, which not only improves the fixed strength, but also increases the probability of complications. In 2009, Santoni et al. proposed the surgical method of fixation with cortical bone trajectory screws to reduce the dependence of screws on bone density [6]. Biomechanical studies have confirmed that cortical bone trajectory screws can significantly improve the fixation strength and stability of internal fixation in osteoporosis samples, and a large number of clinical applications have achieved satisfactory results [8, 9, 29, 30]. Different from thoracolumbar short-segment fixation, the treatment of degenerative scoliosis often requires rotation, compression, and distraction. Finite element analysis found that the anti-rotation ability of cortical bone trajectory screw fixed only in the middle and posterior column could not fully meet the needs of surgery. However, the special screw path of cortical bone trajectory screw allows it to be used as a supplement to the pedicle screw in the same vertebral pedicle. Dual-trajectory internal fixation can significantly improve the strength and stability of fixation [29]. As early as in 2013, Japanese scholar Professor Masaki Ueno et al. [31] reported the case of dual-track internal fixation for the treatment of degenerative scoliosis complicated with osteoporosis. Considering that the patient had severe osteoporosis (T = -4.0), the surgeon adopted L1-S1 dual locus fixation, and the balance of coronal and sagittal plane was restored after surgery. The team of Professor Hu Huiqiang [32], a Chinese scholar, conducted an attempt to correct degenerative scoliosis using a cortical screw satellite rod combined with pedicle screw internal fixation. The team followed 11 patients with degenerative scoliosis who underwent satellite stick surgery with cortical screws for an average of 33 months. There was no significant difference in coronal and sagittal balance at the last follow-up compared with immediately after surgery. It has been confirmed that cortical screw fixation combined with pedicle screw fixation combined with satellite rod orthopedic distal fixation to S1 long-segment lumbosacral fusion can enhance the strength of spinal pelvis fixation and achieve better clinical efficacy in the treatment of degenerative scoliosis. The use of MTA technique in the treatment of degenerative scoliosis with osteoporosis has clear safety and efficacy. Compared with Professor Masaki Ueno's fixed segmental double-trajectory internal fixation, MTA technique selectively inserts cortical bone screws or sacral wing screws on the basis of pedicle screw fixation, which not only ensures the reliability of internal fixation, but also saves the number of internal fixations and reduces the cost of surgical fixation consumables, thereby reducing in the difficulty of surgery and the occurrence of potential surgical complications. Pedicle screws in combination with cortical or sacral wing screws can provide a variety of options for increasing the strength of fixation in the clinic, and provide an effective fixation method for both the surgeon and the patient in spinal deformity correction surgery with osteoporosis, spinal tumor resection and reconstruction surgery, and long-segment fixation for lumbosacral deformity. In conclusion, multi-trajectory and multi-anchor fixation technique can effectively improve the strength of pedicle screw fixation, and can be safely and effectively applied in the surgical treatment of adult degenerative spinal deformities with osteoporosis.

The main indications of the MTA technique are lumbosacral 3-column osteotomy, multi-level lumbosacral fusion for osteoporotic elderly patients, spondylolisthesis, and lumbosacral coronal imbalance. Based on past experience, distal fixation to the pelvic was recommended in the situation above to get stronger internal fixation and greater orthodontic strength. As we know, pelvic fixation may cause dysfunction and even seriously affect the patients' quality of life. With the application of the MTA technique, pelvic fixation can be reduced and the sacroiliac joint can be preserved. The MTA technique provides additional orthopedic strength and makes the lumbosacral internal fixation more solid. Meanwhile, CBT screw and sacral wing screw insertion through a medial entry point demands no additional exposure of the wound.

In general, sacropelvic fixation should be considered in any patient with a long construct ending in the sacrum, or patients with associated risk factors for distal fixation loosening or high risk of pseudarthrosis at L5-S1, or those undergoing 3-column osteotomies or vertebral body resections in the low lumbar spine, and those with severe spondylolisthesis or trunk imbalance [33, 34]. High biomechanical load makes the lumbosacral junction difficult to stabilize during fusion and leads to pseudarthrosis and internal fixation failure which are the prevalent complications, and it most commonly occurs at the 3-column osteotomy site or the lumbosacral junction [35, 36]. This reminds us of the need for a more solid instrument to stabilize the L5-S1 junction. The construction of iliac screw and S2AI screw has been the major advancement in spinopelvic fixation, and it demonstrates the excellent biomechanics. However, the drawbacks in the spinopelvic fixation, including iliac screw-associated screw site prominence, wound complication [37, 38], implant loosening [39], and S2AI-associated sacral iliac joints' violation [40], should be carefully considered. Thus, we are trying to put forward an alternative solution for the pelvic fixation in the lumbar sacral surgery to avoid the complications mentioned above. On the other hand, the MTA technique has its limitations and contraindications. Such as, it is not suitable for patients with severe coronal or sagittal trunk imbalance, which demands sacroiliac screws to provide greater corrective force, and it is difficult to implant both PS and CBT screws for patients with lumbar pedicle dysplasia.

4. Conclusion

The MTA technique is a lumbosacral augmentation fixation technique that combines cortical bone trajectory (CBT) screw with sacral alar screw fixation based on the traditional pedicle screw fixation construct. CBT screws were selectively implanted in the lumbar spine and sacral alar screws were inserted on the same side of the sacrum after completing the pedicle screw fixation and interbody fusion. And the screws were then connected with rod(s), which increased the strength of the internal fixation. The technique comes with the following improvements and advantages. First, the satellite rods are fixed with the additional screws, which make the tension to be more dispersed and avoid stress concentration. Second, the interaction between the multi-trajectory screws anchoring on one vertebra makes the screws stronger and reduces the risk of screw loosening. Third, the MTA screw can provide better stability for the anterior column. Fourth, the MTA fixation can not only strengthen the construct, but also provide additional correction force. Fifth, the MTA technique provides an alternative for pelvic fixation, which preserves the motion of sacroiliac joints.

In conclusion, the MTA technique is a safe and effective means to strengthen lumbosacral internal fixation as well as to provide additional correction for patients with lumbar sacral degenerative, deformity, and tumor. This technique can also be taken as a remedial measure if the pedicle screws loosen intraoperatively. And it still needs long-term observation and follow-up to conclude whether the incidence of rod fracture and pseudarthrosis can be reduced.

5. Case presentation

5.1 Case one

It was a 69-year-old female who complained of low back pain for 7 months, aggravated with weakness and pain in the right leg for 1 month. She was diagnosed with T12 and L5 multiple myeloma. Preoperative examinations showed L5 vertebral destruction and the spinal canal compression (white arrow). The L5 vertebrae were resected trans-right-pedicle and T12 was augmented with cement. The lumbar spine was fixed from L3 to S1. The multiple trajectory anchoring (MTA) technique was applied bilaterally to strengthen the internal fixation, which made it possible to avoid fixing the pelvis and made the surgery less invasive. Postoperative computed tomography (CT) scan showed the trajectory of pedicle screw (PS), cortical bone trajectory (CBT) screws, and sacral alar screws (**Figure 2**).

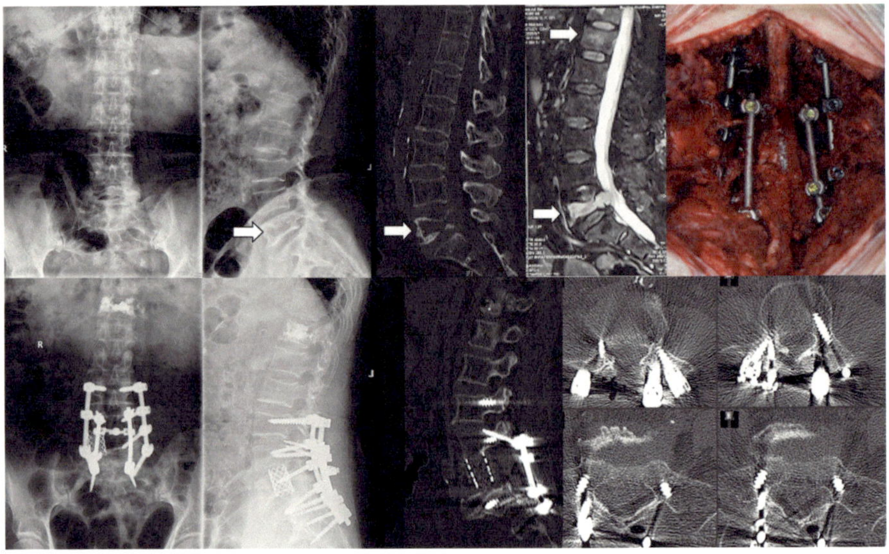

Figure 2.
The application of multiple trajectory anchoring (MTA) technique in the L5 vertebrae resection case.

5.2 Case two

It was a 51-year-old male patient who had severe back pain and radiating right leg pain for 30 years and was diagnosed with congenital scoliosis and lumbar spinal stenosis at L4/5. The scoliosis was generated by the L5 hemivertebrae on the right side (white arrow). L5 hemivertebrae resection and L2 to S1 fusion was performed posteriorly. The multiple trajectory anchoring (MTA) technique was applied to enhance the distraction force on the concave side and strengthen the internal fixation

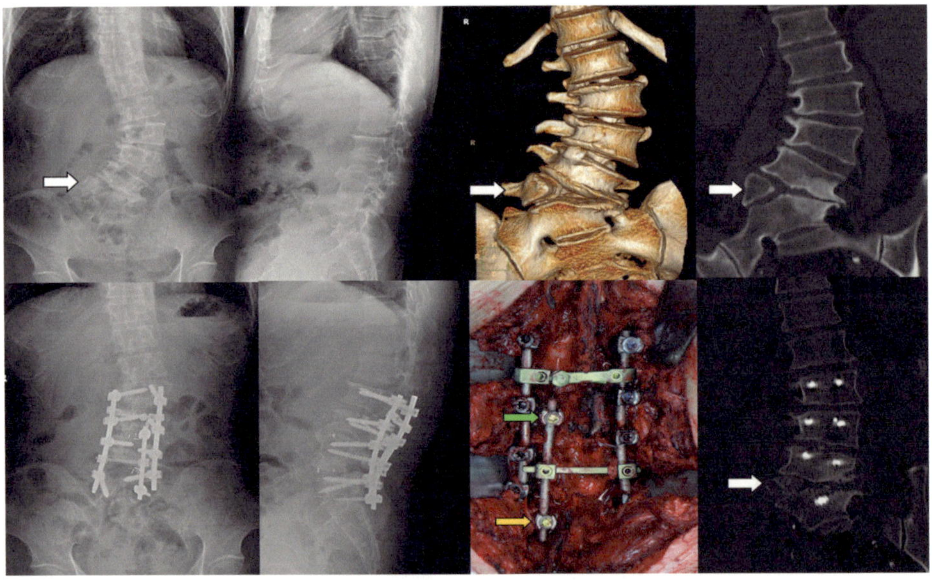

Figure 3.
The application of multiple trajectory anchoring (MTA) technique in the L5 hemivertebrae resection case.

(Green arrow shows the CBT screw and yellow arrow shows the sacral alar screw). The postoperative images showed that the deformity was corrected well with a short-segment operation without fixing down to the pelvis (**Figure 3**).

5.3 Case three

It was a 69-year-old male patient with multi-level lumbar spinal stenosis from L3 to S1. Posterior lumbar decompression and interbody fusion from L3 to S1 was performed. During the surgery, the left pedicle of L5 was fractured due to excessive spinal decompression. In such case, the multiple trajectory anchoring (MTA) technique could be applied by inserting the L4 cortical bone trajectory (CBT) screw and sacral alar screw to enhance the pedicle screw (PS) internal fixation (Green arrow shows the CBT screw and yellow arrow shows the sacral alar screw) (**Figure 4**).

5.4 Case four

It was a 70-year-old male who had severe back pain and left leg pain for 4 months. He was diagnosed with L4 burst fracture and osteoporosis (T score of the bone mineral density was −5.0 in lumbar spine). Posterior L4 corpectomy and L2 to S1 fixation with bone cement augmentation was performed. To prevent internal fixation from loosening, additional fixation was performed using the MTA technique, in which left CBT screw and sacral alar screw were inserted and linked with the rod and connector (Green arrow shows the CBT screw and yellow arrow shows the sacral alar screw) (**Figure 5**).

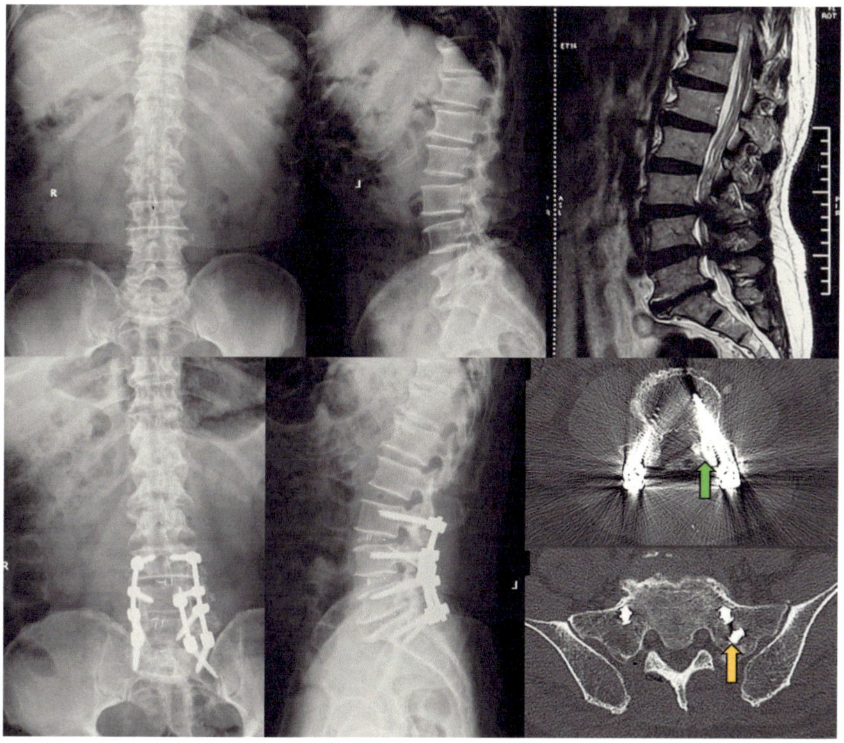

Figure 4.
The application of multiple trajectory anchoring (MTA) technique to reinforce the pedicle screw construction.

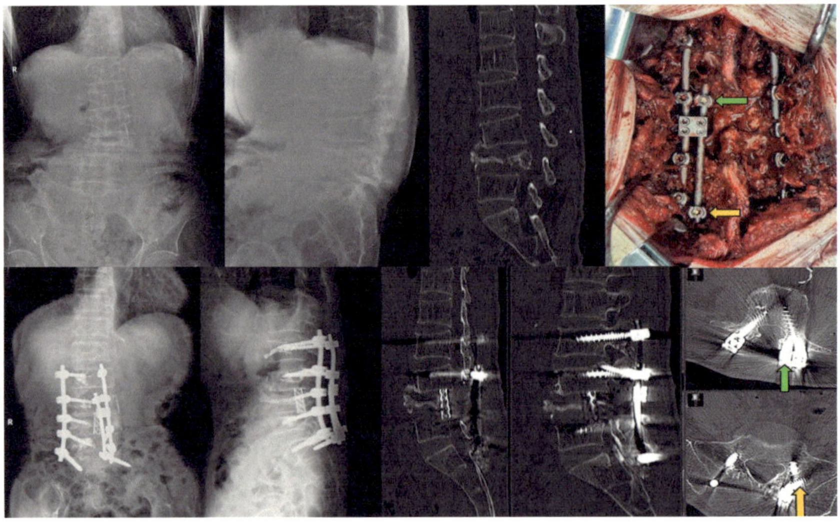

Figure 5.
The application of multiple trajectory anchoring (MTA) technique in the L4 vertebrae resection and severe osteoporotic case.

Author details

Yuzeng Liu*, Yong Hai, Hongtao Ding and Mingzheng Zhao
Spine Surgery Department, Beijing Chaoyang Hospital, Capital Medical University, Beijing, China

*Address all correspondence to: beijingspine2010@163.com

References

[1] Katz JN, Harris MB. Lumbar spinal stenosis. New England Journal of Medicine. 2008;**358**(8):818-825

[2] Lurie J, Tomkins-Lane C. Management of lumbar spinal stenosis. BMJ. 2016;**352**:h6234

[3] Suk S-I et al. Pedicle screw instrumentation in adolescent idiopathic scoliosis (AIS). European Spine Journal. 2012;**21**:13-22

[4] Umeta RS, Avanzi O. Techniques of lumbar-sacral spine fusion in spondylosis: Systematic literature review and meta-analysis of randomized clinical trials. The Spine Journal. 2011;**11**(7):668-676

[5] Wu A-M et al. Lumbar spinal stenosis: An update on the epidemiology, diagnosis and treatment. AME Medical Journal. 2017;**2**

[6] Santoni BG et al. Cortical bone trajectory for lumbar pedicle screws. The Spine Journal. 2009;**9**(5):366-373

[7] Ueno M et al. Posterior corrective fusion using a double-trajectory technique (cortical bone trajectory combined with traditional trajectory) for degenerative lumbar scoliosis with osteoporosis. Journal of Neurosurgery: Spine. 2013;**19**(5):600-607

[8] Matsukawa K et al. In vivo analysis of insertional torque during pedicle screwing using cortical bone trajectory technique. Spine (Phila Pa 1976). 2014;**39**(4):E240-E245

[9] Li HM et al. Biomechanical fixation properties of the cortical bone trajectory in the osteoporotic lumbar spine. World Neurosurgery. 2018;**119**:e717-e727

[10] Wu X et al. A finite-element analysis on biomechanical performance of lumbar cortical bone trajectory versus traditional trajectory screw fixation in osteoporosis. Orthopedic Journal of China. 2018;**26**(12):1126-1131

[11] Hegazy AA, Hegazy RA. Midsagittal anatomy of lumbar lordosis in adult egyptians: MRI study. Anatomy Research International. 2014;**2014**:370852

[12] Sebaaly A et al. Etiology, evaluation, and treatment of failed Back surgery syndrome. Asian Spine Journal. 2018;**12**(3):574-585

[13] Rodriguez A et al. Novel placement of cortical bone trajectory screws in previously instrumented pedicles for adjacent-segment lumbar disease using CT image-guided navigation. Neurosurgical Focus. 2014;**36**(3):E9

[14] Takata Y et al. Hybrid technique of cortical bone trajectory and pedicle screwing for minimally invasive spine reconstruction surgery: A technical note. The Journal of Medical Investigation. 2014;**61**(3-4):388-392

[15] Guevara-Villazón F et al. Multiple-rod constructs in adult spinal deformity surgery for pelvic-fixated long instrumentations: An integral matched cohort analysis. European Spine Journal. 2020;**29**(4):886-895

[16] Hyun SJ et al. Comparison of standard 2-rod constructs to multiple-rod constructs for fixation across 3-column spinal osteotomies. Spine (Phila Pa 1976). 2014;**39**(22):1899-1904

[17] Merrill RK et al. Multi-rod constructs can prevent rod breakage and Pseudarthrosis at the lumbosacral

junction in adult spinal deformity. Global Spine Journal. 2017;**7**(6):514-520

[18] Yamato Y et al. Long additional rod constructs can reduce the incidence of rod fractures following 3-column osteotomy with pelvic fixation in short term. Spine Deformity. 2020;**8**(3):481-490

[19] Hallager DW et al. Use of supplemental short pre-contoured accessory rods and cobalt chrome alloy posterior rods reduces primary rod strain and range of motion across the pedicle subtraction osteotomy level: An In vitro biomechanical study. Spine (Phila Pa 1976). 2016;**41**(7):E388-E395

[20] La Barbera L et al. Biomechanical advantages of supplemental accessory and satellite rods with and without interbody cages implantation for the stabilization of pedicle subtraction osteotomy. European Spine Journal. 2018;**27**(9):2357-2366

[21] Seyed Vosoughi A et al. Optimal satellite rod constructs to mitigate rod failure following pedicle subtraction osteotomy (PSO): A finite element study. The Spine Journal. 2019;**19**(5):931-941

[22] Echt M et al. A systematic review of treatment strategies for the prevention of junctional complications after long-segment fusions in the osteoporotic spine. Global Spine Journal. 2021;**11**(5):792-801

[23] Myung KS, Lee C, Skaggs DL. Early pelvic fixation failure in neuromuscular scoliosis. Journal of Pediatric Orthopedics. 2015;**35**(3):258-265

[24] Shabtai L et al. Sacral alar iliac (SAI) screws fail 75% less frequently than iliac screws in neuromuscular scoliosis. Journal of Pediatric Orthopedics. 2017;**37**(8):e470-e475

[25] Luca A et al. Instrumentation failure following pedicle subtraction osteotomy: The role of rod material, diameter, and multi-rod constructs. European Spine Journal. 2017;**26**(3):764-770

[26] Diebo BG et al. Adult spinal deformity. Lancet. 2019;**394**(10193):160-172

[27] DeWald CJ, Stanley T. Instrumentation-related complications of multilevel fusions for adult spinal deformity patients over age 65: Surgical considerations and treatment options in patients with poor bone quality. Spine (Phila Pa 1976). 2006;**31**(19 Suppl):S144-S151

[28] Lee CK et al. Influence of osteoporosis following spine surgery on reoperation, readmission, and economic costs: An 8-year Nationwide population-based study in Korea. World Neurosurgery. 2021;**149**:e360-e368

[29] Matsukawa K et al. Biomechanical evaluation of cross trajectory technique for pedicle screw insertion: Combined use of traditional trajectory and cortical bone trajectory. Orthopaedic Surgery. 2015;**7**(4):317-323

[30] Sansur CA et al. Biomechanical fixation properties of cortical versus transpedicular screws in the osteoporotic lumbar spine: An in vitro human cadaveric model. Journal of Neurosurgery. Spine. 2016;**25**(4):467-476

[31] Ueno M et al. Posterior corrective fusion using a double-trajectory technique (cortical bone trajectory combined with traditional trajectory) for degenerative lumbar scoliosis with osteoporosis: Technical note. Journal of Neurosurgery. Spine. 2013;**19**(5):600-607

[32] Huiqiang H et al. Cortical bone trajectory and traditional trajectory

combined with satellite rod fixation for degenerative scoliosis. Chinese Journal of Spine and Spinal Cord. 2020;**30**(01):8-12

[33] Jain A et al. Pelvic fixation in adult and pediatric spine surgery: Historical perspective, indications, and techniques: AAOS exhibit selection. JBJS. 2015;**97**(18):1521-1528

[34] Shen FH et al. Pelvic fixation for adult scoliosis. European Spine Journal. 2013;**22**:265-275

[35] Kim YJ et al. Pseudarthrosis in long adult spinal deformity instrumentation and fusion to the sacrum: Prevalence and risk factor analysis of 144 cases. Spine (Phila Pa 1976). 2006;**31**(20):2329-2336

[36] Weistroffer JK et al. Complications in long fusions to the sacrum for adult scoliosis: Minimum five-year analysis of fifty patients. Spine (Phila Pa 1976). 2008;**33**(13):1478-1483

[37] De la Garza Ramos R et al. Iliac screw versus S2 alar-iliac screw fixation in adults: A meta-analysis. Journal of Neurosurgery. Spine. 2018;**30**(2):253-258

[38] Keorochana G et al. Comparison of complications and revisions after sacral 2 alar iliac screw and iliac screw fixation for Sacropelvic fixation in pediatric and adult populations: Systematic review and meta-analysis. World Neurosurgery. 2019;**132**:408-420.e1

[39] Ilyas H, Place H, Puryear A. A comparison of early clinical and radiographic complications of iliac screw fixation versus S2 alar iliac (S2AI) fixation in the adult and pediatric populations. Journal of Spinal Disorders & Techniques. 2015;**28**(4):E199-E205

[40] Hasan MY et al. Postoperative complications of S2AI versus iliac screw in spinopelvic fixation: A meta-analysis and recent trends review. The Spine Journal. 2020;**20**(6):964-972

Chapter 17

Rehabilitation in Lumbar Spinal Surgery

Pragya Kumar and Jasmine Kaur Chawla

Abstract

The chapter has elaborated the role of Physical therapy rehabilitation in assessment and management of patients undergoing Lumbar Spinal Surgery pre- and post - operatively. Further need of pre-habilitation in patients undergoing surgery was emphasized to obtain optimal results after surgery. Outcome measures used widely for assessment of patient before spinal surgery and after surgery was discussed to have an overview of recovery process. Phase-wise goals, precautions and rehabilitation protocols were discussed starting from immediate post-operative phase till return to activity/sports. Special emphasis was laid on the importance of home exercise regimen. Recent advances in management of Lumbar spinal surgery post operative cases like Virtual Reality was discussed in the end for upgrading information on achieving better patient outcomes.

Keywords: low back pain, lumbar spinal surgery, assessment, rehabilitation, patient education

1. Introduction

Low back pain (LBP) is one of the leading musculoskeletal problems common in most age groups. The lifetime prevalence of low back pain is reported to be 84% [1]. The most common cause of LBP is nonspecific in nature, that is, either origin of pain in from the structures around lumbar region (muscles, ligaments, intervertebral disc, facets, etc.) or it is centrally mediated (imbalance in sensory processing and descending pain mechanisms) [2]. Guidelines published globally recommend early screening of risk factors leading to LBP including psychosocial components. Based on cause identified administration of multicomponent approach (including rest, hot/cold application, electrotherapy modalities, exercises), prevention strategies (posture and ergonomic modifications) along with behavior modifications were suggested interventions for LBP [1]. In certain LBP pathologies categorized as degenerative lumbar spine disorders (lumbar disc herniation, spondylolisthesis, spinal canal stenosis) efficacy of non-surgical versus surgical intervention is still not clear. The criteria for indicating patient for surgery are – failed conservative treatment, unmanageable pain, worsening of neurological compromise (sensory & motor loss), Cauda equina syndrome. This chapter will give rehabilitation overview pre- and post – operatively for patients with degenerative lumbar spine disorders.

2. Pre - operative phase

"Pre-habilitation" aims to augment functional outcomes by enhancing physical function and perception of pain during & after surgery by education including activity modifications in patients awaiting lumbar surgery. Studies have highlighted the role of pre-habilitation not only improve surgical outcome, but also reduces hospital stay and financial burden as compared to classic post-operative rehabilitation given alone [3].

Patient referred for pre- operative rehabilitation, should undergo thorough evaluation to understand lesion behavior [4]. This includes:

Posture – to identify postural compensations due to pain.

Range of motion (ROM) – Assessment of Lumbar ROM along with hip mobility.

Movements (static and repeated) – Pain response and discomfort felt by patient with LBP on static holding of position as well as on repeated motions.

Strength – Endurance of major muscle groups around lumbar region (Abdominals & Back Extensors) along with myotome assessment (L1 – S1) Recruitment of Transverse Abdominis.

Sensations and reflexes – Alterations in sensation (pin prick, touch, temperature) in dermatomes (L1 – S5) and spinal reflexes (Knee jerk, Ankle jerk, Plantar reflex).

Therapists will identify provocative postures, movements and thus determine directional preference which reduces pain. Irrespective of method of assessment or treatment used, avoid positions that increases intradiscal pressure leading to pain peripheralization.

2.1 Outcome measures

Patient rated outcome measures are commonly used to assess following parameters:

Patient reported function and activity limitation – Oswestry Disability Index (ODI) is 10 item questionnaires about the level of difficulty faced during function and activity with six options in each item. Higher scores indicate more disability [5].

The Roland Morris Disability Questionnaire (RMDQ) – Self rated disability as a result of LBP can be measured by the patient [6].

Pain – Visual analogue scale (VAS) – VAS is a simple tool consisting of 10 cm horizontal line to assess pain intensity [7].

Health related quality of life – SF-36 – It is self-reported measurement of health by patient, comprising of 36 questions under 8 domains [8].

Anxiety and depression – Hospital Anxiety and Depression Scale (HADS) is used to assess nonphysical symptoms of depression (7 questions) and anxiety (7 questions) in LBP patients. Cut off score ≥ 8 indicates the presence of anxiety and depression [9].

Fear Avoidance – Fear Avoidance Belief Questionnaire (FABQ)- It is a 16-item questionnaire with 2 sub-sections – Work subscale and Physical Activity subscale [10]. This scale is widely used in patients with LBP to understand work, ADLs & levels of physical activity are affected due to fear of increasing pain.

Patient reported treatment effects – Patient Enablement Instrument (PEI) – The scale is a patient rated outcome measure to assess containing 6 questions allowing patient to rate enablement to cope with problem after consultation with doctor/rehabilitation specialist [11].

Goals • Patient education • Description of patho-biomechanics of lumbar spine & disc • Education about surgical procedure, expected outcomes, milestones of progression, precautions & contraindications after surgery. • Awareness of body position and mechanics while performing ADLs • Decrease/centralize/abolish pain. • Patient shall demonstrate and practice Transverse Abdominis (TrA) contraction maintaining spine in neutral position in different postures. • Independence in home exercise program (HEP)
Precautions • Avoid prolonged sitting/driving for more than 20 minutes. • Avoid lifting or carrying activities. • Avoid activities requiring repetitive loading of spine (e.g., jogging, running etc)
Rehabilitation protocol • Relative rest • Modalities for pain relief (US, TENS, Ice) • Lumbar stabilization (Tummy Tuck -in) initiated in unloaded position (crook lying) and advanced to loaded position (sitting, standing etc) • Active ROM of lumbar spine (direction determined in examination) to reduce, centralize or abolish pain. • *Repetitions/sets/hold time/rest time – as tolerated by patient.*
(Recreated from Gage T. Lumbar Microdiscectomy. In: Mosca JC, Cahill JB, Tucker CY, editors. Postsurgical Rehabilitation Guidelines for the Orthopedic Clinician. Elsevier; 2006. p, 328.)

Table 1.
Pre-operative rehabilitation protocol for patients undergoing Lumbar surgery.

2.2 Pre-operative rehabilitation protocol

Patient education is an integral part of therapy in surgical cases. Most of the time this aspect has been overlooked resulting in increased apprehensions and confusions regarding surgery, intended outcome and recovery time in patient's as well as caregivers' mind also. Detailed description of patient's problem and possible surgical solutions with help of educational booklet, models or videos should be explained. Proper guidance regarding recovery time, precautions, and exercises to be followed before and after surgery should be discussed [12]. Description of exercises to be performed day-wise/week wise should be given as mentioned in **Table 1**.

3. Overview of surgical procedures

Commonest surgical procedures used in patients with intractable back pian are Lumbar Microdiscectomy (LMD), Instrumented lumbar fusion surgery. LMD is performed in reverse Trendelenburg's position and midline incision (3 to 6 cm) is done over the affected segment. Paraspinal muscles are stripped and retracted to open interspace. Interspinous ligaments are spared, however ligamentum flavum is resected to perform foraminotomy. The nerve root is retracted medially, posterior longitudinal ligament and nucleus present lateral to nerve root are cut to perform nucleotomy. Damage to ligamentum flavum and paraspinal muscles is not repaired, but lumbar fascia is repaired using absorbable sutures [12].

Posterior lumbar interbody fusion (PLIF) was aimed to provide rigid spinal stabilization along with decompression of surrounding neural structures and correction in vertebral alignment. It is a 4-step procedure including Exposure & decompression; Spinal instrumentation & fixation using titanium/steel rods, plates, screws, and/or wires; Anterior column reconstruction & interbody fusion and Internal stabilization and closure of the area. In stage 3 procedures to restore disc height were performed by distraction without increasing tension in neural structures. Complete discectomy was done, and vertebral end plates are scraped till fresh bleeding. Bone graft is prepared by chipped bone from iliac crest or allograft material and placed over vertebral bone without soft tissue interposition [12].

4. Post-operative rehabilitation protocol

Communication with operating surgeons is critical for understanding early precautions and activity restrictions. However, a therapist based on clinical judgment can initiate early rehabilitation after lumbar spinal surgery. Recent evidence has suggested early mobilization encourages patient's positive self-belief and ultimately enhance their ability to return to work and functional independence [4]. Research has shown conflicting findings regarding initiation of rehabilitation immediately after lumbar surgery but none of the studies has reported any adverse effect. Rather supported the fact that early lifting of post operative limitation results in lesser number of problems [13].

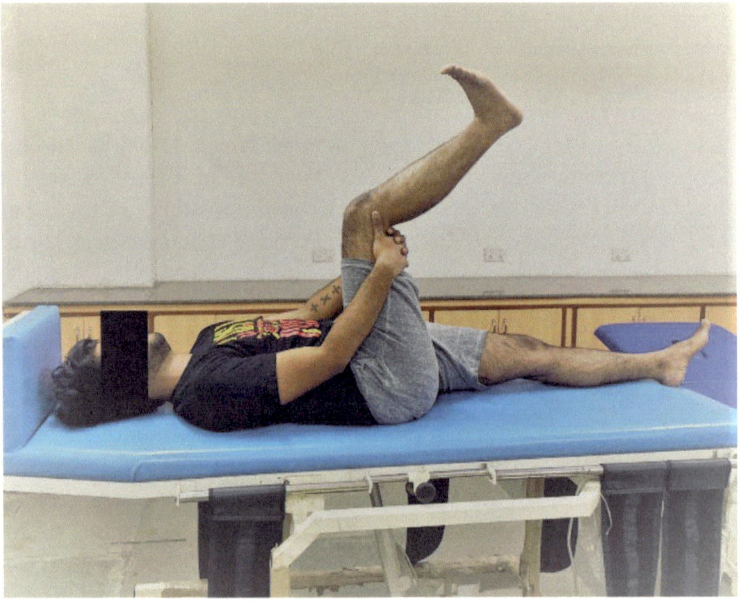

Figure 1.
Sciatic nerve mobilization (with spine supported).

However, initiation of spinal stabilization exercises before and after surgery is key to success in surgical interventions. Studies have suggested that recruitment of lumbar Transversus Abdominis (TA) and Multifidus (MF) muscles is not balanced in patients with long standing LBP as these muscles fine tune the motion at segmental level, thus affecting lumbar stability. Further presence of chronic pain in back in surgical cases along with fear & anxiety in minds of patients undergoing surgery will further inhibit their activation. Thus, activation of these muscles is very much essential to "switch on" stabilization role played by these muscles before as well as after surgery. This can be achieved initially in unloaded position with help of verbal, visual or tactile feedback and gradually progressing to loaded positions to improve motor control [4].

Focus on improving/maintaining range of motion and flexibility of joints adjacent to lumbar spine is important postoperatively. This enables healing at surgical site and simultaneously overall range can be improved. Most of the exercises should be done in supine position after disc surgery to offload the spine. Double Knee to chest exercise helps to stretch thoracolumbar fascia; single knee to chest improve hip mobility & stretch proximal sciatic nerve (**Figure 1**); lower trunk rotation improves blood flow & reduce disc pressure. Repetitions and sets should be decided as per patient's tolerance [4].

Initiation on walking program in immediate post operative phase is widely recommended by surgeons as well as rehabilitation experts [4]. Following lumbar surgery, it has multifaceted role such as:

- Improving overall blood flow – Prevent deep vein thrombosis.
- Promotes cardiovascular fitness.
- Provides nutrition to Intervertebral disc – rhythmic loading & off-loading improves imbibition, nutrition and promotes healing.
- Gentle stretching of sciatic nerve – prevents adhesion formation around nerve and improves blood flow.

The role of neural mobilization in post-surgical cases to prevent risk of nerve root adhesions is crucial. However, the lumbar spine should be maintained in neutral

PHASE I: Postoperative (Day 1–6)
Goals • Protection of surgical site • Pain control • Initiate walking as tolerated. • Independence in performing bed mobility, sit-to-stand and toileting by Day 2
Precautions • Avoid prolonged sitting/driving for more than 20 minutes. • Avoid bending, lifting, and carrying activities (>10 pounds). • Avoid Valsalva maneuver. • Avoid all sporting activities.

Rehabilitation Protocol • Initiate and practice Log rolling transfers while sitting from supine lying (**Figures 2 & 3**). • Basic exercises – abdominal drawing in, gluteal squeezes, ankle foot pumps. Same exercises are suggested for home exercise program after discharge. • Lumbar stabilization in crook lying (**Figure 4**). • Walking session to be initiated with or without support for 5–10 minutes on level surface (1–3 sessions/day as tolerated). Patients are discharged 1–2 days post -operatively.
Criteria for Discharge: • Demonstration of supine to sit transfers by patient. • Gained proper understanding of body mechanics during ADLs (i.e., avoid lumbar flexion. • Independent walking with or without assistive devices. • Demonstrate independence in donning & doffing of lumbar corset
(Recreated from Nigrini CM and Camarillo RM. Lumbar spine Microdiscectomy surgical rehabilitation. In: Brotzman SB and Manske RC editors. Clinical Orthopedic Rehabilitation- An evidence-based approach. 3rd ed. Elsevier Mosby; 2011, p. 326–337)

Table 2.
Immediate Post-operative rehabilitation protocol for patients undergone Lumbar surgery.

position and nerve should be elongated carefully (not more than 6–8% of its length). Dosage depends upon the patient's response. Excessive lengthening of nerve may reduce blood flow resulting in ischemic pain [4, 12]. The rehabilitation in immediate post operative phase is mentioned in **Table 2**.

Table 3 depicts rehabilitation protocol in after immediate post- operative phase [4, 12].

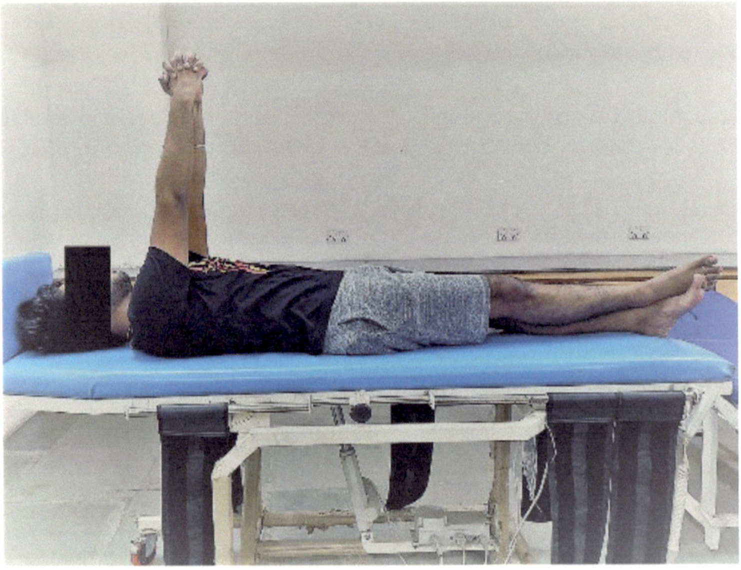

Figure 2.
Log rolling (starting position).

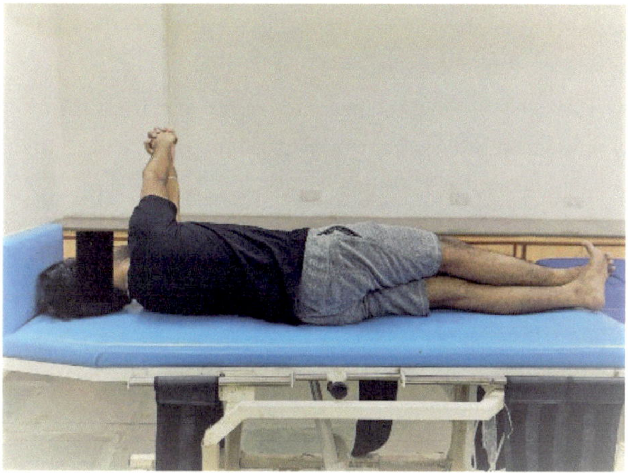

Figure 3.
Log rolling to left side.

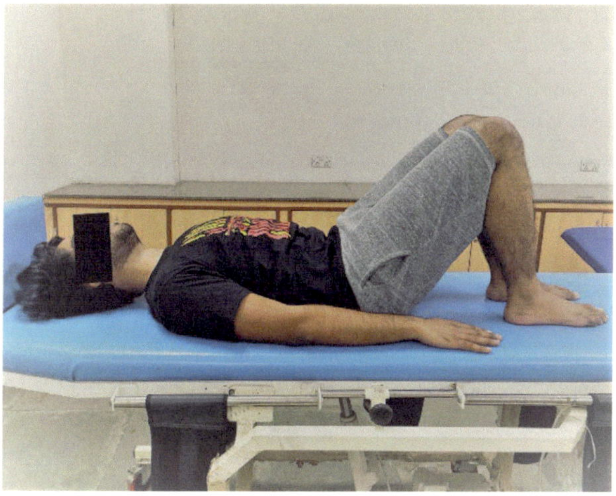

Figure 4.
Lumbar stabilization in crook lying (Transversus abdominis contraction).

PHASE II: PROTECTED MOBILIZATION (Postoperative Week 1–3)

Goals:

- Protection of surgical site
- Pain control
- Improve walking tolerance to 30 minutes.

Precautions

- Avoid prolonged sitting/driving for more than 20 minutes.
- Avoid bending, lifting, and carrying activities (>10 pounds).
- Avoid Valsalva maneuver.
- Avoid sports activities

Rehabilitation protocol

- Relative rest – walking, unloaded cycling.
- Soft tissue mobilization
- Intervention for pain relief (US, TENS, Cryotherapy)
- Lumbar stabilization initiated in supine/prone lying.

Criteria for Progression
Patient can demonstrate:

- Proper sitting postures and body mechanics while transfers
- Lumbar stabilization in unloaded position

PHASE III: NEUTRAL STABILIZATION (Postoperative Week 3–8)

Goals

- Restore Lumbar ROM
- Improve muscle imbalance.
- Improve tolerance to loaded positions.
- Independence in walking without support on level surface
- Return to work (light to moderate) and Activities of Daily living (ADLs).
- Adherence to precautions while during work and ADLs.

Precautions

- Avoid prolonged flexed postures (sitting/driving)
- Avoid activities involving repeated spinal loading (jogging)

Rehabilitation protocol

- Transverse Abdominal exercises in different positions (**Figures** 5 & **6**)
- Progression of bridging exercises (for gluteus maximus)
- Progression of strength training of Hip Abductor (**Figure** 7)
- Initiate active Lumbar ROM - Quadruped rocking (with lumbar flexion & neutral spine) (**Figure 8**), Seated Knee extensions (**Figure 9**) and progress to lumbar active ROM in standing. (**Figure 10**)
- Non-impact lower limb cardiovascular exercises – stationary bicycling, treadmill etc.
- Strength training of upper and lower limb muscles maintaining spine in neutral.

Criteria for Progression

- Full active Lumbar ROM
- Demonstrate proper mechanics while squatting.
- Lower limb muscle strength – 4 out of 5
- Ability to demonstrate neutral spine in loaded positions.

PHASE IV: DYNAMIC STABILIZATION (Postoperative Week 8–14)

Goals

- Demonstrate 5/5 lower limb strength.
- Perform dynamic stabilization without discomfort.
- Able to perform repetitive lumbar spinal motion in all planes.
- Ability to return to actual working situations and perform recreational activities.

For athletes:

- Ability to return to play.

Precautions
Avoid aggravation of symptoms

Rehabilitation protocol • Progression of core stabilization strengthening • Progression of cardiovascular training – initiation of jogging • Progression in strength training • Repetitive motions in directions that centralize pain. • Progress aerobic conditioning
Criteria for Progression • Full pain free active ROM of Lumbar spine • No lower limb neural tension signs • Demonstrates B/L normal flexibility. • Lower extremity strength 5/5. • Good body mechanics in dynamic activities.

Table 3.
Post-operative rehabilitation protocol after discharge for patients undergone Lumbar surgery.

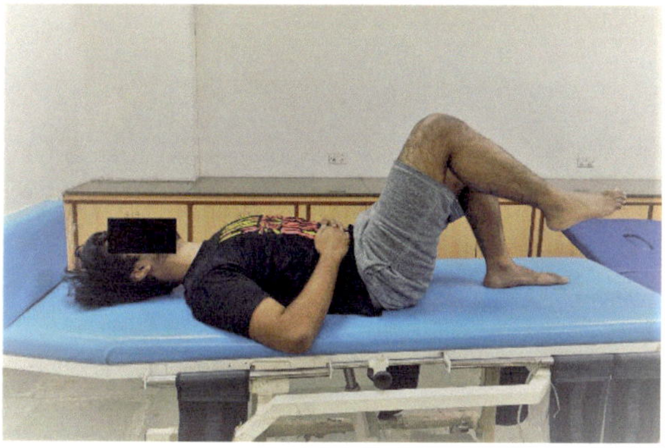

Figure 5.
Transverse abdominis contraction with single leg lift.

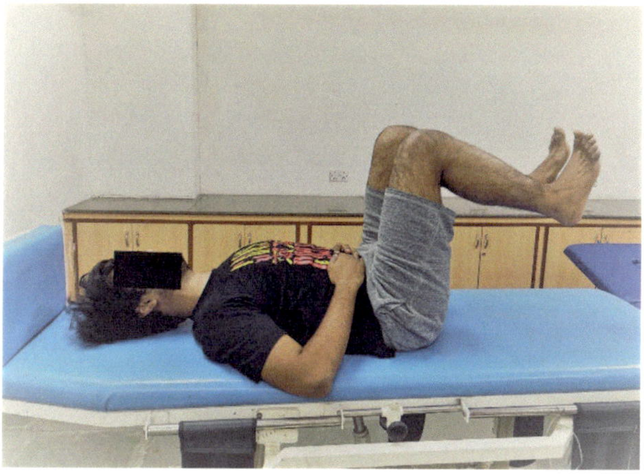

Figure 6.
Transverse abdominis contraction with double leg lift.

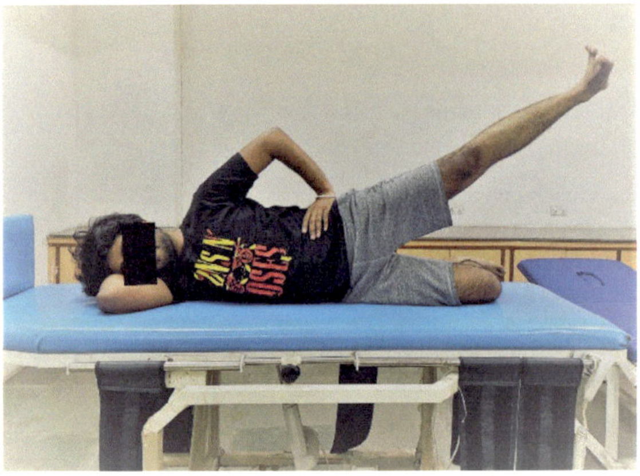

Figure 7.
Hip abductor strengthening (side lying).

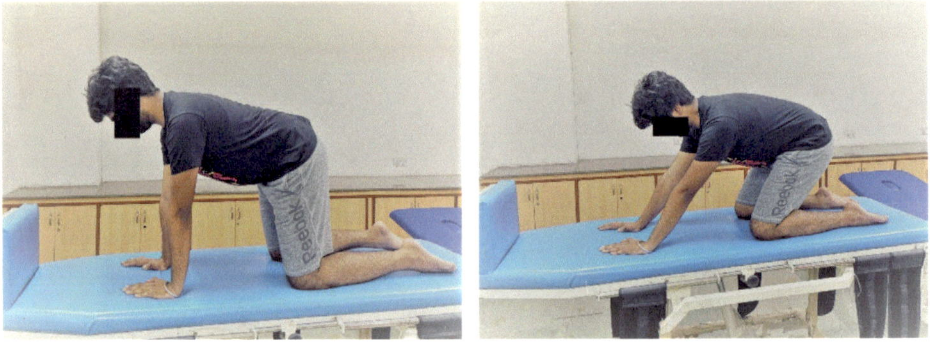

Figure 8.
Quadruped rocking – Starting position (with spine in neutral) & end position.

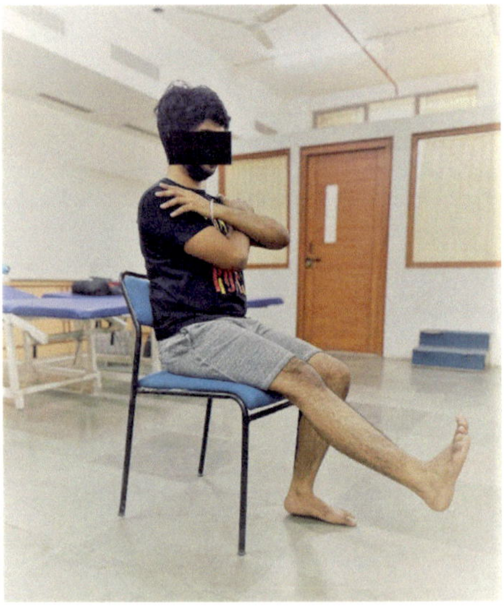

Figure 9.
Seated knee extension (with ankle dorsiflexion).

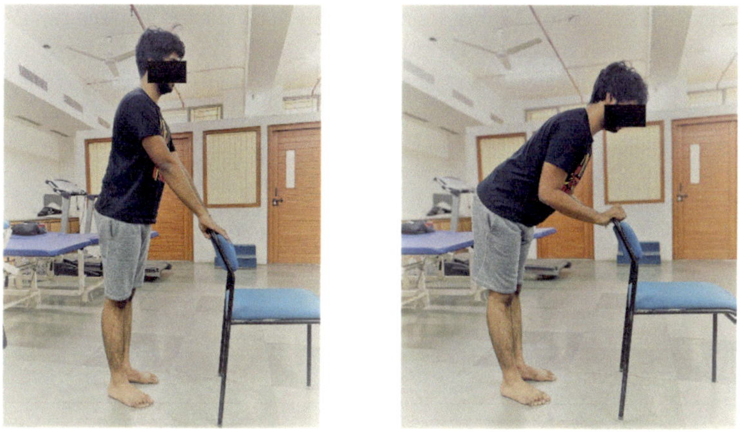

Figure 10.
Standing Lumbar flexion – Starting position (with spine in neutral) & end position.

5. Home exercise program

Limited evidence is available regarding the efficacy of home exercise regimen following lumbar surgery. Experimental study showed that supervised exercises are more effective in reducing pain and disability following lumbar surgery as compared to home-based intervention or no exercises [14]. But sample size of the study was small and adherence rate while exercising at home was not checked. Therefore, emphasis should be laid on improving patient's motivation and involvement of patient in designing home exercise program as per their preferences [13]. Fears in doing exercises at home without supervision should also be dealt with proper patient education as well as opting alternate modes to monitor progress such as telerehabilitation.

6. Recent advances in rehabilitation following Lumbar surgery

The role of virtual reality-based interventions in managing patients after spinal cord injury has been researched well [15] but its application in rehabilitation after spinal surgery is limited. Because of its unique features such as simulation of real-world environment along with ability to capture body's movement, velocity and give visual/auditory/tactile feedbacks makes it a promising rehabilitation tool for management of medical conditions. Recent systematic review has identified promising use of virtual reality in assessment and training following cervical spine surgeries to enhance patient recovery [16] but lacks any experimental fingings. Applicability of virtual reality in management of LBP has been recently discussed [17] but its direct role after lumbar spinal surgery needs to be extensively studied and documented.

7. Conclusions

The chapter has summarized the role of rehabilitation in lumbar surgery. Health care professionals should lay emphasis on pre- operative rehabilitation to ensure early recovery in post operative phase. Proper education and engagement of patients in deciding treatment options is important. Immediate post operative rehabilitation leads to faster reduction in pain and disability. Suitable assessments in phasic manner, following precautions and exercises as recommended will bring better surgical outcomes.

Acknowledgements

No funding involved by any agency.

Conflict of interest

The authors declare no conflict of interest.

Author details

Pragya Kumar* and Jasmine Kaur Chawla
Department of Physiotherapy, Amity Institute of Health Allied Sciences, Amity University, Noida, Uttar Pradesh, India

*Address all correspondence to: pkumar24@amity.edu

References

[1] Lindbäck Y, Tropp H, Enthoven P, Abbott A, Öberg B. PREPARE: Pre-surgery physiotherapy for patients with degenerative lumbar spine disorder: A randomized controlled trial protocol. BMC Musculoskeletal Disorders. 2016;**17**(1):1-8. DOI: 10.1016/j.spinee.2017.12.009

[2] Li W, Gong Y, Liu J, Guo Y, Tang H, Qin S, et al. Peripheral, and central pathological mechanisms of chronic low back pain: A narrative review. Journal of Pain Research. 2021;**14**:1483-1494. DOI: 10.2147/JPR.S306280

[3] Delgado-López PD, Rodríguez-Salazar A, Castilla-Díez JM. "Prehabilitation" in degenerative spine surgery: A literature review. Neurocirugía (English Edition). 2019;**30**(3):124-132. DOI: 10.1016/j.neucie.2018.11.002

[4] Nigrini CM, Camarillo RM. Lumbar spine microdiscectomy surgical rehabilitation. In: Brotzman SB, Manske RC, editors. Clinical Orthopaedic Rehabilitation: An Evidence-Based Approach. Printed in United States of America. Elsevier Health Sciences. Elsevier; 2011. p. 538

[5] Vianin M. Psychometric properties and clinical usefulness of the Oswestry disability index. Journal of Chiropractic Medicine. 2008;**7**(4):161-163. DOI: 10.1016/j.jcm.2008.07.001

[6] Stratford PW, Binkley J, Solomon P, Finch E, Gill C, Moreland J. Defining the minimum level of detectable change for the Roland-Morris questionnaire. Physical Therapy. 1996;**76**(4):359-365. DOI: 10.1093/ptj/76.4.359

[7] Weigl K, Forstner T. Design of paper-based visual analogue scale items. Educational and Psychological Measurement. 2021;**81**(3):595-611. DOI: 10.1177/0013164420952118

[8] Ware JE Jr, Sherbourne CD. The MOS 36-item short-form health survey (SF-36): I. conceptual framework and item selection. Medical Care. 1992;**30**:473-483

[9] Snaith RP. The hospital anxiety and depression scale. Health and Quality of Life Outcomes. 2003;**1**(1):1-4. DOI: 10.1093/occmed/kqu024

[10] Waddell G, Newton M, Henderson I, Somerville D, Main CJ. A fear-avoidance beliefs questionnaire (FABQ) and the role of fear-avoidance beliefs in chronic low back pain and disability. Pain. 1993;**52**(2):157-168. DOI: 10.1016/0304-3959(93)90127-B

[11] Tolvanen E, Koskela TH, Kosunen E. Comparison of the patient enablement instrument (PEI) with two single-item measures among Finnish health care Centre patients. BMC Health Services Research. 2019;**19**(1):1. DOI: 10.1186/s12913-019-4182-2

[12] Lumbar GT. Microdiscectomy. In: Cioppa-Mosca J, Cahill JB, Tucker CY, editors. Postsurgical Rehabilitation Guidelines for the Orthopedic Clinician. Elsevier Health Sciences. St. Louis, Missouri: Elsevier; 2006. pp. 326-337

[13] Oosterhuis T, Costa LO, Maher CG, de Vet HC, van Tulder MW, Ostelo RW. Rehabilitation after lumbar disc surgery. Cochrane Database of Systematic Reviews. 2014;**2014**(3):CD003007. DOI: 10.1002/14651858.CD003007.pub3

[14] Filiz M, Cakmak A, Ozcan E. The effectiveness of exercise programmes after lumbar disc surgery: A

randomized controlled study. Clinical Rehabilitation. 2005;**19**(1):4-11. DOI: 10.1191/0269215505cr836oa

[15] Walia S, Kumar P, Kataria C. Effect of virtual reality training on standing balance in individuals with incomplete spinal cord injury. Comparative Exercise Physiology. 2023;**19**(1):41-48. DOI: 10.3920/CEP220031

[16] Yan C, Wu T, Huang K, He J, Liu H, Hong Y, et al. The application of virtual reality in cervical spinal surgery: A review. World Neurosurgery. 2021;**145**:108-113. DOI: 10.1016/j.wneu.2020.09.040

[17] Bordeleau M, Stamenkovic A, Tardif PA, Thomas J. The use of virtual reality in back pain rehabilitation: A systematic review and meta-analysis. The Journal of Pain. 2022;**23**(2):175-195. DOI: 10.1016/j.jpain.2021.08.001